D1666082

全国高等中医药院校外国进修生教材

University Textbooks of Traditional Chinese Medicine
for Overseas Advanced Students

方 剂 学

Chinese Medical Formulae

主 编　杨育周

Chief Editor　Yang Yuzhou

人 民 卫 生 出 版 社

People's Medical Publishing House

方 剂 学

主　　编：杨育周
出版发行：人民卫生出版社(中继线 67616688)
地　　址：(100078)北京市丰台区方庄芳群园 3 区 3 号楼
网　　址：http://www.pmph.com
E - mail：pmph @ pmph.com
印　　刷：北京人卫印刷厂
经　　销：新华书店
开　　本：787×1092　1/16　印张：22
字　　数：483 千字
版　　次：2001 年 5 月第 1 版　2001 年 5 月第 1 版第 1 次印刷
印　　数：00 001—4 000
标准书号：ISBN 7-117-04302-4/R·4303
定　　价：40.50 元

全国高等中医药院校外国进修生教材
总编辑委员会

University Textbooks of Traditional Chinese Medicine for Overseas Advanced Students

Editorial Committee

Consultants   (in the order of the strokes of Chinese surname)

Wang Yanbin	Wei Guikang	Pi Chiheng	Liu Zhongde
Du Jian	Li Anbang	Li Renxian	Li Mingfu
Zhang Shiqing	Xiao Luwei	Chen Dashun	Fan Yongsheng
Shang Zhichang	Jin Zhijia	Zheng Shouzeng	Meng Nanhua
Xiang Ping	Li Delin	Gao Erxin	Kang Suobin
Sui Dianjun	Xie Jianqun	Dai Ximeng	

Director   Wu Xiufen

Deputy Directors   Li Daosheng Peng Bo

Committee Members   (in the order of the strokes of Chinese surname)

Yu Tiecheng	Feng Zhaosheng	Wang Daokun	Zhu Changren
Liu Degui	Liu Yi	Qi Nan	Lu Yuehua
Su Hua	Li Candong	Li Mingjun	Yang Gongfu
Zhang Yisheng	Zhang Tianfeng	Zhang Xinzhong	Zhang Shuzhen
Tu Ya	Fang Jiayi	Zhao Shuqing	Zhao Yi
Rao Hong	Shi Jianming	Jiang Minjie	He Youshun
Gu Jiazhu	Chai Kefu	Huang Qingxian	Huang Qinhan
Ciu Hongjiang	Zeng Fuhai		

方 剂 学

主　编　杨育周（天津中医学院）

副主编　王秀莲（天津中医学院）
　　　　钱聚义（天津中医学院）
　　　　柴可夫（浙江中医学院）

编　委　徐　立（天津中医学院）
　　　　周　洁（天津中医学院）
　　　　沙明荣（天津中医学院）
　　　　刘　毅（天津中医学院）
　　　　彭　勃（河南中医学院）
　　　　吴秀芬（北京中医药大学）
　　　　于　越（天津中医学院）
　　　　王　彭（天津中医学院）

编　审　戴锡孟（天津中医学院）

主　译　储利荣（天津中医学院）

译　者　徐　立（天津中医学院）
　　　　关启升（天津中医学院）
　　　　王建军（天津中医学院）

CHINESE MEDICAL FORMULAE

Chief Editor Yang Yuzhou (Tianjin College of Traditional Chinese Medicine)

Vice Chief Editors Wang Xiulian (Tianjin College of Traditional Chinese Medicine)

Qian Juyi (Tianjin College of Traditional Chinese Medicine)

Chai Kefu (Zhejiang College of Traditional Chinese Medicine)

Editors Xu Li (Tianjin College of Traditional Chinese Medicine)

Zhou Jie (Tianjin College of Traditional Chinese Medicine)

Sha Mingrong (Tianjin College of Traditional Chinese Medicine)

Liu Yi (Tianjin College of Traditional Chinese Medicine)

Peng Bo (Henan College of Traditional Chinese Medicine)

Wu Xiufen (Beijing University of Traditional Chinese Medicine)

Yu Yue (Tianjin College of Traditional Chinese Medicine)

Wang Peng (Tianjin College of Traditional Chinese Medicine)

Chief Reviser Dai Ximeng (Tianjin College of Traditional Chinese Medicine)

Chief Translator Chu Lirong (Tianjin College of Traditional Chinese Medicine)

Translators Xu Li (Tianjin College of Traditional Chinese Medicine)

Guan Qisheng (Tianjin College of Traditional Chinese Medicine)

Wang Jianjun (Tianjin College of Traditional Chinese Medicine)

前　言

随着世界范围内中医药热潮的涌动，前来我国学习、研究中医药学的各国留学生（进修生）日益增多。已经形成了一支学习、继承、传播、发展中医药事业不可忽视的力量。为了适应中医药学高水平国际交流形势的迫切需要，在上级有关领导部门的支持下，1995年在全国中医药高等教育国际交流与合作学会年会上，由北京中医药大学、广州中医药大学、河南中医学院、浙江中医学院等21所中医药高等院校发起协作编写这套英汉对照"全国高等中医药院校外国进修生教材"，以期为促进中医药学科体系的弘扬传播，为进一步拓展高等中医药教育的国际交流与合作的事业做出应有的贡献。

本套系列教材采取英汉对照形式，包括《中医基础学》、《中医诊断学》、《中药学》、《方剂学》、《中医内科学》、《针灸学》、《推拿学》七本。分别由浙江中医学院、北京中医药大学、福建中医学院、天津中医学院、河南中医学院和广州中医药大学和北京针灸骨伤学院担任主编单位。为确保本教材的编写质量，协编院校成立了教材编写委员会，由北京中医药大学国际学院院长吴秀芬教授任主任，广州中医药大学李道生教授、河南中医学院副院长彭勃教授任副主任，负责组织协调本套教材的中英文编写、翻译及审订、审校工作。

本套教材的编写原则是既坚持中医药学体系的系统性、科学性、独特性和实践性，又注意到阅读对象在学习时间、语言及民族文化心理等方面的特殊性，在确保教学内容的深度、广度的前提下，努力坚持文字简约、通顺易懂，篇幅精练、阐述明确、利于实用。

本套教材编写过程中基本按照教学大纲要求，并参照高等中医药院校五版（部分六版）教材和高等中医药院校外国进修生教材的主要内容，注重协调学术发展中的继承与创新、理论与实践的关系。各书主编及作者均为多年从事高等中医药对外教育第一线的教师，具有大量的实践经验和教学体会，善于针对留学生（进修生）特点进行教学。可以说是一套较为成熟的、结合中医药理论与对外教学实际的、实用性较强的系列教材。

在本套教材的英译工作中各校专家投入了大量精力，为尽可能统一规范英译中医名词术语问题，1996年底在福建中医学院专门召开各书主要英译人员会议。各书在中文定稿时均专门召开主编、副主编审稿会，严格复审、终审，反复斟酌修改。充分注意到留学生语言及文化差异等特点。

中医药学走向世界，尤其是中医药学传统理论走向世界，面临着从实践技能的介绍到思维模式的沟通等等不同层面上的"跨文化传播"问题。因此，本系列教材经过全体编写人员和英译人员的不懈努力，也仅仅是为这一长期目标进行一些初步的探索。限于条件及水平，不足之处敬待使用者指出，以便不断促进高等中医药院校留学生教学工作的深入和提高。

全国中医药高等教育国际交流与合作学会
英汉对照全国高等中医药院校外国进修生教材编委会

PREFACE

Alongside the worldwide enormous upsurge of interest in traditional Chinese medicine more and more overseas (advanced) students come to China to pursue it, and they have become a force not to be ignored in study, inheritance, dissemination and development of traditional Chinese medicine. To meet the urgent high-leveled international exchange in this area, there arose an idea to compile a series of English-Chinese college textbooks of traditional Chinese medicine for overseas students on the 1995 annual meeting of the National Association of TCM Overseas Higher Education & Exahcnge.

The motion was put forward by 21 universities and college of TCM headed by the Beijing University of TCM, Guangzhou University of TCM, Henan College of TCM, Zhejiang College of TCM, etc. with the support of the authority concerned. It is expected the series of textbooks will push dissemination of the scientific system of TCM and make due contribution to international exchange and cooperation in traditional Chinese medical education.

In bilingual form, the series includes seven textbooks, namely: Basic Theory of Traditional Chinese Medicine, Traditional Chinese Diagnostics, Chinese Materia Medica, Chinese Medical Formulae, Traditional Chinese Internal Medicine, Acupuncture-Moxibustion and Tuinaology.

The following six universities and colleges of TCM located in Zhejiang province, Beijing, Fujian province, Tianjin, Henan province and Guangzhou assume the responsibility for the chief editors. To ensure the quality an editorial committee has been established chaired by Prof. Wu Xiufeng, Dean of the International School, Beijing University of TCM. The vice-chairmen are Prof. Li Daosheng, Guangzhou University of TCM and Prof. Peng Bo, Vice-president of the Henan College of TCM. They are in charge of coordination of the compilation, translation and editing.

The series adheres to the systematic scientific and practical nature and uniqueness of the traditional Chinese medical theory, and the specific characteristics of the readers' language, national, cultural psychology and their time spent on study. Predicated on the depth and breadth of the knowledge we advocate simple language easy to understand, limited space, clear exposition and practical usage.

In compilation the series is almost based on the requirement of the syllabus with reference to the mainstay of the Textbooks for Students of Colleges of TCM (6th edition) and the Textbooks for Foreign Advanced Students in association with inheritance and creation, theory and practice in academic progress. The chief editors and authors are faculty members of these universities and colleges engaged in education for foreign students for years. They have accumulated a wealth of experience in teaching of overseas students in accordance with their special characteristics. The series can be regarded as a well-thought-out, practical textbooks which combine the theory of TCM with experience in external teaching.

Great energies have been devoted to the English version. To standardize the Chinese medical terms a special meeting was called for the translators at the Fujian College of TCM at the end of 1996. Chief and deputy-chief editors have gone over the manuscripts and given their comments and suggestions. The series has gone through repeated revision and final revision and the characteristics of the foreign students' language and cultural difference are constantly stressed.

Introduction of traditional Chinese medical therapy, especially its theory to the world is actually a kind of cross-culture dissemination in different levels, from healing art to mode of thinking. With the efforts of the compiling staff and translators it is only a preliminary probe for the long-standing goal.

Because of the present condition and level, the editors hope that readers will comment on the shortcomings of the series to help promote the advance of TCM education for foreign students.

Editorial Committee,
University Textbooks of Traditional Chinese Medicine for
Overseas Advanced Students, National Association of TCM
Overseas Higher Education & Exchange

编 写 说 明

本《方剂学》是英汉对照"全国高等中医药院校外国进修生教材"系列的分册,是针对来华留学生学习方剂的需要而编写的。

该书分为三部分:绪言部分简介了方剂学发展简史;总论部分以方剂学基本理论为主要内容;各论部分按治法分为 20 章,选入主方 153 首,附方 42 首。

在《方剂学》的编写过程中,内容上突出了教材的系统性和科学性,方剂的选择上注意针对性和实用性,以具有典型组方原则、临床常用的方剂作为每类方剂的主方,并将方剂的使用与临床进行了有机结合。文字方面,针对留学生的语言特点,力求简而明,通俗易懂,译文准确流畅。

由于水平有限,书中可能有不少缺点和遗漏之处,敬请国内外同道在使用过程中提出批评指正。

编 者
2001 年 3 月

FOREWORD

Chinese Medical Formulae is one book of English-Chinese Series of College Textbooks of Traditional Chinese Medicine for Overseas Students. It is specially compiled for overseas students to study Chinese herbal prescriptions.

The book is divided into three parts: The first part, Introduction, is the brief history of Chinese medical formulae; the second part, Generalities, is the basic theory of Chinese medical formulae; and the third part, Particulars, is the individual prescriptions which are divided into 20 chapters according to treatment methods and contains 153 main prescriptions and 42 appended prescriptions.

During the compilation, we systematically and scientifically organized the contents of the book and collected practical formulas. Taking the prescriptions of typical composing principles and the commonly used prescriptions as the main formulas, we organically combined the application of prescriptions with clinical practice. As for the language and translated text, we tried to make them concise, accurate, smooth and easy to understand so as to be most suitable for overseas students.

Because of our limited level, there may be some defects and omissions in the book, we welcome criticism and corrections from colleagues in China and abroad.

Author

March, 2001

目　录

CONTENTS

2 Heat-Clearing Prescriptions ·· (131)

绪言

方剂，是在辨证求因、确定治法的基础上，按照一定的组方原则选择药物组成的。方剂学则是研究阐明方剂理论及其运用的一门学科。

方剂的历史悠久。早在原始社会时期，我们的祖先就已经使用单味药物治疗疾病了，在实践过程中逐步认识到几味药物合起来使用疗效更佳，由此而形成了方剂的雏形。1979 年长沙市马王堆三号汉墓中发现的《五十二病方》可以说是中国现存最早的一部方书，其成书年代约在公元前三世纪。

始于战国成于秦汉时期的《黄帝内经》是现存最早的一部中医理论经典著作，此书虽非方剂学专著，但对方剂学的基本理论，如对治则、治法、遣药组方和配伍宜忌等方面都进行了论述，同时还记载了 13 首方剂及汤、膏、丸、酒等剂型，为方剂学的形成与发展奠定了理论基础。东汉张仲景所著《伤寒杂病论》载方 375 首，不仅有方名、服法，且融理法方药为一体，组方严谨，疗效可靠，被后世誉为"方书之祖"。晋唐时期，方剂学进一步发展，如孙思邈的《千金要方》、《千金翼方》，王焘的《外台秘要》收集了大量方剂，是集唐以前诸方之大成。宋代著名方书《太平圣惠方》，载方 16834 首，《圣济总录》载方近两万首，《太平惠民和剂局方》不仅是中国历史上第一部由官方编制成的药典，也是世界上最早的国家药局方之一。宋代成无己《伤寒明理论》对 20 首方剂进行了解释，开方论之先河。明代《普济方》收方六万余首，是收方最多的方书。吴崑的《医方考》是历史上第一部详细释方的专著，它的问世，是方剂学发展史上的一个转折，由重在收集转变为重在释方。清代，随着温病学派的崛起，创造了许多治疗温热病的方剂，使得方剂学的内容更加充实完善。

中华人民共和国成立以后，对方书进行了大量搜集、注释、点校工作，通过临床和实验研究，进一步探讨了方剂的作用机理，筛选了众多的有效方剂，进行了剂型改革，使方剂学的发展呈现出更加广阔的前景。

总之，方剂学是在历代医家广泛实践的基础上逐步发展起来的，是中医辨证论治体系的重要组成部分，也是临床各科的基础，因此学习方剂学必须强调是在中医理论的指导下学习。在学习方剂学的过程中，要注意掌握组方规律，即设计一首方剂首先依据临床辨证，确立治法原则，而后根据立法，选药用方；要注意方义分析，即解释方义必须以理法为指导，结合功效、主治病证全面分析，并且在分析一首方剂时，既要看到单味药的治疗作用，又要重视药物配伍应用的协同作用，进而真正学到立法组方的理论知识和技能。

上篇 总 论

1 组方原则

方剂不是具有相同作用的药物的拼凑，其组成有严格的原则性。"方从法出"及"主、辅、佐、使"的配伍组成，是遣药组方必须遵循的原则。

"方从法出"说明了方剂与治法的关系。方剂的组成是在辨证立法的基础上进行的，先立法，后组方，以法统方。治法是遣药组方的依据，而组成的方剂是体现和完成治法的手段，方中寓法，不含治法的方剂是不存在的，治法与方剂相互依存密不可分。

"主、辅、佐、使"是方剂的配伍原则。按此原则配伍，能发挥最佳疗效。

主药：是针对病因或主证起主要治疗作用的药物，是每个方剂中的核心。

辅药：有两种意义。(1)辅助主药治疗主证，加强主药疗效。(2)针对兼证起主要治疗作用。

佐药：有3种意义。(1)协助主药、辅药起治疗作用。(2)消除或缓解主药、辅药的药物毒性。(3)反佐作用。即病邪甚，可能拒药，配伍与君药性味相反又能在治疗中起相成作用的药物。

使药：有两种意义。(1)引经药，即引方中诸药到达病所的药物。(2)调和药，具有调和方中诸药作用的药物。

综上所述，可知主药是一个方中的主导，必不可少，而且用量宜大。而其它药物不一定完全具备，要视病情需要进行选择，如主药无毒或作用不峻猛，就不需要用消除、减弱毒性或制其猛烈之性的佐制药。在方剂的配伍中，有的是主辅相配，有的主佐相合，有的主使同用，还有的单用主药，当然也有的主辅佐使俱备，如麻黄汤。这些不同的配伍形式，主要取决于治法，依据于病情。

2 组成变化

　　方剂的组成既有严格的原则性，又有很大的灵活性。灵活性主要是根据病证的变化，进行药味加减、药量变化以及剂型的更换。只有把原则性和灵活性在临床运用中统一起来，才能方证相符，提高疗效。

2.1　药味加减变化

　　指在一首方剂的主证不变的情况下，随着次要症状及兼证的不同，对该方剂除主药以外的其它药物进行增减。如桂枝汤主治风寒表虚证，若患者兼有咳喘，在桂枝汤的基础上加用厚朴、杏仁，名桂枝加厚朴杏子汤。又如麻黄汤主治外感风寒表实证，重在发汗解表。若外感风寒，所伤在肺而出现鼻塞声重，咳嗽痰多等证，以宣肺解表为主，用麻黄汤去掉桂枝，名三拗汤。这种药味加减的变化，体现了组方的灵活性。

2.2　药量增减变化

　　指组成方剂的药物不改变，而药量发生改变，方剂的作用也随之发生变化。其结果有的是原来的作用不变，增加了其他作用，有的是主要作用发生了变化。如四逆汤与通脉四逆汤二方药物组成相同，只是四逆汤中附子、干姜用量较小，其功用主要是回阳救逆。而通脉四逆汤，附子、干姜用量较大，其功用是回阳逐阴，通脉救逆。由于功效不同，主治证亦有不同。前方主治阴盛阳微所致四肢厥逆，恶寒蜷卧、下利、脉微弱等，后方则用于阴盛格阳所致四肢厥逆，下利清谷，脉微欲绝的证候。

2.3　剂型更换的变化

　　同一方剂，由于剂型不同，其治疗作用也不同。剂型的更换主要是根据病情决定的。一般认为汤剂作用快，力量大；而丸、散剂作用缓而持久。如理中汤与理中丸，药味完全相同，均治中焦虚寒、腹痛、自利或便溏不成形等，只是由于剂型不同而其功用有别，理中汤适用于病证重急者，而理中丸适用于病情较轻者。

　　以上3种变化，在临床上可以分别运用，也可以合并运用，灵活掌握方剂的组成变化，就能使辨证施治达到预期的目的。

3 剂型与煎服法

3.1 剂型

方剂的剂型有汤剂、散剂、丸剂、膏剂、丹剂、酒剂、茶剂、药露、锭剂、饼剂、条剂、线剂、灸剂、糖浆剂、片剂、冲服剂、针剂等等。临床最常用的是汤剂、丸剂。现介绍如下：

3.1.1 汤剂

把药物配齐后，用水或黄酒，或水酒各半浸透后，再煎煮一定时间，然后去渣取汤，称为汤剂。汤剂的特点是吸收快，力量强，便于根据病情及病人体质状况灵活加减。一般做内服用，也可以灌肠、外洗。汤剂是临床最常用的剂型。

3.1.2 丸剂

将药物研成细末，用蜜、水、或米糊、或面糊、或酒、或醋、或药汁、或蜂蜡等作为赋型剂制成的圆形固体剂型。丸剂的特点是吸收缓慢，药力持久，服用方便，一般适用于慢性和虚弱性疾病。临床最常用的是蜜丸和水丸。

蜜丸：是将药物研成细粉，用炼过的蜂蜜作赋型剂制成丸。

水丸：是将药物研成细粉，用冷开水或酒、醋、或其中部分煎汁等湿润、粘合作用，用人工或机械制成的小丸。

3.2 煎法

煎药前，先将药物放入陶瓷砂锅内，加冷水漫过药面，浸透后再煎煮。开始用武火，煎沸后用文火。煎药时不宜频频打开锅盖，以防气味走失。对解表药、清热药、芳香类药，宜武火急煎，以免药性挥发，药效降低。对于厚味滋补药，宜文火缓煎，使药效尽出。对于一些有毒性的药物，宜慢火久煎，以减低毒性。

对于某些特殊药物应采取特殊煎煮方法，处方时要注明。现介绍几种特殊煎法：

3.2.1 先煎

介壳类、矿石类药物，应打碎先煎，煮沸后约 10～20 分钟，再下其它药。对于泥砂较多的药物如灶心土等也应先煎，取汁澄清，再以其汁代水煎煮其它药物。

3.2.2 后下

气味芳香，有效成分容易挥发的药物，宜在其它药即将煎好时投放；煎 4～5 分钟即可，如薄荷、砂仁等。

3.2.3 包煎

有些药物煎后药液混浊，或服药时对咽喉有刺激，应用纱布包好，再放入锅内煎，如辛夷、旋覆花等。

3.2.4 另炖

为了尽量保存某些贵重药物的有效成分，减少同时煎药被其它药物吸收，可另炖或另煎，如将人参、切成小片，放入盖盅内，隔水炖2～3小时。对于贵重又难于煎出气味的药物，如羚羊角也应另煎。

3.2.5 溶化（烊化）

对于胶质、粘性大而且易溶的药物，应单独加温溶化，再加入去渣的药液中微煮或趁热搅拌，溶解后服用，如阿胶、鹿角胶等。

3.2.6 冲服

散剂、丹剂、小丸、自然汁以及某些芳香或贵重药物，需要冲服，如麝香、三七末等。

3.3 服法

服药方法当否，直接影响着疗效。服法包括服药时间和服药方法。

3.3.1 服药时间

一般补养药宜饭前服用；对胃肠道有刺激的药宜饭后服；杀虫药及泻下药宜空腹服；安神药宜睡前服。急性病不狙时间，及时服药。慢性病服丸、散、膏、酒者应定时。一般药可每日早晚各1次，有的可1日数次，也有的可代茶频服。

3.3.2 服药方法

汤剂一般温服，1剂药可分为2服或分3服。解表药除温服外，还应注意服后温覆取微汗。热证用寒药时，可以冷服。寒证服热药可以热服。如系真热假寒，宜寒药热服；如系真寒假热，则宜热药冷服。对于呕吐不止者，宜加入少许姜汁，或嚼少许陈皮，或少服、频服。对于昏迷病人，或牙关紧闭者，可采用鼻饲给药方法。

下篇 各 论

1 解表剂

凡是以解表药为主组成，具有发汗、解肌、透疹作用，用以解除表证的方剂，统称为解表剂。解表剂的适应证是表证。

根据表证有风寒、风热之别，患者的体质有虚实之异，故将解表剂分为辛温解表，辛凉解表，扶正解表 3 类。

使用解表剂需注意煎煮时间不宜过长，以免有效成分挥发，治疗作用减弱。服药后要避风保暖取微汗。

1.1 辛温解表

辛温解表剂适用于外感风寒表证，以恶寒发热、头项强痛、肢体酸痛、无汗或有汗、脉浮紧或浮缓为主证。

麻 黄 汤
《伤寒论》

【组成】 麻黄（去节）6g 桂枝 4g 杏仁（去皮尖）9g 甘草（炙）3g

【用法】 水煎服，服后覆盖衣被取微汗。

【功效】 发汗解表，宣肺平喘。

【主治】 外感风寒，恶寒发热，头痛身痛，骨节酸痛，无汗，口不渴，或伴有喘促气逆，舌苔薄白而润，脉浮紧。

【方解】 用麻黄苦辛温，发汗解表，宣肺平喘，为方中主药；用桂枝辛甘温，温经通阳，振奋营卫，有助于营卫赴表抗邪，为辅药；杏仁苦辛温，宣肃肺气，为佐药；炙甘草调和诸药，且缓解麻黄、桂枝相合的峻烈之性，为使药。四药配伍，共收散寒解表，宣肺平喘之功。

【按语】

（1）本方为辛温发汗峻剂，临床适用于外感风寒表实证，以发热恶寒、无汗而喘、脉浮紧为辨证要点。现代医学中的感冒、流感、支气管炎、支气管哮喘有上述见症者，可用本方加减治疗。

（2）风寒表虚证，风热表证及素体营血不足，正气虚弱者禁用。

【附方】

（1）麻黄加术汤《金匮要略》 即麻黄汤原方加白术 12g。功能发汗解表，散寒祛湿。用治寒湿伤于肌表,身体烦痛者。

(2) 麻黄杏仁薏苡甘草汤《金匮要略》 麻黄 6g 杏仁 6g 薏苡仁 15g 炙甘草 3g。功能解表祛湿。用治风湿在表,一身尽痛,下午发热加剧者。

(3) 三拗汤《太平惠民和剂局方》 即麻黄汤减去桂枝。功能宣肺解表,用治外感风邪,鼻塞声重,语音不出,咳嗽痰多,胸满气短,头痛身痛等。

桂 枝 汤
《伤寒论》

【组成】 桂枝 9g 芍药 9g 炙甘草 6g 生姜 3 片 大枣 4 枚

【用法】 水煎温服,服后可喝少量开水或热稀粥,冬季盖被保温,以助药力。禁食油腻生冷。

【功效】 解肌发表,调和营卫。

【主治】 外感风邪,发热头痛,汗出恶风,鼻鸣干呕,苔白不渴,脉浮缓或浮弱。

【方解】 用桂枝辛温,解肌发表,外散风邪,为方中主药;用芍药苦酸,敛阴和营,与桂枝相伍,调和营卫为辅药;生姜辛温,既助桂枝解肌,又能和胃止呕;大枣甘平,与生姜配伍,可助桂、芍调和营卫之功,共为佐药;炙甘草益气和中,调和诸药,为使药。诸药配伍,共收解肌和里之功。

【按语】

(1) 本方适用于外感风寒表虚证,以发热恶风,汗出,脉缓为辨证要点。临床上亦可用于产后、病后、内科杂病中出现的发热自汗出,脉浮弱者。对于妊娠恶阻属营卫不和,气血不调者亦有良效。

(2) 表实无汗或有里热者不宜使用。

【附方】

桂枝加厚朴杏子汤《伤寒论》 即桂枝汤原方加厚朴、杏仁各 6g。功能解肌发表,下气平喘。用治宿有喘病复感风寒而见桂枝汤证者,或表证未解而微喘者。

葛 根 汤
《伤寒论》

【组成】 葛根 12g 麻黄 9g 生姜 9g 桂枝 6g 白芍 6g 炙甘草 6g 大枣 4 枚

【用法】 水煎温服,覆被取微似汗出。

【功效】 发表解肌。

【主治】 外感风寒,项背强几几,无汗恶风者,或下利或呕,脉浮。

【方解】 本方实为桂枝汤加麻黄、葛根组成。葛根甘辛凉入脾胃经,可解阳明肌表之邪,以除项背强几几,为方中主药;麻黄配桂枝汤发太阳经之汗,以散风寒而解表。诸药配伍,共治太阳阳明合病诸证。

【按语】

(1) 本方适用于外感风寒表实证的项背强急,以无汗恶风为辨证要点。颈椎病、肩周炎表现后头隐痛,项背牵强,肩臂疼痛酸麻者,可用本方加减治疗。

(2) 汗出恶风者禁用。

【附方】

桂枝加葛根汤《伤寒论》 即葛根汤去麻黄。功能解肌舒筋。用治太阳病,项背强痛,汗出恶风者。

苏羌达表汤
《重订通俗伤寒论》

【组成】 苏叶6g 防风3g 杏仁6g 羌活3g 白芷3g 橘红3g 生姜3g 茯苓皮6g

【用法】 水煎温服。

【功效】 发汗解表除湿。

【主治】 外感风寒兼湿证,头痛项强,鼻塞流涕,身体重痛,发热恶寒或恶风,无汗,脉浮。

【方解】 用苏叶辛温,羌活苦辛温,辛散在表风寒湿邪,共为方中主药;用辛温之白芷、防风助主药祛风解表胜湿止痛,为辅药;用杏仁、橘红轻苦微辛,宣肺理气燥湿,为佐药;用生姜、茯苓皮辛淡发散祛湿,共为使药。诸药配伍,共收发汗解表,祛湿之功。

【按语】

(1) 本方应用于外感风寒湿证,以身体疼痛,无汗为主证。流感、风湿性关节炎属于风寒湿在表者,可加减应用。

(2) 临床使用可根据病情,适当加重药物用量,注意不要久煎。

(3) 茯苓皮可用茯苓代之,用治一般伤风感冒亦可酌减或不用。

1.2 辛凉解表

辛凉解表剂适用于外感风热证。以发热微恶风寒,头痛咽痛、口渴、脉浮数为主证。

桑 菊 饮
《温病条辨》

【组成】 桑叶7.5g 菊花3g 杏仁6g 连翘5g 薄荷2.4g 桔梗6g 甘草2.4g 苇根6g

【用法】 水煎服,日2服。

【功效】 疏风清热,宣肺止咳。

【主治】 外感风热初起,身热不甚,咳嗽,口微渴,咽干或咽痛。

【方解】 用菊花辛凉、桑叶甘寒,清透肺络,疏散上焦风热,为方中主药;薄荷辛凉宣散,助桑叶、菊花疏解上焦风热;杏仁、桔梗一升一降宣肺止咳,共为辅药;连翘清热透表,苇根清热生津,为佐药;甘草调和诸药,为使药,且与桔梗配伍可利咽喉。诸药配伍,共奏疏风清热,止咳之功。

【按语】

流感、急性支气管炎,属于风热者,可用本方加减治疗。另外,用本方加白蒺藜、决明子、夏枯草可治流行性结膜炎。加牛蒡子、生地、玄参、板蓝根、山豆根、土牛膝等可治疗急性扁桃体炎。

银翘散
《温病条辨》

【组成】 银花9g 连翘9g 桔梗6g 薄荷6g 竹叶4g 生甘草5g 荆芥5g 淡豆豉5g 牛蒡子9g 芦根9g

【用法】 水煎服，日2服。

【功效】 辛凉解表，透热解毒。

【主治】 外感风热初起，发热微恶风寒，无汗或有汗不畅，头痛口渴，咳嗽咽痛，苔薄白或薄黄，舌边尖红，脉浮数。

【方解】 用银花、连翘甘寒芳香，辛凉透表，清热解毒，为方中主药；用荆芥、豆豉助主药开皮毛而逐邪，二药虽为辛温之品，但配入辛凉药物之中，无温燥之弊，而有增强透邪之功；薄荷辛凉，疏散风热，三药并为辅药；牛蒡子、桔梗、甘草宣肺祛痰利咽；竹叶、芦根清热生津止渴，为佐药，且生甘草调和诸药。诸药配伍，共收辛凉透表，清热解毒之功。

【按语】

(1) 临床适用于流感、急性扁桃体炎、麻疹初期、流行性脑膜炎初起有风热表证者；也可酌加清热解毒药，用于疮痈初起有风热表证者。

(2) 头痛、恶寒发热、口不渴、脉不数者，不宜用本方。

清解汤
《医学衷中参西录》

【组成】 薄荷叶12g 蝉蜕9g 生石膏18g 甘草5g

【用法】 水煎服，薄荷叶后下。

【功效】 透表清热。

【主治】 外感风热，头痛、周身骨节酸痛，肌肤壮热，背微恶寒无汗，脉浮滑。

【方解】 用薄荷辛凉，疏散在表的风热，为方中主药；用蝉蜕甘寒，助主药凉散风热。石膏辛寒，清散肺胃之热，共为辅药；石膏配伍薄荷、蝉蜕达表之药，使内热由表而散；甘草调和诸药为使药。四药配伍，共收解表清热之功。

【按语】

(1) 感冒、流感属于外感风热而见上述症状者可用本方治疗。

(2) 外感风寒所致周身关节疼痛忌用。

1.3 扶正解表

扶正解表剂适用于体虚外感之证，由于体虚有气虚、阳虚、阴虚的不同，故有益气解表，助阳解表和滋阴解表之别。

人参败毒散
《太平惠民和剂局方》

【组成】 人参6g（或党参9g） 枳壳6g 桔梗6g 柴胡6g 前胡6g 羌活6g 独

活 6g　川芎 6g　茯苓 6g　甘草 6g　生姜 2 片　薄荷 3g

【用法】　水煎服，日 2 服。

【功效】　益气解表，散风祛湿

【主治】　气虚之人外感风寒湿邪，症见头痛项强，憎寒壮热，肢体酸痛，鼻塞声重，胸膈满闷，咳嗽有痰，舌苔白腻，脉浮无力。

【方解】　用羌活、独活辛温，辛散一身上下之风寒湿邪而止周身疼痛，为方中主药；川芎活血祛风，柴胡辛散解肌，助主药祛邪止痛，为辅药；前胡、枳壳理气化痰，桔梗、茯苓宣肺利湿，四药合用利肺气，除痰湿，止咳嗽；人参、甘草益气扶正以祛邪，为佐药；生姜、薄荷发散风寒，宣解表邪，皆为佐使之药。诸药配伍，共奏益气解表、散风除湿之功。

【按语】

（1）本方亦适用于痢疾初起，正气虚而表里俱寒者。

（2）使用本方，人参的用量可据病人的情况加减，但不能完全去掉。无表证，邪已入里化热的痢疾忌用。

麻黄附子细辛汤
《伤寒论》

【组成】　麻黄 6g　附子 9g　细辛 3g

【用法】　水煎温服。

【功效】　助阳解表。

【主治】　素体阳虚外感风寒，症见恶寒发热，寒重热轻，神疲欲卧，舌苔水滑，脉沉细。

【方解】　用麻黄辛温发汗，解在表的风寒之邪；附子辛热，温一身之阳气；细辛通彻表里，内助附子散少阴寒邪，外助麻黄解在表之寒邪。三药配合，共奏助阳解表之功。

【按语】

（1）虚寒性头痛、咽痛，亦可用本方治疗。

（2）本方适用于阳虚而兼外感者，但阳虚程度不宜过重。若下利清谷，脉微欲绝的阳气衰微之证，不宜使用本方。

加减葳蕤汤
《通俗伤寒论》

【组成】　葳蕤（玉竹）9g　淡豆豉 9g　生葱白 6g　桔梗 5g　白薇 3g　薄荷 5g　炙甘草 1.5g　红枣 2 枚

【用法】　水煎温服。

【功效】　滋阴清热，发汗解表。

【主治】　素体阴虚，感受外邪。头痛身热，微恶风寒，无汗或有汗不多，咳嗽心烦，咽干口渴，舌赤脉数。

【方解】　用葳蕤甘平，滋阴养液，以助汗源，润肺燥，为方中主药；豆豉、薄荷、葱白、桔梗解表宣肺，止咳利咽，且疏散外邪，共为辅药；白薇助葳蕤养阴清热，除烦止渴，甘草、大枣甘润增液共为佐药。诸药配伍，解表发汗而不伤阴，滋阴而不留邪，共奏滋阴解表之功。

【按语】

(1) 本方除用于阴虚体弱的感冒外，还可用于冬温咳嗽，咽干痰结，以及肺结核患者，复感外邪，有阴伤之象者。

(2) 感冒无阴虚之象，或挟痰湿者禁用。

小结

解表剂共选主方 10 首，根据其功用分为辛温解表、辛凉解表、扶正解表 3 类。

(1) 辛温解表 麻黄汤发汗之力较强，且具宣肺平喘之功，适用于外感风寒，无汗而喘的表实证。桂枝汤发汗之力较逊，善于解肌和营，适用于外感风寒，汗出恶风的表虚证。葛根汤长于发汗解肌，适用于外感风寒，项背强几几，无汗恶风者。而苏羌达表汤发汗解表兼以祛湿，适用于外感风寒挟湿证。

(2) 辛凉解表 银翘散、桑菊饮均为治疗风热表证的常用方剂。银翘散疏表之力较大，且长于清热解毒，适用于热重寒轻、咳嗽咽痛、口渴等证。而桑菊饮解表力小，长于宣肺止咳，适用于风热袭肺，咳而微发热者。清解汤辛凉透表兼具清里热之功，适用于外感风热，周身关节酸痛，肌肤壮热者。

(3) 扶正解表 人参败毒散益气解表，适用于气虚而外感风寒湿邪者。麻黄附子细辛汤助阳解表，适用于阳虚外感风寒者。加减葳蕤汤养阴解表，适用于阴虚外感风热者。

复习思考题

(1) 试比较麻黄汤、桂枝汤组成、功效、主治的异同。

(2) 试述银翘散、桑菊饮的异同点。

(3) 扶正解表方剂分为哪几类，各自代表方剂是什么？

(4) 人参败毒散的组方意义是什么？

2 清热剂

以清热药为主要组成，具有清热、泻火、解毒、凉血的作用，用于治疗里热证的方剂，统称为清热剂。

里热证有在气分、血分、脏腑的不同，又有实热、虚热的区别，将清热剂分为清气分热、清营凉血、气血两清、清热解毒、清脏腑热、清虚热6类。

清热剂的适应证是外无表邪、里无结实的里热证。使用时要注意辨别热证的虚实，区分所在脏腑，并根据患者热势轻重、体质情况，适时、适量的应用，务求切中病机，并注意防止过度损伤脾胃。

2.1 清气分热

清气分热的方剂适用于热在气分、热盛伤津见壮热、烦渴、汗出、脉洪大等证，或热炽气分，扰及胸膈，或热病后余热未清，见心烦不安等证。

白 虎 汤
《伤寒论》

【组成】 石膏30g 知母9g 甘草3g 粳米9g

【用法】 上药用水同煎，煎至米熟汤成，去药渣温服。

【功效】 清热生津，除烦止渴。

【主治】 阳明气分热盛，壮热汗出，面赤烦渴，脉洪大有力或滑数。

【方解】 用石膏辛甘大寒，清阳明气分之实热，为主药；知母苦甘寒，清热生津除烦，为辅药；甘草、粳米益胃护津，且防石膏、知母过寒伤胃，共为佐使。四药配伍，共奏清热生津，除烦止渴之功。

【按语】

(1) 本方以身热、汗出、口渴、脉洪大为使用依据。流脑、乙脑、流感、肺炎、中暑、小儿麻疹等凡具备上述症状者均可使用。系统性红斑狼疮高热、风湿热高热、细菌感染用抗生素无效的高热，亦可用本方加减治疗。

(2) 凡恶寒不罢、口不渴、无汗，或虽有汗而面色㿠白，脉虽大而重按无力者，不可使用原方。

【附方】

(1) 白虎加人参汤《伤寒论》 即白虎汤加人参（党参）。功能清热益气生津。用治热盛于里，津气两伤，或暑病见有津气两伤，身热而渴，汗出背微恶寒，脉洪大而芤。

(2) 白虎加苍术汤《类证活人书》 即白虎汤加苍术。功能清热祛湿。用治壮热、汗出、胸痞、舌红苔腻。

栀子豉汤
《伤寒论》

【组成】 栀子 10g 豆豉 10g

【用法】 水煎服。

【功效】 清热除烦。

【主治】 身热，心烦不眠，舌红苔微黄或黄腻，脉数。

【方解】 用栀子苦寒，清热泻火除烦；豆豉辛甘微苦，宣透胸膈郁热，二药合用，清透郁热而除烦。

【按语】

(1) 临床凡邪热在气分而出现发热不恶寒、无汗、心烦不眠者，即可应用本方。

(2) 若兼少气者加甘草 6g，兼呕者加生姜 9g。

(3) 方中栀子苦寒，损伤中阳，若平日脾阳素虚，大便溏薄者，不可服用本方。

凉 膈 散
《太平惠民和剂局方》

【组成】 川大黄 朴硝 甘草各 600g 山栀子仁 薄荷（去梗） 黄芩各 300g 连翘 125g

【用法】 上药共为粗末，每服 6g，加竹叶 3g，蜜少许，水煎服。亦可作汤剂煎服。

【功效】 泻热通便，清上泄下。

【主治】 中上二焦邪郁生热，胸膈结热。身热口渴，胸膈烦热，面赤唇焦，口舌生疮，或咽痛吐衄，便秘溲赤，舌苔黄，脉滑数。

【方解】 用连翘、薄荷、竹叶辛凉，清宣胸膈之热；栀子、黄芩苦寒泄热兼以解毒；酒大黄、芒硝通腑导热下行；甘草、白蜜缓急润燥。诸药配合，共奏清上泄下之功。

【按语】

(1) 急性胆囊炎，胆石症以及乙型脑炎、流脑具有发热、烦躁、便秘者，牙痛齿衄，口疮，咽喉肿痛，扁桃体炎，颈淋巴结肿大，均可用本方加味治疗。

(2) 无实热者忌用。

2.2 清营凉血

清营凉血的方剂，具有清营透热、凉血散瘀、清热解毒的作用，适用于热入营分证、热入血分证。

清 营 汤
《温病条辨》

【组成】 犀角 2g（水牛角代） 生地 15g 元参 9g 竹叶 3g 麦冬 9g 丹参 6g 黄连 5g 银花 9g 连翘 6g

【用法】 水煎服，1 日 3 服。

【功效】 清营透热,养阴活血。

【主治】 热邪传营。身热夜甚,神烦少寐,时谵语,口干不欲饮,或斑疹隐隐,舌红绛,脉细数。

【方解】 用水牛角咸寒、生地甘寒清营凉血解毒,为方中主药;元参咸寒、麦冬甘寒养阴清热为辅药;佐以银花、连翘、黄连、竹叶清热解毒,透邪于外,使邪热转出气分而解,丹参助主药清热凉血,活血散瘀,防止瘀热互结,且引诸药入心而清热,为使药。诸药合用,共收清营解毒、透热养阴之功。

【按语】

(1) 乙脑、流脑、中暑、败血证或其他热性病而见营分证者均可用本方治疗。

(2) 使用本方须以舌红绛为依据。若舌绛而苔白滑或白腻忌用。

(3) 犀角现皆用水牛角 30～60g 先煎代替。

犀角地黄汤
《备急千金要方》

【组成】 犀角 3g(水牛角代)　生地 30g　芍药 12g　丹皮 9g

【用法】 水煎服。

【功效】 清热凉血,解毒散瘀。

【主治】 热入血分。①热甚动血,出现吐血、衄血、便血、溲血以及斑色紫黑等。②蓄血,善忘如狂,漱水不欲咽,胸中烦痛,大便色黑而易解。③热扰心营,出现神昏谵语,或昏狂谵妄,舌绛起刺。

【方解】 用水牛角清心凉血解毒,为方中主药;生地清热凉血,一可助主药清解血分热毒,增强止血之功,一可养血滋阴,为辅药;芍药、丹皮凉血散瘀,共为佐使药,四药配伍,共奏凉血止血,活血散瘀之功。

【按语】

(1) 肝昏迷、尿毒症出血、各种败血证、疔疮走黄以及血液病的出血属于血热者,均可用本方治疗。支气管扩张、大叶性肺炎表现为热证咳血者,亦可用本方治疗。

(2) 犀角现用水牛角 30～60g 先煎代替。

2.3　气营（血）两清

气血两清的方剂,适用于既有气分证,又有营血分证的所谓"气血两燔证"。

加减玉女煎
《温病条辨》

【组成】 石膏 90g　知母 12g　元参 12g　生地 18g　麦冬 18g

【用法】 水煎服。

【功效】 清气凉血,养阴生津。

【主治】 气营两燔。壮热口渴,头痛,烦躁,肌肤发斑,舌绛苔黄,脉数。

【方解】 重用石膏伍知母清气泄热生津,仿白虎之义;生地、麦冬、玄参即增液汤,滋营阴而清营热。诸药合用,共奏清气凉营,养阴生津之效。

【按语】

（1）本方适用于外感热病，邪热炽盛，气营两燔之证。临床亦可加减用于急性口腔炎、舌炎而见口舌糜烂者。

（2）本方寒凉滋润，大便稀软者，不宜使用。

<h2 style="text-align:center">清瘟败毒饮</h2>
《疫疹一得》

【组成】　生石膏60g　生地30g　犀角（水牛角30g代替）　黄芩　栀子　知母　赤芍　玄参　连翘　丹皮各10g　黄连、桔梗、竹叶各6g　甘草3g

【用法】　水牛角、石膏先煎，再入群药。

【功效】　清热解毒，凉血泻火。

【主治】　温热疫毒，充斥内外，气血两燔。高热神昏，头痛如劈，大渴引饮，口干咽痛，或吐血、衄血，或外发斑疹，或四肢抽搐，或厥逆，脉沉数，或沉细数，或浮大而数，舌绛唇焦。

【方解】　本方是取白虎汤、黄连解毒汤、犀角地黄汤三方之义组合而成，具有诸方综合协同作用。其中，重用石膏配知母、甘草，清热保津，取白虎汤之义；黄芩、黄连、栀子泻三焦实火，仿黄连解毒汤之义；水牛角、生地、芍药、丹皮即犀角地黄汤凉血止血，解毒化斑；玄参、连翘、桔梗、甘草润喉利咽止痛，竹叶清心利尿，导热下行。诸药配伍泻火，凉血解毒，共奏气血两清之功。

【按语】

（1）乙脑、流脑、败血症、出血热等出现气血两燔者，常用本方治疗。

（2）本方药性大寒，非热毒极盛者，不可使用。

（3）本方用量为临床一般用量。

2.4　清热解毒

清热解毒的方剂，具有清热、泻火、解毒的作用，适用于火毒内盛及风热疫毒之证。

<h2 style="text-align:center">黄连解毒汤</h2>
《外台秘要》引崔氏方

【组成】　黄连9g　栀子9g　黄芩6g　黄柏6g

【用法】　水煎服，1日2服。

【功效】　泻火解毒。

【主治】　一切实热火毒，炽盛三焦。高热烦躁，口燥咽干，或神志错乱；或热病吐血、衄血、发斑，身热下利，湿热黄疸；外科疮痈疔毒，舌红苔黄，脉数。

【方解】　方中之药均为苦寒之品，用黄连泻上焦心火，兼泻中焦胃火，为主药；黄芩泻上焦肺火，为辅药；黄柏泻下焦之火，为佐药；栀子通泻三焦之火，导热下行，为使药。四药合用，苦寒直折，共奏清热泻火解毒之功。

【按语】

（1）脓毒血症、痢疾、肺炎等属于火热毒甚者均可用本方治疗。用于治疗脓疮疔毒，除内服外，亦可研末外敷。

（2）本方药物均苦寒之品，适用于火热之毒亢盛而阴液未伤者。注意久服易伤脾胃。热邪伤阴者不宜服用。

普济消毒饮
《东垣试效方》

【组成】 黄芩 黄连各15g 甘草 陈皮 玄参 桔梗 柴胡各6g 牛蒡子 连翘 薄荷 马勃 板蓝根各3g 升麻 僵蚕各2g

【用法】 上药为末，汤调，时时服之，或蜜拌为丸，噙化。或水煎服。

【功效】 疏风散邪，清热解毒。

【主治】 流行性热病。恶寒发热，头面红肿灼赤，目不能开，咽喉肿痛，烦躁不安，舌红苔黄，脉数有力。

【方解】 用黄芩、黄连苦寒，直折上焦心肺之热毒，为方中主药；用牛蒡子、薄荷、连翘、僵蚕辛凉，疏散上焦头面风热，为辅药；玄参、马勃、板蓝根、桔梗、甘草清解咽喉之热毒，陈皮理气疏壅，以散邪结，为佐药；升麻、柴胡疏散郁热，并协助诸药上达头面，为使药。诸药配伍，共奏清热解毒，疏风消肿之功。

【按语】

（1）颜面丹毒、流行性腮腺炎、急性扁桃体炎以及头面痈疮肿毒，有上述症状者，均可使用本方加减治疗。

（2）本方药物苦寒辛散，宜中病即止，以防过用伤阴。

（3）便秘者可加大黄。

升 降 散
《伤寒温疫条辨》

【组成】 僵蚕6g 蝉蜕3g 姜黄6g 大黄12g

【用法】 原方为细末，合研匀，分2～4次，用黄酒蜂蜜调匀冷服。现代亦作汤剂，水煎服。

【功效】 宣郁、泄热、解毒。

【主治】 温病表里三焦大热。憎寒壮热，或头痛，烦渴引饮，或咽喉肿痛，或身面红肿，或胸膈胀满等。

【方解】 用大黄苦寒，入气入血，借阳明谷道，降泻于内；僵蚕辛苦，清热解毒散结；蝉衣甘寒，散风凉肝，与僵蚕同用，轻清走上，透邪于外，皆为方中主药，为攻药；用姜黄辛散温通，入气走血，开泄气血之郁结为辅佐药。四药配伍，共奏宣郁开结、泄热解毒之功。

【按语】

本方配伍特点是升降并施，苦凉清泄，适用于温病郁热为主的病证。乙型脑炎、急性扁桃体炎、腮腺炎、肺炎、咽炎、胆道感染以及急性传染性肝炎等热病，均可用升降散加味治疗。

2.5 清脏腑热

清脏腑热的方剂,适用于邪热在不同脏腑而产生的不同的火热证候。

导 赤 散
《小儿药证直诀》

【组成】 生地 15g 木通 6g 竹叶 9g 甘草梢 3g

【用法】 水煎服。

【功效】 清心利尿。

【主治】 心经热盛,心烦口渴,渴欲冷饮,面赤,口舌生疮;或心热下移小肠,小便短黄,尿时刺痛,舌红脉数。

【方解】 用生地甘寒,清热凉血养阴,为方中主药;用木通苦寒、竹叶甘淡寒,上清心降火除烦,下利水通淋,导热下行,共为辅药;甘草清热解毒,调和诸药,为使药。诸药配伍,共奏清心养阴,导热下泄之功。

【按语】

(1) 口腔炎、肾盂肾炎、膀胱炎、小儿鹅口疮等属于心经热盛者,可用本方加减治疗。

(2) 本方以口舌生疮、小便短赤涩痛、舌红脉数为辨证要点。属于湿热蕴结膀胱的小便不利则忌用。

(3) 原方用生地、木通、生甘草梢各等份,为末,每服 10g,入竹叶 1.5g,水煎,食后温服。

龙胆泻肝汤
《医方集解》

【组成】 龙胆草 6g 柴胡 6g 泽泻 12g 车前子 9g 木通 9g 黄芩 9g 栀子 9g 当归 3g 生地 9g 生甘草 6g

【用法】 水煎服,1 日 2 服。

【功效】 泻肝胆实火,清下焦湿热。

【主治】 肝胆实火上扰,症见胁痛、口苦、目赤、耳聋耳肿、头痛;肝经湿热下注,小便淋浊、阴痒、阴肿、妇女带下等。

【方解】 用龙胆草苦寒,泻肝胆实火,清肝经湿热,为方中主药;黄芩、栀子苦寒,助主药清热泻火,为辅药;泽泻、木通、车前子清热利湿,助主药清利肝胆湿热;当归、生地养血益阴和肝,意在泻中有补,去邪不伤正,俱为佐药;柴胡疏肝,引诸药入肝胆;甘草调和诸药,为使药。诸药配伍,泻中有补,利中有滋,泻实火,利湿热而不伤阴血。

【按语】

(1) 现代常用本方治疗急性结膜炎、急性中耳炎、急性肝炎、急性胆囊炎属于肝经实火者以及急性肾盂肾炎、膀胱炎、尿道炎、急性盆腔炎、外阴炎、睾丸炎等属于肝经湿热下注者。

（2）本方药物苦寒，易损伤脾胃，要中病即止，不宜久服。

【附方】

泻青丸《小儿药证直诀》　龙胆草、栀子、大黄、川芎、当归、羌活、防风各等份，为末，蜜为丸。功能清肝泻火。用治肝胆郁火，夜卧不安，烦躁易怒，目赤肿痛，溲赤便秘，脉洪实，以及小儿急惊，热盛抽搐等。

麻杏石甘汤
《伤寒论》

【组成】　麻黄 6g　杏仁 9g　生石膏 18g　炙甘草 6g

【用法】　生石膏先煎，纳诸药，1 日 2 服。

【功效】　清宣肺热。

【主治】　肺热咳喘。身热，喘咳气急，甚或鼻煽，口渴，有汗或无汗，舌苔薄白或黄，脉滑数。

【方解】　用麻黄辛温，宣肺平喘；石膏辛寒，清泄肺热；二药相伍，两辛相加，寒温相抵，变辛温为辛凉，开壅清热，共为方中主药。杏仁降气平喘，为辅药；生甘草调和诸药为使药，且与石膏配伍，生津止渴。四药配伍，共收辛凉宣泄清肺平喘之功。

【按语】

（1）上呼吸道感染、肺炎、急性支气管炎、慢性支气管炎急性发作、大叶性肺炎、支气管肺炎以及小儿麻疹合并肺炎等病证属于肺热壅盛者均可用本方治疗。

（2）恶寒发热、口不渴、咳喘痰多者，不宜应用本方。

（3）本方石膏的用量，临床一般无汗而喘者，石膏可 2 倍于麻黄；汗出而喘者，石膏可 3～5 倍于麻黄。

泻 白 散
《小儿药证直诀》

【组成】　桑白皮 9g　地骨皮 9g　甘草 3g　粳米 6g

【用法】　水煎服。

【功效】　清肺泻热，止咳平喘。

【主治】　肺热咳嗽，甚则气喘，皮肤蒸热或发热，下午尤甚，舌红苔黄，脉细数。

【方解】　用桑白皮甘寒，泻肺热而止咳平喘，为方中主药；地骨皮甘淡寒，泻肺中伏火，兼退虚热，为辅药；甘草、粳米益胃和中以扶肺气，共为佐使。四药配伍，共奏清泻肺热，止咳平喘之功。

【按语】

（1）支气管炎、麻疹肺炎、肺结核等表现为肺热见症者可以用本方治疗。

（2）外感风寒引起的咳嗽或虚寒性咳嗽不宜使用。

（3）原方用地骨皮、桑白皮各 30g，炙甘草 3g，锉末，入粳米一撮，水煎服。

清 胃 散
《脾胃论》

【组成】 生地 12g 当归 6g 黄连 3g 丹皮 9g 升麻 3g

【用法】 水煎服。

【功效】 清胃凉血。

【主治】 胃火上攻，牙痛牵引头脑痛，面颊发热，或牙宣出血；或牙龈溃烂；或唇舌颊腮肿痛；或口气热臭，口舌干燥，舌红苔黄，脉数。

【方解】 用黄连苦寒，清泻胃火，为方中主药；生地、丹皮清热凉血滋阴，为辅药；当归养血和血，有助于消肿止痛，为佐药；升麻散火解毒，与黄连配伍，升降相宜，使上炎之火得以泄降，使内郁之火得以解散，并为阳明引经药，为使药。诸药配伍，共奏清胃凉血之功。

【按语】

(1) 三叉神经痛、口腔炎、牙周炎属于胃火上攻者，皆可用本方治疗。

(2) 风寒牙痛或肾虚火上炎的牙痛、牙宣出血，不宜使用。

芍 药 汤
《保命集》

【组成】 芍药 20g 当归 9g 黄芩 9g 黄连 6g 大黄 9g 木香 6g 槟榔 6g 官桂 3g 甘草 6g

【用法】 水煎 2 次分服。

【功效】 调和气血，清热解毒。

【主治】 胃肠湿热，下痢腹痛，大便脓血，里急后重，肛门灼热，舌苔黄腻。

【方解】 用芍药苦酸寒、当归甘辛，调和营血，止腹痛，治下痢脓血，为方中主药；大黄、黄芩、黄连苦寒清热燥湿解毒，且通导积滞治痢，为辅药；木香、槟榔行气导滞，为佐药；甘草调中缓急，反佐一味辛热的肉桂，以防大黄、黄芩、黄连苦寒伤阳，冰伏湿热，共为使药。诸药配伍，"行血"与"调气"共施，寒热并投，兼以通因通用，便脓自愈，后重自除。

【按语】

(1) 本方是一首清泄肠胃湿热，调气和血止痢的专用方剂。细菌性痢疾、阿米巴痢疾、过敏性结肠炎、急性肠炎见有泻下不爽，里急后重等属于湿热者，均可用本方治疗。

(2) 痢疾初起有表证者，不宜用此方。

白 头 翁 汤
《伤寒论》

【组成】 白头翁 15g 黄柏 12g 黄连 5g 秦皮 12g

【用法】 水煎温服。

【功效】 清热解毒，凉血止痢。

【主治】 热痢。腹痛，里急后重，肛门灼热，便下脓血，赤多白少，渴欲饮水，脉弦数。

【方解】 用白头翁苦寒清热解毒，凉血止痢，为方中主药；黄连、黄柏苦寒清热，助主药清热解毒止痢；秦皮味苦性寒而涩，收涩止痢，共为辅佐药；四药配伍，使热清而毒解，痢止而后重自除。

【按语】

（1）本方是治疗热毒血痢的专方。临床常用于治疗急、慢性痢疾，阿米巴痢疾、细菌性痢疾，见有热毒炽盛，下痢脓血者。

（2）血虚热痢或热痢伤阴者，用本方加阿胶、甘草，名白头翁甘草阿胶汤。

左 金 丸
《丹溪心法》

【组成】 黄连180g 吴茱萸30g

【用法】 为末，水泛为丸。现代多作汤剂，按原方比例酌减。

【功效】 清肝泻火，降逆止呕。

【主治】 肝火犯胃，胁肋胀痛，胃中嘈杂，呕吐吞酸，口苦，脘痞嗳气，舌红苔黄，脉弦数。

【方解】 用黄连以泻心肝之火，为方中主药；用吴茱萸辛散温通，以疏达气机，开散郁结，且能降逆止呕，为佐使药，二药相伍，一寒一热，辛开苦降，疏散郁火，共奏清肝泻火，降逆止呕之功。

【按语】

（1）本方常用于急、慢性胃炎而见肝火犯胃者。如胃热而兼肝气不和者，可合四逆散加减，以加强疏肝和胃的功效。

（2）注意本方黄连与吴茱萸的用量比例是6:1。

2.6 清虚热

清退虚热的方剂，适用于热病后期，余邪未尽，阴液已伤的邪留阴分证，或肝肾阴虚而致的骨蒸潮热以及久热不退的虚热证。

青蒿鳖甲汤
《温病条辨》

【组成】 青蒿6g 鳖甲15g 生地12g 知母6g 丹皮9g

【用法】 以水5杯，煮取2杯，1日2服。

【功效】 滋阴透热。

【主治】 温病后期，阴液耗伤，余邪留伏阴分。夜热早凉，热退无汗，能食形瘦，舌红少苔，脉沉细略数。

【方解】 用鳖甲咸寒，滋阴清热，青蒿苦寒芳香，清热透络，引邪外出，二药配伍，滋阴清热，内清外透，使阴分邪热外达，共为方中主药；生地甘凉，知母苦寒，助鳖甲养阴清热，丹皮泄血中伏热，助青蒿透络，共为辅佐药。诸药配伍，滋中有清，清中能透，标本兼顾，共奏滋阴透热之效。

【按语】

小儿夏季热、不明原因的久热不退以及慢性肾盂肾炎、肾结核、低热不退属于阴虚有热者均可用本方加减治疗。

清 骨 散
《证治准绳》

【组成】 银柴胡 5g　鳖甲　地骨皮　知母　秦艽　青蒿　胡黄连各 3g　炙甘草 2g

【用法】 水煎 2 次分服。

【功效】 清虚热，退骨蒸。

【主治】 阴虚内热，骨蒸劳热。午后夜间潮热，手足心热，心烦口干，舌红少苔，脉细数或虚数。

【方解】 用银柴胡甘寒，清骨蒸虚劳之热，为方中主药；胡黄连、知母、地骨皮三药苦甘寒，入阴分退虚火，共为辅药；青蒿、秦艽透伏热，鳖甲滋阴清热，甘草调和诸药，共为佐使药。诸药配伍，共奏清虚热退骨蒸之功。

【按语】

(1) 本方侧重于清骨蒸之热，兼以滋阴透热。结核病、某些慢性疾病过程中出现的低热、潮热、手足心热等阴虚程度较轻，而热象较重者可用本方加减治疗。

(2) 阴虚较重，而潮热不太严重者，不宜使用原方。

(3) 方中鳖甲临床可用 9～18g，先煎。

小结

清热剂共选主方 20 首，根据其功用分为清气分热、清营凉血、气营（血）两清、清热解毒、清脏腑热、清虚热 6 类。

(1) 清气分热　白虎汤功用是清热生津，主治阳明热盛，壮热、汗出、口渴、脉洪大，为治气分热盛证的代表方剂；栀子豉汤具有清热除烦之功，以热邪初入气分、心烦不眠为主证；凉膈散能清泄膈热，且兼泻下之功，适用于热灼胸膈，烦躁不安，口舌生疮，便秘等。

(2) 清营凉血　清营汤具有清营透热、养阴活血之功，主要治疗邪入营分，身热夜甚，时有谵语，斑疹隐隐等证。犀角地黄汤则具有清热解毒、凉血散瘀之功，治疗热入血分，迫血妄行之证。

(3) 气营（血）两清　加减玉女煎、清瘟败毒饮均具气营（血）两清之功，适用于气分证未罢，又见营血分证的“气血两燔证”。加减玉女煎药力较轻，适用于气营两伤的轻证；而清瘟败毒饮清气凉血、泻火解毒并进，适用于毒邪充斥内外，气血两燔的重证。

(4) 清热解毒　黄连解毒汤、普济消毒饮、升降散均有清热解毒之功。黄连解毒汤以苦寒泻火解毒为主，主治三焦火毒热盛证。普济消毒饮则兼具疏风散邪之功，主治风热疫毒发于头面之证。升降散升降并施，兼具宣郁泄热之功，适用于郁热为主的热毒证。

（5）清脏腑热 本类方剂是按照脏腑邪热偏盛的不同分别使用的。导赤散的功用是清心利尿，主治心经有火。龙胆泻肝汤功用是泻肝胆实火，清下焦湿热，主治肝胆实火上扰、肝经湿热下注证。左金丸功用是清泄肝火，降逆止呕，主治肝火犯胃。麻杏石甘汤功用是清宣肺热，主治风热壅肺的咳喘。而泻白散的功用是清泻肺热，主治肺有伏火郁热所致的咳喘，二者虽都有清肺热之功，但前者侧重于清宣，后者侧重于清泻。清胃散的功用是清胃凉血，主治胃有积热，循经上扰的牙痛或牙宣出血等证。白头翁汤和芍药汤均有清热解毒之功，都能治疗痢疾，白头翁汤兼有凉血止痢之功，适用于赤多白少的热毒痢，而芍药汤以调气和血为主，适用于赤白相兼的湿热痢。

（6）清虚热 青蒿鳖甲汤和清骨散均有滋阴退热之功，均能治疗虚热证。青蒿鳖甲汤养阴与透热并重，主治温病后期，邪伏阴分证；而清骨散则以清虚热为主，兼以滋阴透热，主治虚劳骨蒸。

复习思考题

（1）清热剂分哪几类？其适应证各是什么？

（2）试述白虎汤的组成、功用及主治，并分析其方义。

（3）试述清营汤的组成、功用及主治，并说明配伍银花、连翘、竹叶、黄连等气分药的作用。

（4）试述黄连解毒汤的组成、功用、主治，并分析其方义。

（5）龙胆泻肝汤的组成、功用及主治是什么？为什么使用补养阴血的生地、当归？

（6）白头翁汤与芍药汤均为治痢的代表方剂，二方在功用、主治上有何不同？

（7）青蒿鳖甲汤由哪些药物组成？试分析其方义。

3 祛暑剂

凡以祛暑药为主组成，具有祛除暑邪的作用，用于治疗暑病的一类方剂，统称为祛暑剂。

根据暑邪致病具有易耗气伤津、易挟湿、或又兼表寒的特点，将祛暑剂分为祛暑解表、清暑利湿、清暑益气 3 类。

使用祛暑剂需注意，祛暑不宜过于寒凉，以免助湿；配伍祛湿之品不宜过于温燥，以免伤津。

3.1 祛暑解表

祛暑解表剂适用于暑湿内伏，复感风寒者。

香 薷 饮
《太平惠民和剂局方》

【组成】 香薷 9g　白扁豆 6g　厚朴 6g

【用法】 水煎服，或加酒少量同煎。

【功效】 祛暑解表，化湿和中。

【主治】 暑热季节，贪凉饮冷，外感于寒，内伤于湿所致头痛，恶寒发热，无汗，或腹满吐泻，舌苔白腻，脉浮等证。

【方解】 用香薷芳香辛温，发汗解表，祛暑化湿，为方中主药；用厚朴辛温理气，除满化湿为辅药；白扁豆甘淡入中焦，消脾胃之暑湿，降浊而升清为佐使药。三药配伍，共收祛暑解表，化湿和中之功。

【按语】

(1) 本方药性偏温，主治夏令感寒兼湿之证，以恶寒无汗为辨证要点。临床适用于夏季流感、胃肠炎等病见上述症状者。

(2) 发热有汗，虽有恶寒，本方亦不宜使用。

【附方】

新加香薷饮《温病条辨》 即本方加银花、连翘各 9g。功能祛暑解表，清热化湿。用治暑湿兼寒邪外束，症见恶寒发热无汗，头身疼痛，口渴面赤，舌苔白腻，脉浮而数者。

3.2 祛暑利湿

祛暑利湿剂适用于暑热挟湿证。

六 一 散
《伤寒直格》

【组成】 滑石 180g　甘草 30g

【用法】 为细末，每服 10g，包煎，或温开水调下，每日 2～3 次。亦常加入其它方药中煎服。

【功效】 祛暑利湿。

【主治】 暑湿之证，身热烦渴，小便不利或泄泻。

【方解】 用滑石性寒，味甘淡，质重而体滑，清热利湿，使三焦湿热从小便而解，为方中主药；生甘草清热和中，与滑石同用，可加强清解暑热之功，又可缓滑石之寒凉太过。二药相伍，使内蕴之暑湿下解，则热可退，渴可止。

【按语】

（1）本方用于暑湿证，以身热口渴、心烦、小便短赤为辨证要点。临床亦常用本方加味治疗湿热淋证，小便涩痛或砂淋等证。

（2）滑石 6 倍于甘草，故名六一散。因此临床应用本方，应注意其药量比例。

【附方】

（1）益元散《伤寒直格》 即六一散加辰砂、灯心汤调服。功能清心祛暑，安神。用治暑湿证兼心悸怔忡、失眠多梦者。

（2）碧玉散《伤寒直格》 即六一散加青黛。功能祛暑清热。用治暑湿证兼见咽痛目赤，口舌生疮等肝胆郁热见症者。

（3）鸡苏散《伤寒直格》 即六一散加薄荷。功能疏风祛暑，用治暑湿证兼微恶风寒、头痛头胀、咳嗽不爽者。

3.3 清暑益气

清暑益气剂适用于暑热灼伤气津之证。

王氏清暑益气汤
《温热经纬》

【组成】 西洋参 5g 石斛 15g 麦冬 9g 黄连 3g 竹叶 6g 荷梗 15g 知母 6g 甘草 3g 粳米 15g 西瓜翠衣 30g

【用法】 水煎服。

【功效】 清热涤暑，益气生津。

【主治】 暑伤津气证。身热息高，心烦口渴，汗多溺黄，体倦神疲，脉虚无力。

【方解】 用西瓜翠衣甘凉，清热透暑，止渴利小便，西洋参甘寒，益气生津止渴，共为方中主药；荷梗助西瓜翠衣清热解暑，石斛、麦冬甘寒，助西洋参养阴清热，共为辅药；知母苦寒质润，滋阴泻火，竹叶甘淡寒，清热除烦，黄连苦寒泻火，三药共为佐药；甘草、粳米益气和中，为使药。诸药配伍，使暑热消除，气阴得复。

【按语】

（1）本方用于夏月感受暑热，伤津耗气之证，以体倦少气、口渴汗多、脉虚数为辨证要点。临床亦用本方加减治疗小儿夏季热久热不退而气津不足者。

（2）本方中因有养阴滋腻之品，暑病挟湿耗伤气津者应加减使用本方。

【附方】

清暑益气汤《脾胃论》 黄芪 6g 苍术 升麻 炒曲 白术 麦门冬 黄柏 葛根

泽泻　五味子各3g　人参　橘皮各1.5g　当归　青皮　炙甘草各1g 水煎服。功能清暑益气生津，健脾除湿。用治平素气虚，复感受暑湿，头疼身热，口渴自汗，四肢困倦，不思饮食，胸满身重，小便黄赤，大便溏薄，苔腻脉虚者。

小结

祛暑剂选主方3首，按功用分为祛暑解表、祛暑利湿、清暑益气3类。

（1）祛暑解表　香薷饮具有祛暑解表、化湿和中之功，适用于夏月感寒兼湿之证。

（2）祛暑利湿　六一散为祛暑利湿剂的基础方，主治暑邪挟湿证。

（3）清暑益气　王氏清暑益气汤具有清热涤暑，益气生津之功，主治暑伤津气证。

复习思考题

（1）香薷饮主治何病？其发病机理是什么？由什么药物组成？其常见的加减变化方剂是什么？

（2）六一散常见变化方有哪些？其组成、功效、主治证各是什么？

（3）简述王氏清暑益气汤方义。

4 祛寒剂

凡以温热药为主组成，具有温里助阳，散寒通脉的作用，用于治疗里寒证的方剂，统称为祛寒剂，亦称温里剂。

里寒证的成因有外寒直中脏腑经脉和素体阳虚，寒自内生的不同。不论外寒直中，还是里寒内生，均以温里祛寒立法。根据温里剂的不同作用及里寒证的轻重，所伤的部位不同，将祛寒剂分为温中祛寒、温经散寒和回阳救逆 3 类。

祛寒剂多为辛温燥热之品，真热假寒之热厥证绝对禁用，故临床应用时必须详辨真假寒热。再者，辛热之品多有伤阴之弊，临床使用要注意中病即止。

4.1 温中祛寒

温中祛寒剂适用于中焦虚寒证。

理中丸（汤）
《伤寒论》

【组成】 人参 6g　干姜 5g　白术 9g　炙甘草 6g

【用法】 现代多用作汤剂，水煎服。

【功效】 温中祛寒，补气健脾。

【主治】 脾胃虚寒，腹痛泄泻，呕吐食少，口不渴，舌淡白，脉沉细或迟缓。

【方解】 用干姜辛热，温中祛里寒，为方中主药；用人参甘温补气健脾，为辅药；用白术健脾燥湿，以助脾胃升清降浊，受纳运化之功能，为佐药；炙甘草益气和中，为使药。四药相伍，共奏温中祛寒，补气健脾之功。

【按语】

（1）本方是治疗中焦虚寒证的代表方剂。临床适用于慢性痢疾、慢性胃肠炎，消化不良，胃肠功能减弱，以及胃、十二指肠溃疡属于脾胃虚寒者。亦常加减应用于胸痹、小儿慢惊风以及妇女功能性子宫出血属于脾胃虚寒者。

（2）以蜜为丸，作用和缓，适用于病情较轻者，若病情较急者，宜汤剂。

【附方】

附子理中丸（汤）《阎氏小儿方论》　即本方加附子。功能温阳祛寒，益气健脾。用治脾胃虚寒，下利不止，脉微，手足不温等证。

小 建 中 汤
《伤寒论》

【组成】 白芍 18g　桂枝 9g　炙甘草 6g　生姜 9g　大枣 4 枚　饴糖 30g

【用法】 前 5 味药水煎 2 次，取汁，兑入饴糖，分 2 次温服。

【功效】 温中补虚，和里缓急。

【主治】 脾胃虚寒，腹中时痛，喜温喜按，得温得按痛减，舌淡苔白，脉细弦而缓。或气血两虚，心悸虚烦不眠，面色无华，四肢酸楚等证。

【方解】 用饴糖甘温质润益脾气，养脾阴，温中焦，缓肝急，为方中主药；用桂枝，温阳气，白芍益阴血，为辅药；炙甘草助桂枝、饴糖甘温益气，合白芍，酸甘化阴，益肝滋脾，缓急止痛，为佐药；生姜、大枣补脾和营，亦为佐药。诸药配伍，辛甘化阳，酸甘化阴，共奏温中补虚，和里缓急之功。

【按语】

(1) 胃溃疡、十二指肠溃疡、肠痉挛等属于虚寒性腹痛者，以及慢性肝炎、慢性腹膜炎、神经衰弱而见上述症状者，均可用本方治疗。

(2) 注意方中饴糖须重用；白芍用量大于桂枝1倍。

【附方】

(1) 黄芪建中汤《金匮要略》 即小建中汤加黄芪。功能温中补气。用治虚劳里急诸不足。

(2) 当归建中汤《千金翼方》 即小建中汤加当归。功能温补气血，用治产后气血两虚，小腹绞痛不止，倦怠少气，或内脏虚寒，小腹时痛，痛引腹背者。

大 建 中 汤
《金匮要略》

【组成】 川椒3g 干姜4.5g 人参6g 饴糖30g

【用法】 前3味水煎，取汁，兑入饴糖，分2次温服。

【功效】 温中补虚，降逆止痛。

【主治】 中阳虚衰，阴寒内盛。心胸大寒痛，呕不能食，上下攻撑，不可触近，或腹中漉漉有声，苔白滑，脉弦迟或细紧。

【方解】 用饴糖甘温，温阳补中，缓急止痛，为方中主药；人参（党参）甘温，大补元气，助饴糖补中扶正，为辅药；川椒入肝，干姜入脾胃，皆为辛热温通之品，疏通厥阴气机，温中散寒，共为佐使，四药合用，共奏温中补虚，散寒降逆止痛之功。

【按语】

(1) 本方临床可用于肠痉挛、肠疝痛等所致的腹中绞痛属中焦阳虚者。

(2) 服本方后需注意盖被卧床休息，忌生冷硬食。

(3) 人参可用党参代替。

吴 茱 萸 汤
《伤寒论》

【组成】 吴茱萸6g 人参6g 大枣4枚 生姜20g

【用法】 水煎服。

【功效】 温肝暖胃，降逆止呕，

【主治】 肝寒胃虚，浊阴上逆所致之胃痛，巅顶痛，或呕吐涎沫，或吐利，或干呕等证。

【方解】 用吴茱萸辛苦燥热，温肝暖胃，散寒降浊，为方中主药；用生姜辛散寒邪，暖胃止呕，为辅药；用人参、大枣甘温，补中益气为佐使。四药合用，共奏温中补虚，温肝降逆之功。

【按语】

(1) 临床用于慢性胃炎，神经性头痛，耳源性眩晕，或妊娠呕吐属于肝寒胃虚者。

(2) 呕吐吞酸有寒热之不同，属于肝胃有热者禁用。使用本方需以舌质不红，苔白滑，脉细迟或弦细不数为辨证要点。

4.2 温经散寒

温经散寒剂适用于阳虚血弱，经络有寒的病证。

当归四逆汤
《伤寒论》

【组成】 当归9g 白芍9g 桂枝9g 细辛3g 炙甘草6g 通草6g 大枣4枚

【用法】 水煎服。

【功效】 温经散寒，养血通脉。

【主治】 (1) 阳气不足而又血虚，外受寒邪所致之手足厥冷，舌淡苔白，脉沉细或脉细欲绝者。(2) 寒入经络，腰、股、腿、足疼痛。

【方解】 用当归甘温而辛，入肝温通血脉，养血补血为方中主药；用白芍和营"通血痹"，桂枝入血通阳，细辛辛散温通，直入三阴，通阳散寒，共为辅药，伍当归可内疏厥阴，外和营卫；用通草清泄郁伏之阳热，为佐药；用大枣、甘草，补益中焦，振奋生化之源为使药。诸药合用，共奏温经散寒，养血通脉之功。

【按语】

(1) 本方适用于阳虚血虚复感寒邪的四肢厥冷，肢体疼痛，以及妇女月经不调，腰腹冷痛，寒疝等证。

(2) 血栓闭塞性脉管炎，雷诺氏症以及动脉炎，无脉症等属于血虚有寒者，均可使用。

(3) 原方细辛用量同桂枝，临床可据病情酌定，不必拘泥3g，方中通草可用木通。

4.3 回阳救逆

回阳救逆剂适用于阴盛阳微之证。

四 逆 汤
《伤寒论》

【组成】 生附子5~10g 干姜6~9g 炙甘草6g

【用法】 水煎服。若服药呕吐，可冷服。

【功效】 回阳救逆。

【主治】 阳气衰微，阴寒内盛，四肢逆冷，神疲欲寐，腹中冷痛，下利清谷，苔白滑，脉沉或微细欲绝。

【方解】 用附子辛热，通行十二经，振奋周身之阳气，为方中主药；用干姜辛热，温中散寒，助主药增强回阳之力，为辅药；用甘草甘温补中，既有益气之功，又可缓附子、干姜辛烈之性，为佐药。三药配伍，共奏回阳救逆之功。

【按语】

(1) 本方是回阳救逆的重要方剂，也是中医的急救方之一。适用于各种疾病发展到阳气虚脱的严重阶段。心肌梗死合并休克、脑血管意外出现昏迷、大出血引起的肢冷、汗出、休克，以及心力衰竭属于亡阳证者，均可用本方加减治疗。

(2) 本方适用于阳虚阴盛的四肢厥逆症。而阳气内郁，不能外达的四肢厥逆（热厥），不宜使用本方。

【附方】

通脉四逆汤《伤寒论》 即四逆汤原方增大生附子（15g），干姜（9～12g）用量，功能回阳通脉，主治少阴病，下利清谷，里寒外热，手足厥逆，脉微欲绝，身反不恶寒，其人面色赤，或利止，脉不出等证。

参 附 汤
《妇人良方》

【组成】 人参 12g 炮附子 9g

【用法】 人参另炖，熟附子水煎，取汁合服。

【功效】 回阳益气固脱。

【主治】 阳气暴脱，手足逆冷，汗出气短，呼吸微弱，关尺脉微等。

【方解】 用人参甘温，大补元气，为方中主药；附子辛热，温壮真阳，为辅佐药；二药配伍，益气与回阳同用，大温大补，方简而效捷。

【按语】

(1) 对于心力衰竭出现的休克、妇人产后、或经来暴崩，或外疡溃脓而致血脱亡阳证，均可用本方救治。

(2) 本方亦为救急方之一，宜中病即止。

小结

祛寒剂选主方 7 首，按功用分为温中祛寒、温经散寒、回阳救逆 3 类。

(1) 温中散寒 本类方剂适用于中焦虚寒证。理中丸温中祛寒，兼益气健脾之功，是治疗中焦虚寒、腹痛吐利的主方；小建中汤、大建中汤均有温中补虚、祛寒止痛之功。小建中汤偏于温阳养阴、缓急止痛，以补虚为主，治疗阴阳两虚，偏于阳虚的腹痛等；而大建中汤偏于温阳祛寒，降逆止痛，以祛邪为主，主要治疗中焦虚寒、阴寒内盛的心胸大寒痛；吴茱萸温中补虚、降逆止呕，以治阴寒上逆的呕吐头痛为主。

(2) 温经散寒 当归四逆汤是温经散寒的代表方剂，适用于阳虚血弱，经络有寒的手足厥冷证。

(3) 回阳救逆 四逆汤、参附汤均为回阳救逆的急救方，适用于阳气衰微、阴寒内盛的四肢厥逆、恶寒蜷卧、吐利腹痛等证。而四逆汤专于回阳以治疗阴寒内盛，阳气欲脱为主。参附汤兼有益气之功。其救急之力大而速，治疗正气大亏、阳气暴脱者。

复习思考题

(1) 试述理中丸的组成、功用及主治。

(2) 简述吴茱萸汤的方义。

(3) 试述当归四逆汤的组成、功用、主治。

(4) 试述四逆汤、参附汤组成、功用、主治的异同。

5 祛湿剂

凡以祛湿药为主组成，具有化湿利水，通淋泄浊作用，治疗水湿病证的一类方剂，统称为祛湿剂。

根据湿邪的部位以及偏热、偏寒的不同，将祛湿剂分为燥湿和胃、清热祛湿、温化水湿、祛风胜湿、利水渗湿 5 类。

使用祛湿剂，当注意先辨别病变的上下内外，病情的虚实及偏寒、偏热，有针对性地选择。因"气行则水行，气滞则水停"，故同时要注意调整脏腑功能，注意理气药的配伍应用。对于病后体弱者及孕妇水肿要慎用祛湿剂。

5.1 燥湿和胃

燥湿和胃剂适用于湿困中焦脾胃的病证。

藿香正气散
《太平惠民和剂局方》

【组成】 大腹皮 白芷 紫苏 茯苓各30g 半夏曲 白术 陈皮 厚朴 苦桔梗各60g 藿香90g 甘草75g

【用法】 上为细末，每服6g，用生姜3片，大枣1枚，水煎服。

【功效】 解表化湿，理气和中。

【主治】 外感风寒，内伤湿滞，呕吐泄泻，恶寒发热，头痛胸闷，肠鸣腹痛，舌苔白腻。

【方解】 用藿香辛温芳香，解表和中，辟秽化浊，为方中主药；紫苏、白芷亦为辛温芳香之品，助藿香解表散寒，芳香化浊，为辅药；半夏曲、陈皮、厚朴、大腹皮，辛开苦降，行气燥湿，降逆止呕，消胀除满；白术、茯苓益气健脾，渗湿止泻；桔梗宣开肺气，以利水道，共为佐药；生姜、大枣、甘草调和脾胃，调和药性。诸药合用，共奏外散风寒、内化湿浊、理气和中之功。

【按语】

(1) 胃肠型感冒、急性胃肠炎属于表寒里湿者用本方治疗。特别是夏季感冒，导致胃肠不和者，效果更佳。对于夏秋季感受暑湿秽浊之气而致猝然闷乱烦躁，甚至神昏耳聋的中暑病证，以及水土不服的吐泻均可使用。

(2) 本方辛香温燥药较多，适用于湿滞脾胃而偏寒者。若内热较盛，或阴虚无湿邪者忌用。

(3) 本方现今市售有水剂和软胶囊剂，携带服用便捷。亦可作汤剂水煎服，参考剂量：藿香12g 茯苓12g 紫苏9g 大腹皮9g 炒白术9g 半夏曲9g 白芷6g 陈皮6g 厚朴5g 桔梗5g 炙甘草3g。

平 胃 散
《太平惠民和剂局方》

【主成】 苍术 15g　厚朴（姜汁炒）9g　陈皮 9g　炙甘草 5g

【用法】 上为细末，每服 6g，生姜 3 片、大枣 2 枚，水煎服。或为汤剂，水煎服。

【功效】 燥湿运脾，行气和胃。

【主治】 湿困中焦，脾胃不和。脘腹胀满，不思饮食，恶心呕逆，口淡乏味，大便溏薄，身体倦惰嗜卧，苔白厚腻，脉缓。

【方解】 用苍术苦温，燥湿运脾，为方中主药；厚朴苦辛温，行气燥湿，消胀除满，为辅药；陈皮气香性温，能行能降，理气化湿和胃，为佐药；炙甘草益中焦，和诸药；姜、枣调和脾胃，共为使药。诸药配伍，共奏化湿浊，调气机，健脾和胃之功。

【按语】

(1) 本方药物配伍特点辛、燥、苦并用，能散、能消、能化，是治疗中焦湿滞证的代表方剂。慢性胃炎、胃下垂、胃神经官能症的脘部胀满作痛，以及急性胃肠炎出现上述症状者，可用本方加减治疗。对于初到气候潮湿之地，感受山岚瘴雾，水土不服者亦可应用。

(2) 本方适用于实证，不可以原方作为健脾补虚之品常服。脾虚无湿，或阴虚者，以及孕妇不宜服用。

5.2　清热祛湿

清热祛湿剂适用于外感湿热，或湿热内盛、或湿热下注等证。

茵 陈 蒿 汤
《伤寒论》

【组成】 茵陈 30g　栀子 15g　大黄 9g

【用法】 水煎服，先煎茵陈。

【功效】 清热，利湿，退黄。

【主治】 湿热黄疸。发热，面目全身俱黄，黄色鲜明，大便不畅，小便黄赤，胸腹胀满，口干，舌苔黄腻，脉滑数或沉实。

【方解】 用茵陈苦寒，清热利湿退黄，为方中主药；栀子苦寒泻火，通利三焦，使湿热从小便而解，为辅药；大黄苦寒沉降，泻热逐瘀，使湿热从大便而下，为佐药。三药合用，入气入血，共奏清热利湿退黄之功。

【按语】

(1) 急性传染性黄疸性肝炎、胆囊炎、胆石症、急性胰腺炎等，属于湿热证者可用本方加减治疗。对于早期肝硬化，或肝癌早期出现的黄疸，亦可应用本方。

(2) 阴黄证不宜使用。

二 妙 散
《丹溪心法》

【组成】 苍术 15g 黄柏 15g

【用法】 上 2 味研成细末，或水泛为丸，每服 5g，温水送下。或为汤剂水煎服。

【主治】 湿热下注引起的下肢痿软无力，足膝红肿热痛，或下部湿疮，或湿热带下、淋浊等症，舌苔黄腻。

【方解】 用黄柏苦寒，清热燥湿；苍术苦温燥湿。二药配伍可使热去湿除。

【按语】

（1）本方是治疗下焦湿热的常用方。风湿性关节炎、脚气病、外阴炎、阴囊湿疹等，属于下焦湿热者，均可用本方加减。

（2）下焦寒湿证不宜使用本方。

【附方】

三妙丸《医学正传》 黄柏 120g 苍术 180g 川牛膝 60g 为末，面糊为丸，如梧桐子，每服五、七十丸，空心姜、盐汤下。功能清热燥湿。用治湿热下注，两脚麻木，或如火烙之热。

三 仁 汤
《温病条辨》

【组成】 杏仁 15g 滑石 18g 白通草 6g 白蔻仁 6g 竹叶 6g 厚朴 6g 生薏仁 18g 半夏 9g

【用法】 水煎服。

【功效】 宣畅气机，清热利湿。

【主治】 湿温初起，恶寒少汗，身重肢倦，头重如裹，胸闷脘痞，午后身热，苔白腻，脉弦细而濡。

【方解】 用杏仁苦辛温，宣开上焦肺气，白蔻仁芳香，化湿行气宽中，薏苡仁甘淡，渗利湿热，共为方中主药；滑石、通草、竹叶甘寒淡渗，助薏苡仁清利湿热，为辅药；半夏、厚朴行气化湿除满，为佐药。诸药配伍，共奏宣上畅中渗下，利湿清热之功。

【按语】

（1）肠伤寒、胃肠炎、肾盂肾炎，属于湿重于热，阻滞气机者，可用本方加减治疗。对于输液后出现的身重、胸闷、苔白腻等症亦可使用。

（2）湿温病，热重于湿者不宜原方使用。

八 正 散
《太平惠民和剂局方》

【组成】 瞿麦 木通 萹蓄 车前子 生山栀 熟大黄 甘草各 500g

【用法】 上为散，每服 6～9g，灯心草 1.5g，水煎服。亦可作汤剂，水煎服。

【功效】 清热泻火，利尿通淋。

【主治】 湿热淋证。热淋、血淋、石淋，小便涩痛，淋漓不畅，甚或癃闭不通，小腹胀急，口渴心烦，舌苔黄腻，脉滑数。

【方解】 用瞿麦、萹蓄苦寒，利水通便，清利下焦湿热，为方中主药；用车前子、滑石、灯心、木通，清热利湿，通淋利窍，为辅药；栀子、大黄苦寒清热泻火，为佐药；甘草调和诸药，且缓急止尿道涩痛。诸药配伍，共奏清热泻火，利水通淋之功。

【按语】

(1) 膀胱炎、尿道炎、泌尿道结石、急性肾炎、肾盂肾炎，属于下焦湿热者，均可用本方加减治疗。对于膀胱癌出现热淋症状，亦可用本方加减治疗。

(2) 本方以苦寒通利药为主，适用于湿热淋证。如淋证日久，正气已虚者不宜应用。

5.3 温化水湿

温化水湿剂适用于湿从寒化和阳不化水的水肿等证。

真 武 汤
《伤寒论》

【组成】 附子 9g　茯苓 9g　白芍 9g　白术 6g　生姜 9g

【用法】 水煎服。

【功效】 温阳利水。

【主治】 脾肾阳虚，水气内停。小便不利，四肢沉重疼痛，肢体浮肿，腹痛下利，苔白不渴，脉沉。

【方解】 用附子辛热，温补脾肾阳气，为方中主药；茯苓、白术、健脾利水，为辅药；白芍缓急止痛，且利小便，为佐药；生姜辛而微温，辛散水气，为使药。诸药配伍共奏温肾逐寒，扶脾利水之功。

【按语】

(1) 慢性肠炎、心源性水肿、肾炎水肿、耳源性眩晕、慢性肝病浮肿，属于脾肾阳虚者，均可用本方加减治疗。

(2) 注意方中附子要熟用。

5.4 祛风胜湿

祛风胜湿剂适用于风湿痹痛。

桂枝芍药知母汤
《金匮要略》

【组成】 桂枝 12g　白芍 9g　知母 12g　生姜 15g　白术 15g　防风 12g　麻黄 6g　附片 6g　炙甘草 6g

【用法】 水煎服。

【功效】 祛风湿，清热止痹痛。

【主治】 风寒湿痹，郁而化热，寒热错杂。全身关节疼痛、肿大，并伴有灼热，身体羸瘦衰弱，头眩短气等。

【方解】 用桂枝、麻黄、防风辛温，温散风寒，为主药；用附子辛热，白术苦温，助主药温经散寒祛湿，为辅药；芍药、知母清热和阴，且防主辅药过于燥热，为佐药；生姜、甘草调胃和中，为使药。诸药配伍，共奏祛风除湿、清热止痛之功。

【按语】

(1) 本方主治风寒湿痹，邪初化热之证。类风湿性关节炎、强直性脊柱炎可用此方加减治疗。

(2) 本方药物配伍特点寒热并用，临床需要根据病情加减。若关节掣痛难以屈伸，得热则轻者，应重用辛热的附子、麻黄、桂枝；若疼痛部位灼热较重者，则应重用芍药、知母、甘草等，并加用生地、忍冬藤、生石膏等品。

独活寄生汤
《千金方》

【组成】 独活 9g 桑寄生 秦艽 防风 细辛 当归 川芎 生地黄 牛膝 杜仲 茯苓 桂心 人参 芍药 甘草各 6g

【用法】 水煎服，每日 3 次分服。

【功效】 祛风湿，止痹痛，益肝肾，补气血。

【主治】 肝肾不足，气血两亏的风湿痹痛。腰膝冷痛，酸软无力，屈伸不利或麻木不仁，畏寒喜温，心悸气短，舌淡苔白，脉细弱。

【方解】 用独活辛苦温，入肾经，祛下焦及筋骨间的风寒湿，为方中主药；用细辛、防风辛温，秦艽苦辛微寒，祛风湿止痹痛；桑寄生、杜仲、牛膝祛风湿，补肝肾，健腰膝，共为辅药；人参、茯苓、当归、生地、川芎、白芍补益气血，桂心温通血脉，共为佐药；甘草调和诸药，为使药；诸药配伍，共奏祛风湿，止痹痛，益肝肾，补气血之功。

【按语】

(1) 本方扶正与祛邪兼顾，主治痹证日久，正虚邪实者，以腰膝冷痛，舌淡苔白，脉细弱为辨证要点。风湿性关节炎、腰肌劳损、坐骨神经痛、骨质增生等属于肝肾两虚，气血不足者可用本方加减治疗。对于妇女素有腰腿疼痛，妊娠数月，症状加重者亦可用本方治疗。

(2) 细辛用量 2～3g 为宜。

5.5 利水渗湿

利水渗湿剂适用于水湿壅盛所致的癃闭、淋浊、水肿、泄泻等证。

五 苓 散
《伤寒论》

【组成】 茯苓 9g 猪苓 9g 泽泻 15g 白术 9g 桂枝 6g

【用法】 上为散，每服 3～6g，或作汤剂水煎服。

【功效】　利水渗湿，温阳化气。

【主治】　外有表证，水湿内停。头痛、发热、小便不利，或烦渴欲饮，水入即吐，苔白腻，脉浮。水湿内停的水肿、身重、小便不利或泄泻以及暑湿吐泻等。

【方解】　用泽泻甘淡寒，利水渗湿，为方中主药；茯苓、猪苓甘淡平，淡渗利湿，为辅药；白术健脾燥湿，助土制水，桂枝温阳化气行水，共为佐使。诸药配伍，共奏健脾祛湿、化气利水之功。

【按语】

(1) 本方常用于肾炎水肿、胃肠炎吐泻、心脏病、肝硬化出现的小便不利等症。也可以用于腹部手术后，排尿功能障碍，膀胱括约肌痉挛引起的尿潴留。

(2) 注意阴虚小便不利者忌用。

五 皮 饮
《华氏中藏经》

【组成】　茯苓皮　陈皮　生姜皮　大腹皮　桑白皮各9g

【用法】　水煎服。

【功效】　健脾理气，利水消肿。

【主治】　脾虚湿盛，头面四肢水肿，心腹胀满，上气喘息，小便不利，以及妊娠水肿，苔白腻，脉沉缓。

【方解】　用茯苓皮甘淡平，利湿健脾调中，为方中主药；陈皮芳香化湿，理气和中，为辅药；桑白皮肃降肺气，通调水道，下输膀胱，大腹皮行气消胀利水，生姜皮辛散水气，共为佐使。诸药配伍，共奏健脾利水，理气消肿之功。

【按语】

本方为治皮水之剂，适用于水肿部位较表浅，水肿较轻者。对于慢性肾炎水肿、心脏病水肿属于脾虚气滞水停者，以及早期肝硬化腹水，均可使用。

猪 苓 汤
《伤寒论》

【组成】　猪苓　茯苓　泽泻　阿胶（烊化）　滑石各9g

【用法】　水煎服。

【功效】　利水清热养阴。

【主治】　水热互结，小便不利，发热，心烦不眠，或淋病，尿血，小便涩痛，小腹胀满等。

【方解】　用猪苓甘淡，渗利水湿，为方中主药；茯苓健脾利水，泽泻、滑石甘淡寒，利湿泻热，共为辅药；阿胶滋肾水，防渗利药物伤阴，为佐使药。诸药配伍，利水不伤阴，滋阴不敛邪，共奏利水清热养阴之功。

【按语】

泌尿系感染，尿路结石，肾炎，膀胱炎引起的尿急、尿痛、尿血，属于水热互结伤阴者，用本方加减治疗。

小结

去湿剂选主方 12 首，按其功用分为燥湿和胃、清热祛湿、温化水湿、祛风胜湿、利水渗湿 5 类。

（1）燥湿和胃　平胃散、藿香正气散均有燥湿和胃之功，平胃散专于燥湿行气，是治疗湿滞脾胃的主方；藿香正气散兼具外散风寒之功，是治疗外感风寒，内伤湿滞证的常用方。

（2）清热祛湿　茵陈蒿汤功于清热利湿退黄，是治疗阳黄证的专方。二妙散清热燥湿，是治疗湿热下注的下肢痿软，湿疮带下等证的基础方。八正散，清热泻火，利尿通淋，是治疗湿热下注所致淋证的代表方剂。三仁汤宣畅气机，清利湿热，是治疗湿温初起，湿重于热的常用方剂。

（3）温化水湿　真武汤温阳利水，是治疗阳虚水停的常用方，以周身浮肿，小便不利，或四肢沉重疼痛为主证。

（4）祛风胜湿　桂枝芍药知母汤功于祛风湿清热止痛，适用于风寒湿痹，邪初化热，关节疼痛肿大伴灼热之证。而独活寄生汤祛风湿、止痹痛、益肝肾、补气血，主治肝肾不足，气血两亏的腰膝冷痛，酸软无力证。

（5）利水渗湿　五苓散与猪苓汤同为淡渗利水之剂，均治小便不利证。而五苓散兼具温阳化气解表之功，适用于太阳表邪随经入之蓄水证。猪苓汤兼具清热养阴之功，适用于水热互结，热邪伤阴之证。五皮饮能健脾理气，利水消肿，适用于脾虚湿盛之身面浮肿。

复习思考题

（1）燥湿和胃剂适用于哪些病证？平胃散的组成意义和主治症是什么？
（2）试述茵陈蒿汤的功用、主治及组方意义。
（3）三仁汤主治何证？试述其功用及组成意义。
（4）五苓散与猪苓汤在组方意义和适应证方面有何异同？
（5）独活寄生汤的组成是什么？主治何种类型的痹证？
（6）试述真武汤的主治、功用及组方意义。

6 祛痰剂

凡是以祛痰药为主组成，具有消除痰饮作用，用于治疗各种痰病的方剂，统称为祛痰剂。

根据痰的性质有湿痰、热痰、风痰等不同，将祛痰剂分为温化痰饮、清热化痰、治风化痰及攻逐痰涎 4 类。

使用祛痰剂要注意配伍理气药，因气顺痰消。另外，祛痰药属于行消之品，不宜久服，中病即止。

6.1 温化痰饮

温化痰饮剂适用于湿痰与寒痰所致的病证。

二 陈 汤
《太平惠民和剂局方》

【组成】 半夏 15g　橘红 15g　茯苓 9g　炙甘草 5g　生姜 3g　乌梅 1 枚

【用法】 水煎服。一般可不用乌梅。

【功效】 燥湿化痰，理气和中。

【主治】 湿痰证，咳嗽痰多，恶心呕逆，胸膈满闷，头眩心悸，舌苔白润或薄腻，脉滑。

【方解】 用半夏辛温，燥湿化痰、降逆止呕，为方中主药；用橘红辛苦温，理气燥湿化痰，为辅药；茯苓健脾渗湿，使湿无所聚，痰无由生，为佐药；炙甘草和中健脾，生姜降逆化痰，且制半夏毒性，用少量乌梅收敛肺气，共为使药。诸药配伍，共奏燥湿化痰、理气和中之功。

【按语】 本方是治疗湿痰之主方，可加减治疗各种痰证。临床常用于治疗慢性支气管炎、肺气肿、慢性胃炎、耳源性眩晕、脑血管意外及妊娠恶阻、多寐证、小儿流涎等属湿痰病证者。对于嗜酒之人手臂重痛麻木等证，亦可加味使用。

【附方】

（1）金水六君煎《景岳全书》 即二陈汤加当归、熟地。功能滋阴化痰。用治肺肾虚寒，水湿上泛为痰，湿痰内盛，咳逆多痰，或年迈阴虚，血气不足，外受风寒，咳嗽呕恶，多痰喘急，舌苔白厚腻，脉滑等。

（2）苓术二陈煎《景岳全书》 即二陈汤加猪苓、白术、泽泻、干姜。功能健脾化痰。温中疏滞，化气行水。用治脾胃虚寒，四肢倦怠，精神疲倦，咳嗽吐白稀痰等症。

（3）温胆汤《千金方》 即二陈汤减乌梅加竹茹、枳实、大枣。功能理气化痰，清胆和胃。用治胆胃不和，痰热内扰。虚烦不眠，口苦胸闷，呃逆呕吐，或惊悸不宁，癫痫等。

小 青 龙 汤
《伤寒论》

【组成】 麻黄 9g 白芍 9g 细辛 3g 干姜 6g 炙甘草 6g 桂枝 9g 半夏 9g 五味子 3g

【用法】 水煎服。

【功效】 解表蠲饮，止咳平喘。

【主治】 外感风寒，内有痰饮。恶寒发热，无汗咳喘，咳痰清稀而多，或身体痛重，头面四肢浮肿，舌苔白润，脉浮。

【方解】 用麻黄、桂枝辛温，解表发汗，除外寒宣肺气而为方中主药；用干姜、细辛辛热，温肺化饮，且助主药解表，为辅药；五味子敛气，白芍护阴，半夏祛痰和胃散结，均为佐药；炙甘草益气和中，调和诸药，为使药。诸药配伍，共奏外散风寒，内去水饮，止咳平喘之功。

【按语】

(1) 本方是一首发汗祛痰剂。感冒、流感及慢性支气管炎、支气管哮喘、肺气肿等病合并外感，出现外寒内饮者，皆可用本方加减治疗。

(2) 干咳无痰或痰少而粘，痰黄而稠者忌用。

【附方】

射干麻黄汤《金匮要略》 射干 6g 麻黄 9g 生姜 9g 细辛 3g 紫菀 6g 款冬花 6g 半夏 9g 五味子 3g 大枣 3 枚。功能宣肺祛痰，下气止咳。用治咳逆上气，喉中有水鸡声者。

苓桂术甘汤
《金匮要略》

【组成】 茯苓 12g 桂枝 9g 白术 6g 炙甘草 6g

【用法】 水煎服。

【功效】 健脾渗湿，温化痰饮。

【主治】 中阳不足之痰饮病。胸胁胀满，咳嗽短气，心悸目眩，舌苔白滑，脉弦滑。

【方解】 用茯苓甘淡，健脾利水渗湿，为方中主药；桂枝辛温，温阳化饮，助膀胱气化以利水，为辅药；白术苦甘温，益气健脾燥湿，以去生痰之源，为佐药；炙甘草益气和中，为使药。诸药配伍，共奏健脾渗湿，温化痰饮之功。

【按语】

(1) 本方的配伍特点是温而不热，利而不峻，是治疗痰饮的平和之剂。慢性支气管炎、支气管哮喘、胸膜炎、胸腔积液属脾虚有痰者，以及脾虚湿胜的泄泻均可用本方加减治疗。

(2) 本方药性偏温，痰饮偏热者不宜使用。

6.2 清热化痰

清热化痰剂适用于热痰证。

清气化痰丸
《医方考》

【组成】 胆南星　姜半夏各45g　瓜蒌仁　陈皮　黄芩　杏仁　枳实　茯苓各30g。

【用法】 共为细末，姜汁为丸，每服6g，亦可作汤剂水煎服，原方用量酌减。

【功效】 清热化痰，理气止咳。

【主治】 痰热内结，咳嗽，痰黄粘稠难出，气急呕恶，胸膈满闷，小便短赤，舌红苔黄腻，脉滑数。

【方解】 用胆南星苦寒，清热化痰，为方中主药；黄芩苦寒，瓜蒌甘寒，降肺火，化痰热，为辅药；陈皮、枳实疏理气机，消痰散结；茯苓、半夏健脾和中，祛湿化痰；杏仁宣利肺气止咳，共为佐使，诸药配伍，共奏清热化痰，理气止咳之功。

【按语】

（1）本方是治疗热痰的常用方剂，重点在于清气、顺气而达除痰的目的。肺炎、慢性支气管炎，属痰热内阻者，可用本方治疗。

（2）寒痰、燥痰禁用。

小 陷 胸 汤
《伤寒论》

【组成】 黄连6g　半夏12g　瓜蒌实30g

【用法】 水煎服。

【功效】 清热化痰，宽胸散结。

【主治】 痰热互结心下，胸脘痞闷，按之则痛，或咳痰黄稠，苔黄腻，脉浮滑或滑数。

【方解】 用瓜蒌实甘寒，清热化痰，宽胸利气，为方中主药；用黄连苦寒，泄热降火，除心下之痞为辅药；用半夏辛开心下之痞结，与黄连同用则辛开苦降，三药合用，共奏清热涤痰，散结开痞宽胸之功。

【按语】

（1）本方配伍特点辛开苦降，是治疗痰热阻结心下的常用方剂。临床以心下不舒，按之痛为诊断要点。渗出性胸膜炎、支气管肺炎、胆囊炎、急性胃炎属于痰热互结心下者，均可用本方加减治疗。

（2）小陷胸汤运用于胸脘有痰热实邪者，以舌苔黄腻有根为使用依据，若苔黄腻而刮之即去者，属中气虚而兼挟湿热，不宜使用。

6.3 治风化痰

治风化痰剂适用于风痰证，风痰有内外之分，内风生痰宜熄风化痰；外风生痰，宜疏风化痰。

半夏白术天麻汤
《医学心悟》

【组成】 半夏9g 茯苓6g 白术15g 橘红6g 天麻6g 甘草4g 生姜1片 大枣2枚

【用法】 水煎服。

【功效】 化痰熄风，健脾燥湿。

【主治】 风痰上扰，眩晕头痛，胸闷呕恶，苔白腻，脉弦滑。

【方解】 用半夏辛温，燥湿化痰，降逆止呕。天麻平肝熄风，二药为治风痰要药，为方中主药；白术、茯苓健脾燥湿，橘红理气化痰，为辅药；生姜、大枣、甘草调和脾胃，调和诸药，为佐使药。诸药配伍，共奏化痰熄风止晕之功。

【按语】

(1) 耳源性眩晕、神经衰弱头晕、头痛兼胃肠症状者，脑动脉硬化、脑血管意外等表现为风痰上扰者，均可用本方加减治疗。

(2) 肝阳上亢引起的头晕头痛禁用本方。

止 嗽 散
《医学心悟》

【组成】 百部9g 白前9g 紫菀9g 陈皮6g 荆芥6g 甘草4.5g 桔梗9g

【用法】 水煎服。

【功效】 止咳化痰，疏表宣肺。

【主治】 外感咳嗽，咽痒，咯痰不爽，或有轻微恶寒发热，舌苔薄白等。

【方解】 用百部、白前、紫菀辛苦、甘平，止咳化痰，共为方中主药；桔梗苦辛平，宣肺祛痰，橘红理气化痰，为辅药；荆芥疏风解表，为佐药；甘草调和诸药，与桔梗配伍，利咽喉，为使药。诸药配伍，共奏止咳化痰、疏表宣肺之功。

【按语】

(1) 本方药性平和，长于止咳化痰，临床可治疗多种咳嗽，使用时可根据咳嗽偏寒偏热的不同进行加减。感冒、流感、急性支气管炎属风邪犯肺者均可使用。

(2) 阴虚咳嗽不宜使用。

6.4 攻逐痰涎

攻逐痰涎剂适用于痰涎壅盛于里的实证。

控 涎 丹
《三因极一病证方论》

【组成】 甘遂60g 大戟60g 白芥子60g。

【用法】 上药共为细末，糊丸梧桐子大，食后临卧，姜汤送下5～7丸。

【功效】 祛痰逐饮。

【主治】 痰涎伏留胸膈上下，突然胸背、手足、腰胯、颈项痛不可忍，筋骨牵引疼痛，游走不定，或手足重浊冷痛，或神志昏倦多睡，或饮食无味，或痰多流涎等。

【方解】 用大戟苦辛寒，逐泄脏腑之水湿，用甘遂苦甘寒，攻破经隧之水湿，用白芥子辛温，驱散皮里膜外之痰气，三药配伍，共奏攻逐痰涎、水饮之功。

【按语】

（1）气管炎、肺炎痰涎壅盛者、早期肝硬化腹水、以及瘰疬、痰核、附骨疽有上述见症者均可使用本方。

（2）大便平素溏泻及体虚之人不宜使用。

小结

祛痰剂选主方 8 首，根据其功用分为温化痰饮、清热化痰、治风化痰和攻逐痰涎 4 类。

（1）温化痰饮 温化痰饮剂用治湿痰、寒痰证。其中二陈汤具有燥湿化痰、理气和中之功，是治疗湿痰证的基础方。主要治疗湿痰内阻，咳嗽、呕恶、眩晕等。苓桂术甘汤健脾渗湿、温化痰饮，是治疗中阳不足，湿聚成痰的代表方剂。小青龙汤有温肺散寒平喘的作用，适用于素有痰饮，复感外寒而诱发的咳喘。

（2）清热化痰 清气化痰丸具有清热化痰、理气止咳之功，用治痰热内结、咳痰色黄粘稠之证。而小陷胸汤清热化痰，兼具宽胸散结之功，适用于痰热互结心下的小结胸证。

（3）治风化痰 半夏白术天麻汤燥湿化痰，平肝息风，善治风痰上扰的眩晕头痛。而止嗽散止咳化痰、疏表宣肺，是治疗外感咳嗽的常用方剂。

（4）攻逐痰饮 控涎丹具有祛痰逐饮之功，改丸剂应用，其力较缓，用治痰涎水饮停于胸膈，而见胸胁隐痛、舌苔粘腻、脉弦滑等证。

复习思考题

（1）祛痰剂分为几类，各适宜何种痰证？

（2）试述二陈汤的组成，主治病证及其方义。

（3）苓桂术甘的功用、主治是什么？

（4）试述清气化痰丸的组成、功用、主治，并说明方中配伍理气药的意义？

（5）半夏白术天麻汤治疗何种眩晕头痛？试述其组成方义。

（6）止嗽散与桑菊饮均可用于外感咳嗽，其功用、主治有何不同？

7 和解剂

凡是有和解或调和作用，用于治疗少阳病或肝脾不和、肠胃不和病证的方剂，统称为和解剂。

根据和解剂的作用，分为和解少阳，调和肝脾，调和肠胃3类。

7.1 和解少阳

和解少阳剂适用于邪在半表半里的少阳病。

小 柴 胡 汤
《伤寒论》

【组成】 柴胡12g 黄芩9g 人参6g 半夏9g 炙甘草5g 生姜9g 大枣4枚。

【用法】 水煎服。

【功效】 和解少阳。

【主治】 少阳病，寒热往来，胸胁苦满，不欲饮食，心烦喜呕，口苦咽干，目眩，苔白脉弦。

【方解】 用柴胡苦辛微寒，轻清升散，疏邪透表，为方中主药；黄芩苦寒清泄，为辅药；二药配伍，一散一清，共解少阳之邪。半夏和胃降逆止呕。人参、甘草味甘和中，益气扶正，以助邪气外出，为佐药；生姜、大枣辛甘，调和营卫，为使药。诸药配伍，以祛邪为主，兼顾正气，共奏和解少阳之功。

【按语】 本方是治疗少阳病的代表方剂，临床对各种杂病，如疟疾、黄疸、慢性肝炎以及产后或经期感受外邪，热入血室等证均可使用。

蒿芩清胆汤
《重订通俗伤寒论》

【组成】 青蒿6g 黄芩9g 竹茹9g 制半夏5g 赤茯苓9g 枳壳5g 陈皮5g 碧玉散9g（包）

【用法】 水煎服。

【功效】 清胆利湿，和胃化痰。

【主治】 少阳湿热，胆胃不和。寒热如疟，热重寒轻，胸闷呕恶，口苦吞酸或呕黄涎，舌红苔白腻，脉数而右滑左弦者。

【方解】 用青蒿苦寒芳香，清透少阳邪热，为方中主药；黄芩苦寒，清泄少阳胆火，为辅药；竹茹清热化痰，除烦止呕，陈皮、半夏、枳壳理气化湿，和胃降逆，共为佐药；赤茯苓、碧玉散清利湿热，导热下行，为使药。诸药同用，共奏清胆利湿，和胃化痰，透达少阳，邪热外解之功。

【按语】

急性胆囊炎、急慢性肝炎、慢性胰腺炎、胃炎出现胆经湿热者，可用本方加减治疗。另外，对于肝胃不和的呕吐，痰湿中阻的眩晕，肝胆湿热扰于阴分的夜汗，痰热所致的心悸、失眠亦可使用。

7.2 调和肝脾

调和肝脾剂适用于肝脾不和证。

四 逆 散
《伤寒论》

【组成】 柴胡 6g　枳实 6g　白芍 9g　炙甘草 6g

【用法】 水煎服。

【功效】 透邪解郁，疏肝理脾。

【主治】 邪热内郁，手足厥冷，或脘腹疼痛，或泄利下重。

【方解】 用柴胡苦辛微寒，疏肝解郁，调和气机，使郁热外达，为方中主药；用枳实苦泻，下气破结，为辅药，与柴胡相伍，升降调气；白芍益阴和里缓急止痛，为佐药；炙甘草调和诸药，配白芍柔肝和脾，为使药。诸药配伍，共奏透热解郁，调和肝脾之功。

【按语】

（1）慢性肝炎、肋间神经痛、胃炎、胆道疾病、胸膜炎、急性胰腺炎等表现为肝郁气滞者，均可用本方治疗。

（2）阳虚阴寒内盛所致四肢厥冷者禁用。

逍 遥 散
《太平惠民和剂局方》

【组成】 柴胡 9g　当归 9g　白芍 9g　白术 9g　茯苓 12g　炙甘草 5g　薄荷 2g　煨姜 2g

【用法】 水煎服。

【功效】 疏肝解郁，健脾养血。

【主治】 肝郁血虚，脾不健运，两胁疼痛，目眩头痛，口燥咽干，神疲食少，或往来寒热，或月经不调，乳房作胀，舌淡红，脉弦而虚。

【方解】 用柴胡苦辛微寒，疏肝解郁，为方中主药；用当归甘辛温、白芍苦酸微寒，养血和血柔肝；用茯苓、白术、炙甘草、煨姜健脾和中益气，为辅药；薄荷助柴胡疏散肝郁，为使药。诸药配伍，共奏疏肝解郁，健脾和营之功。

【按语】

本方肝脾并调，气血兼顾，为调和肝脾的常用方剂。慢性肝炎、慢性胃炎、胸膜炎、神经衰弱，以及妇女经期紧张症、妇女不孕证属于肝郁血虚者，均可使用。它如肺结核浸润期的潮热盗汗、中心性视网膜脉络膜病变、婴幼儿高烧后双目失明，诊为球后神经炎者，亦可加味使用。

【附方】

（1）加味逍遥丸《内科摘要》　即本方加丹皮、栀子。功能疏肝健脾，和血调经。

用治肝脾血虚，化生火热，或烦躁易怒，或自汗盗汗，或头痛目涩，或少腹坠胀，小便涩痛等。

（2）黑逍遥散《医略六书·女科摘要》 即本方加生地或熟地。功能疏肝健脾，养血调经，用治肝脾血虚，临经腹痛，脉弦虚。

痛 泻 要 方
《景岳全书》

【组成】 炒白术 9g 炒白芍 6g 陈皮 4.5g 防风 6g

【用法】 水煎服。

【功效】 补脾泻肝。

【主治】 肝旺脾虚，肠鸣腹痛，大便泄泻，泻后腹痛不去，每因情绪影响诱发加重，舌苔薄白，脉弦。

【方解】 用白术苦甘温，健脾燥湿止泻，为方中主药；白芍味酸微寒，养血泻肝止痛，为辅药；陈皮理气醒脾以助运化，防风散肝舒脾胜湿，为佐使药。诸药配伍，共奏补脾土，泻肝木，调气机，止痛泻之功。

【按语】

（1）本方适用于肝旺脾虚的泄泻。慢性肠炎，过敏性肠炎、肠功能紊乱、慢性痢疾等病的腹痛泄泻属肝脾不和者，可用本方加减治疗。

（2）肠胃湿热所致的泄泻忌用本方。

7.3 调和肠胃

调和肠胃适用于肠胃不和、寒热错杂、升降失司所致的痞、满、吐、利等证。

半夏泻心汤
《伤寒论》

【组成】 半夏 9g 黄芩 6g 黄连 3g 干姜 6g 人参 6g 炙甘草 6g 大枣 4 枚。

【用法】 水煎服。

【功效】 和胃降逆，开结散痞。

【主治】 肠胃不和，寒热互结，心下痞硬不痛，干呕或呕吐，肠鸣下利，舌苔薄黄而腻。

【方解】 用半夏、干姜辛温散寒，用黄芩、黄连苦寒泄热燥湿，用人参、大枣、甘草甘温益气补虚。诸药配伍，寒热并用，辛开苦降，补气和中，共奏和胃降逆，开结除痞之功。

【按语】

本方是治疗中虚上热下寒心下痞满，呕吐泄泻的代表方剂。急性胃肠炎、慢性肠炎有上述症状者，均可加减使用。

【附方】

（1）生姜泻心汤《伤寒论》 即半夏泻心汤减干姜用量为 2g，加生姜 12g（一方无人参）。功能和胃消痞、散结除水。用治水热互结，心下痞硬，肠鸣下利，干噫食臭，腹中雷鸣者。

（2）甘草泻心汤《伤寒论》 即半夏泻心汤加甘草用量为9g。功能益气和胃，消痞止呕。用治胃气虚弱，腹中雷鸣下利，水谷不化，心下痞硬而满，干呕心烦不得安者。

（3）黄连汤《伤寒论》 黄连5g 炙甘草6g 干姜5g 桂枝5g 人参3g 半夏9g 大枣4枚。功能平调寒热，和胃降逆。用治胸中有热，胃中有寒，胸中烦热，痞闷不畅，气上冲逆，欲呕吐，腹中痛，或肠鸣泄泻，舌苔白滑，脉弦。

小结

和解剂选主方6首，根据其功用分为和解少阳，调和肝脾，调和肠胃3类。

（1）和解少阳 小柴胡汤为和解少阳主方。长于和解少阳，并祛邪扶正，主治寒热往来，胸胁苦满，心烦喜呕等少阳证。蒿芩清胆汤以清胆利湿为主，并能和胃化痰，适用于邪犯少阳，兼痰湿内阻，寒热起伏，热重寒轻，胸膈胀闷，呕吐或吐黄涎而粘等证。

（2）调和肝脾 四逆散、逍遥散、痛泄要方均有调和肝脾的作用，用治肝脾不和证。四逆散兼有解郁透邪之功，主治阳气内郁所致的四肢厥冷，腹痛下利等证；逍遥散养血疏肝，健脾和营，适用于肝郁血虚所致的两胁作痛，食少神疲，月经不调等证；痛泄要方则补脾平肝，适用于肝旺脾虚所致的腹痛泄泻。

（3）调和肠胃 半夏泻心汤是调和肠胃的代表方剂，具有辛开苦降、寒热并用、调整肠胃之功，适用于寒热错杂、升降失常的痞闷、呕吐、腹痛、腹泻等证。

复习思考题

（1）什么叫和解剂？和解剂分为哪几类？其适应证各是什么？

（2）试述小柴胡汤的组成，功用、主治病证及其方义。

（3）试述四逆散、逍遥散的组成，功用及其主治，并分析二方的区别。

（4）痛泻要方证在病机、症状上有何特点？方中为什么用防风？

（5）试述半夏泻心汤组成，功用、主治，并列举出衍化方。

8 泻下剂

凡以泻下药物为主组成，具有通导大便、排除肠胃积滞、攻逐水饮寒积的作用，用以治疗里实证的方剂，统称为泻下剂。

根据里实证有热结、寒结、燥结、水结的不同，将泻下剂分为寒下、温下、润下和攻逐水饮 4 类。

泻下剂易伤胃气，治疗里实证，中病即止，不可过用。年老体弱、津血不足、孕妇、产后，即使有实邪，亦不可单独使用。

8.1 寒下

寒下剂适用于里热与积滞互结的实证。

大 承 气 汤
《伤寒论》

【组成】 大黄 12g 厚朴 15g 枳实 12g 芒硝 9g

【用法】 水煎服，先煎厚朴、枳实，去渣内大黄，再去渣，溶服芒硝。

【功效】 峻下热结。

【主治】 阳明腑实证，大便不通，脘腹痞满，腹痛拒按，甚至潮热谵语，手足濈然汗出，舌苔焦黄起刺，或焦黑燥裂，脉沉实。或下利稀水，臭秽难闻，脐腹疼痛，按之有块。以及里实证的热厥、痉病和发狂等。

【方解】 用大黄苦寒，泻热通便，荡涤肠胃积滞结热，为方中主药；用芒硝咸寒软坚润燥，为辅药；厚朴、枳实行气除满，消痞散结，协助主药通下阳明腑气，推荡肠胃积滞，共为佐使。诸药配伍，共奏峻下热结之功。

【按语】

(1) 本方的辨证要点是痞、满、燥、实、坚俱备。急性单纯性肠梗阻、粘连性肠梗阻、急性胆囊炎、急性阑尾炎属阳明腑实证者，均可用本方加减治疗。对于某些热病中的高热、神昏、痉厥、发狂而胃肠燥实者，也可用本方加减治疗。

(2) 胃肠无结热者不宜使用。

【附方】

(1) 小承气汤《伤寒论》 大黄 12g 厚朴 6g 枳实 9g。功能轻下热结。用治阳明腑实轻证，大便秘结，潮热，腹中痛，脉沉滑；或痢疾初起，腹中胀痛，或脘腹胀痛，里急后重等。

(2) 调胃承气汤《伤寒论》 大黄 12g 炙甘草 6g 芒硝 12g。功能缓下热结。用治阳明胃肠燥热。大便不通，口渴心烦，蒸蒸发热等。以及胃肠燥热而致的发斑吐衄、牙龈咽喉肿痛等。

8.2 温下

温下剂适用于寒冷积滞于胃肠的里实证。

大黄附子汤
《金匮要略》

【组成】 大黄 6g 炮附子 9g 细辛 3g

【用法】 水煎服。

【功效】 温阳散寒，泻结行滞。

【主治】 寒积里实。腹痛便秘，胁下偏痛，发热，手足厥逆，舌苔白腻，脉紧弦。

【方解】 用附子辛热，温阳祛寒，为方中主药；用细辛辛温，除寒散结，大黄苦寒攻下积滞，为辅佐药。大黄与附子、细辛配伍，去苦寒之性而存攻下之用。三药配伍，共奏温下之功。

【按语】

(1) 本方适用于寒实积滞所致的便秘。急性阑尾炎、肠梗阻属虚寒型者，可用本方加减治疗。

(2) 注意大黄用量不宜超过附子。

8.3 润下

润下剂适用于津枯血虚，胃肠燥热的便秘。

麻子仁丸
《伤寒论》

【组成】 麻子仁 500g 芍药 250g 枳实 250g 大黄 500g 厚朴 250g 杏仁 250g

【用法】 上药共为细末，炼蜜为丸，如梧桐子大，每次 10 丸，每日 1～2 次，温开水送服。或按原方比例酌减，作汤剂煎服。

【功效】 润肠通便，泄热行气。

【主治】 肠胃燥热，大便秘结，脘腹胀满，腹中疼痛，或痔疮便秘。

【方解】 用麻子仁甘平质润，润肠通便，为方中主药；杏仁性苦微温，降气润肠，白蜜、芍药养阴润燥滑肠；大黄泻热通便，枳实、厚朴行气破结除满，共为辅佐。诸药配伍，共奏润肠泄热，行气通便之功。

【按语】

(1) 本方属于缓下剂，痔疮便秘、肛裂及习惯性便秘属于津液不足，兼胃肠燥热者可以使用。

(2) 年老体弱，或津枯血燥，而内无邪热的便秘以及孕妇应慎用。

增液承气汤
《温病条辨》

【组成】 玄参 30g 麦冬 24g 生地 24g 大黄 9g 芒硝 4.5g

【用法】 水煎服，不下再服。

【功效】 滋阴增液，泄热通便。

【主治】 热结阴亏，燥屎不行，下之不通，口渴，咽燥，舌红苔黄少津。

【方解】 用玄参、麦冬、生地甘咸寒，滋阴增液，以壮水清热，益肺润肠，为方中主药；大黄、芒硝软坚润燥，泄热通便，为辅佐药。诸药配伍，共奏滋阴泻下之功。

【按语】

本方是一首攻补兼施、增液通便之方。临床除用于热病伤阴的便秘外，亦可用于痔疮日久，或动力性肠梗阻、急性单纯性肠梗阻属于热结阴亏者。

【附方】

新加黄龙汤《温病条辨》 细生地 15g 生甘草 6g 人参 4.5g 生大黄 9g 芒硝 3g 玄参 15g 麦冬 15g 当归 4.5g 海参 2 条 姜汁 6 匙 功能滋阴益气，泻结泄热。用治热结里实，气阴不足。大便秘结，腹中胀满而硬，神疲少气，口干咽燥，唇裂舌焦，苔焦黄或焦黑燥裂。

8.4 逐水

逐水剂适用于水饮壅盛于里的实证。

十枣汤
《伤寒论》

【组成】 大枣 10 枚 甘遂、大戟、芫花各等份。

【用法】 甘遂、大戟、芫花研末，每服 0.5～3g，每日 1 次，纳入枣汤，清晨空腹服用。得下利后，糜粥自养。

【功效】 攻逐水饮。

【主治】 悬饮，胁下有水气，咳唾胸胁引痛，心下痞硬，干呕短气，头痛目眩，或胸背掣痛不得息，舌苔滑，脉沉弦。水肿，肚腹胀大，二便不利，身体壮实者。

【方解】 甘遂善行经遂之水湿，大戟善泄脏腑之水湿，芫花善消胸胁伏饮水湿，三药峻烈，各有专攻，合而用之，逐水饮，除积聚，消肿满；用大枣益气护胃，且缓解三药的毒性。诸药配伍，使下而不伤正，共奏攻逐水饮之功。

【按语】

(1) 肝硬化腹水、渗出性胸膜炎、慢性肾炎所致胸水、腹水或全身水肿，而体质壮实者可以应用。

(2) 本方不宜做煎剂。应严格按用法谨慎使用。如泻后，出现精神疲倦、食欲减退，虽水未尽去，亦应暂停服药，观察后据情况再定。

小结

泻下剂选主方 5 首，根据其功用分为寒下、温下、润下、逐水 4 类。

(1) 寒下 大承气汤具有峻下热结之功，是治疗胃肠实热积滞的主要方剂，适用于"痞、满、燥、实"之证。

(2) 温下 大黄附子汤能温经散寒，泻下寒积，主治素体阳虚，寒实内结的便秘。

（3）润下　麻子仁丸与增液承气汤均为润下剂，治疗肠燥便秘。麻子仁丸润肠通便，兼具泻下热结之功，适用于胃肠燥热的大便秘结，而增液承气汤能滋阴增液，泻热通便，适用于阴亏热结的便秘。

（4）逐水　十枣汤能泻下逐水，主治水肿腹胀实证以及水停胁下的悬饮。

复习思考题

（1）泻下剂如何分类？分述其代表方剂。

（2）大承气汤的配伍意义是什么？

（3）十枣汤主治何证？其病机是什么？为什么方中用大枣？

（4）麻子仁丸和增液承气汤如何区别运用？

9 表里双解剂

凡以解表药配伍泻下药、清热药或温里药，具有表里同治作用，治疗表里同病的方剂，统称为表里双解剂。

根据表里同病的性质不同，将表里双解剂分为解表攻下、解表清里、解表温里三类。

使用表里双解剂需辨别表证与里证的属寒属热，属虚属实等，有针对性地选择方剂。并需注意分清表证与里证的轻重，权衡表药与里药的比例。

9.1 解表攻下

解表攻下剂适用于外有表邪，内有实积的证候。

大 柴 胡 汤
《金匮要略》

【组成】 柴胡15g 黄芩9g 芍药9g 半夏9g 枳实9g 大黄9g 生姜15g 大枣5枚

【用法】 水煎服。

【功用】 和解少阳，内泻热结。

【主治】 心下痞满，按之作痛，往来寒热，郁郁微烦，胸胁苦满，或腹满胀痛，大便不解，或发热，汗出不解，心中痞硬，吐利并作，舌苔黄，脉弦有力。

【方解】 用柴胡苦辛微寒，疏透少阳之邪，为方中主药；黄芩、半夏、生姜助主药和解少阳，为辅药；芍药，大黄，枳实泻阳明热结为佐药；大枣安中，且与生姜配伍调和营卫，为使药。诸药配伍，共奏和解少阳，内泻热结之功。

【按语】

(1) 本方以寒热往来、胸腹疼痛、便秘、舌黄脉弦，为辨证要点。急性单纯性肠梗阻，急性胰腺炎、急性胆囊炎，胆结石常用此方加减治疗。

(2) 注意本方组成，《伤寒论》原方无大黄，《金匮要略》原方有大黄。

防风通圣散
《宣明方论》

【组成】 防风15g 荆芥15g 连翘15g 麻黄15g 薄荷15g 当归15g 川芎15g 炒白芍15g 白术15g 山栀15g 大黄15g 芒硝15g 生石膏30g 黄芩30g 桔梗30g 滑石90g 甘草60g

【用法】 上药共为末，每服6g，加生姜3片，水煎服。丸剂口服每次6g，1日2次。亦可按原方比例酌减用量作汤剂服用。

【功效】 疏风解毒，泻热通便。

【主治】 风热壅盛，表里俱实。憎寒壮热，头痛目眩，口苦咽干，咽喉不利，大便秘结，小便短赤，舌苔黄腻，脉洪数或弦滑。

【方解】 防风、荆芥、麻黄、薄荷疏风解表，使邪从汗解；石膏、黄芩、连翘、桔梗清解肺胃之热；大黄、芒硝泻热通便，山栀、滑石清热利湿，使里热从二便而解。当归、川芎、白芍养血活血。白术健脾燥湿。甘草、生姜和中。诸药配伍。共奏解表通里。疏风清热之功。

【按语】

(1) 流感、急性扁桃体炎、疖痈、败血症、胆囊炎、胰腺炎、阑尾炎、荨麻疹、过敏性紫癜等出现上述症状者均可用本方加减治疗。对于难治性头痛、偏头痛属于实证者亦有效。另外，此方还可以用于减肥和预防脑血管意外。

(2) 本方是汗、清、下三法并用，适用于风热壅盛，表里俱实的证候。虚证头痛，脾胃虚弱，内伤生冷所致的恶寒发热等症，忌用本方。

【附方】

双解散《痈医大圣》 即防风通圣散减麻黄、芒硝、白术、栀子加桂枝组成。功能疏表清热通下。用治风热壅遏，痘疮初起，透而不畅，便结尿赤，以及疮毒内外皆热者。

9.2 解表清里

解表清里剂适用于表证未解，里热已炽的证候。

葛根黄芩黄连汤
《伤寒论》

【组成】 葛根 15g 炙甘草 6g 黄芩 9g 黄连 9g

【用法】 水煎服。

【功效】 解表清热。

【主治】 身热下利，胸腹烦热，口干口渴，自汗气喘，舌红苔黄脉数。

【方解】 用葛根甘辛凉，解肌清热，升清止泻，为方中主药；黄芩黄连苦寒，清热燥湿止泻，为辅药；甘草甘缓和中，调和诸药。诸药配伍，共奏解表清里止泻之功。

【按语】

(1) 急性肠炎、细菌性痢疾出现上述症状者，用本方加减治疗。

(2) 寒湿下利及虚寒下利者，禁用本方。

9.3 解表温里

解表温里剂适用于外有表证，里有寒象的证候。

五 积 散
《太平惠民和剂局方》

【组成】 白芷 川芎 炙甘草 茯苓 当归 肉桂 芍药 半夏各90g 枳壳 陈皮 麻黄各180g 苍术720g 干姜120g 桔梗360g 厚朴120g

【用法】 上药除肉桂、枳壳另为粗末外，余药共为粗末，微火炒之令色变，晾凉，再入肉桂，枳壳末调匀，每服 9g，加生姜 3 片。水煎温服。或按原方比例酌减用量，作为汤剂水煎服。

【功效】 发表散寒，顺气化痰，活血消积。

【主治】 外感风寒，内伤生冷，或素有寒、食、气、血、痰五积。身热无汗，头身疼痛，项背拘急，腹满恶食，呕吐腹痛，或妇女月经不调属寒者。

【方解】 用麻黄、白芷辛温，发汗解表，干姜、肉桂辛热、温里散寒，四药配伍共除内外之寒，为方中主药；苍术、厚朴燥湿健脾，陈皮、半夏、茯苓理气化痰；当归、川芎、白芍活血养血调经以除血积；枳壳、桔梗升降气机，利胸膈除满闷，共为辅佐药；炙甘草和中健脾，调和诸药，为使药。诸药配伍，共奏发汗解表，温里散寒，气血同治，痰食并消之功。

【按语】

（1）凡感冒、风湿性腰腿痛，急慢性胃肠炎、胃痉挛、妇女白带、月经不调等见上述症状者，均可加减使用本方。对于腰腿下腹冷痛、身热无汗，苔滑脉沉迟者亦适用。

（2）本方药物繁杂，临床需随症加减，无表证者去掉解表药。注意苔黄、口渴、心烦、脉数者禁用。

小结

表里双解剂选主方 4 首，根据其功用分为解表攻下、解表清里、解表温里 3 类。

（1）解表攻下　大柴胡汤和解为主，与泻下并用，治疗邪入少阳、热结在里。防风通圣散解表、清热、攻下三法并用，治疗风热壅盛、表里俱实之证。

（2）解表清里　葛根芩连汤具有解表清热止利之功，适用于表邪未解而协热下利者。

（3）解表温里　五积散能解表温中消积，是为寒、食、气、血、痰五积而设，主治外感风寒，内伤生冷之证。

复习思考题

（1）表里双解剂分为几类？各自的适应证及用药配伍规律是什么？

（2）葛根黄芩黄连汤的组成、功用、主治证是什么？为什么以葛根为方中主药？

（3）简述五积散方义。

（4）防风通圣散功效、主治证是什么？

10 补益剂

凡是以补益药为主组成，具有补益人体气血阴阳不足的作用，用于治疗各种虚证的方剂，统称为补益剂。

由于虚证有气虚、血虚、气血两虚、阴虚、阳虚的不同，所以将补益剂分为补气、补血、气血双补、补阴、补阳5类。

补益剂适用于久病体虚，脏腑气血津液不足，机能衰退所致的各种虚证。使用时要注意辨清虚证的真假和轻重缓急，正确运用平补、峻补。而对于正气未虚、邪气亢盛者，不可用补益剂，以免误补留邪、助邪。

10.1 补气

补气的方剂，适用于脾肺气虚而出现的倦怠乏力，脉虚弱等证；或气虚下陷而出现的脱肛、子宫脱垂等证。

四 君 子 汤
《太平惠民和剂局方》

【组成】 人参　白术　茯苓　甘草　各等份。

【用法】 共为细末，每服6克，水煎服。

【功效】 益气健脾。

【主治】 脾胃气虚。面色㿠白，倦怠乏力，语声低微，食少便溏，舌淡苔薄白，脉细缓。

【方解】 用人参甘温，益气补脾养胃，为方中主药；白术苦温，健脾燥湿，为辅药；茯苓甘淡，渗湿健脾，与白术相佐，使健脾祛湿之力更强；炙甘草甘温，益气和中为使药。诸药配伍，共奏益气健脾之功。

【按语】

（1）本方为治疗脾胃气虚证的基础方剂，对于各种原因引起的脾胃气虚、运化乏力均可加减应用。慢性胃肠炎、消化不良、神经衰弱、胃肠功能紊乱等病表现为气虚证者，可用本方加减治疗。

（2）阴虚者、气滞者忌用。

（3）人参临床多用党参代替，亦多作汤剂。可用党参9g，白术9g，茯苓9g，炙甘草6g，水煎服。

参苓白术散
《太平惠民和剂局方》

【组成】 人参、白术、白茯苓、山药、炒甘草各1000g、白扁豆750g、莲子肉、薏苡仁、砂仁、桔梗各500g。

【用法】 共为细末，每服6g，枣汤调下。小儿量依岁数加减服用，也可作汤剂，

— 55 —

按原方比例酌定。

【功效】 益气健脾，和胃渗湿。

【主治】 脾虚湿停。四肢无力，形体消瘦，饮食不化，或吐或泻。胸脘胀闷，面色萎黄，舌淡苔白腻，脉细缓或虚缓。

【方解】 用人参、白术甘苦温补气健脾，为方中主药；用山药、莲子肉甘平，助人参益气补脾，白扁豆、苡仁、茯苓辅助白术健脾渗湿止泻，共为辅药；砂仁、桔梗和胃醒脾，理气宽胸，为佐药；甘草调和诸药，为使药。

【按语】

（1）慢性胃肠炎、贫血、慢性肾炎及妇女带下病等属于脾虚湿停者，均可采用本方治疗。对于肺气虚弱的久咳痰多，亦可用本方治疗以"培土生金"。

（2）阴虚火旺者慎用；气阴两虚或阴虚兼有脾虚者，应酌情使用。

补中益气汤
《脾胃论》

【组成】 黄芪 15g　炙甘草 5g　人参 10g　当归 10g　陈皮 6g　升麻 3g　柴胡 3g　白术 10g

【用法】 水煎服，或作丸剂，每服 10g。

【功效】 补中益气，升阳举陷。

【主治】 脾胃气虚。身热、自汗、渴喜热饮，少气懒言，肢体倦怠乏力，舌淡苔薄白，脉虚软无力。以及用治脱肛、子宫脱垂、久泻、久痢，中气下陷等证。

【方解】 用黄芪补中益气，升阳固表，为方中主药；人参、白术、炙甘草健脾益气，为辅药，与主药配合，增加补中益气之功；陈皮理气和胃，当归养血补虚，共为佐药；升麻、柴胡升阳举陷，为使药。诸药配伍，共奏补中益气，升阳举陷之功。

【按语】

（1）低血压病，慢性胃肠炎，重症肌无力等属于脾胃气虚者，以及脱肛、子宫脱垂、胃下垂、肾下垂、久泻、久痢、眼睑下垂等属气虚下陷者，均可加减使用。

（2）本方为"甘温除热"之剂，可用治气虚发热。阴虚发热及内热炽盛者忌用；病后津气两伤者，亦不得使用。

（3）方中人参，现常用党参代替。

【附方】

升陷汤《医学衷中参西录》　生黄芪 18g　知母 9g　柴胡 3g　桔梗 5g　升麻 3g。功能益气升陷，用治胸中大气下陷。气短不足以息，呼吸困难，或气息将停，危在旦夕，脉沉迟微弱或不调。

生 脉 散
《内外伤辨惑论》

【组成】 人参 10g　麦冬 15g　五味子 6g

【用法】 水煎服。

【功效】 益气生津，敛阴止汗。

【主治】 气阴两伤。体倦乏力，气短懒言，咽干口渴，脉虚细；亦治久咳肺虚，干咳少痰，气短自汗，口干舌燥，脉虚细或虚数。

【方解】 用人参甘温，益气补肺，为方中主药；用麦冬甘寒，养阴清热生津，为辅药；五味子酸温，敛汗生津止渴，为佐使药。诸药配伍，共奏益气生津，敛阴止汗之功。

【按语】

(1) 中暑、慢性支气管炎、肺结核、心脏病等属于气阴两虚者，可使用本方加减治疗。

(2) 外邪未解，或暑病热盛而气阴未伤者，不宜使用。

10.2 补血

补血的方剂，适用于血虚而出现的头晕眼花，心悸怔忡，舌淡脉细数等证。

四 物 汤
《太平惠民和剂局方》

【组成】 熟地 当归 白芍 川芎 各等份。

【用法】 上为细末，每服9克，水煎服。

【功效】 补血调血。

【主治】 血虚血滞。头晕目眩，心悸失眠，面色无华，妇女月经不调，经少或经闭，舌淡，脉细弦或细涩，以及产后恶露不下，结生瘕聚，少腹坚痛等。

【方解】 用熟地甘温厚味，滋阴养血，为方中主药；当归可补血养肝，和血调经，为辅药；白芍养血柔肝和营，为佐药；川芎活血行气，调畅气血，为使药，四药相伍，补血不滞血，行血不破血，补中有散，散中有收，共收补血调血之功。

【按语】

(1) 营养不良、贫血、植物神经紊乱、更年期综合征、妇女月经不调、胎前产后等病症属于血虚血滞者，均可用本方加减治疗。

(2) 凡平素脾胃气虚，食少便溏者，不宜应用本方。

当归补血汤
《内伤外感辨惑论》

【组成】 黄芪30g 当归6g

【用法】 水煎服。

【功效】 补气生血。

【主治】 劳倦内伤，气弱血虚，阳浮外越，肌热面赤，烦渴欲饮，脉洪大而虚，以及妇女经期、产后血虚发热头痛。或疮疡溃后，久不愈合。

【方解】 用黄芪甘温大补脾肺之气，以资气血生化之源，为方中主药；用当归甘辛温养血和营，为辅药。两药配伍，"阳生阴长""气旺血生"，共奏补气生血之功。

【按语】

(1) 各种贫血、过敏性紫癜等属气弱血虚者，均可伍用本方加减治疗。

（2）阴虚潮热忌用本方。

归 脾 汤
《济生方》

【组成】 白术　茯神　黄芪　龙眼肉　酸枣仁各30g　人参　木香各15g　炙甘草8g　当归　远志各3g

【用法】 共为粗末，每服12g，加生姜5片、大枣1枚，水煎服；或作丸剂，每丸10g，温开水送服。

【功效】 益气补血，健脾养心

【主治】 心脾两虚。心悸怔忡，食少体倦，面色萎黄，舌淡苔薄白，脉细缓。脾不统血。便血，皮下紫癜，妇女崩漏，月经先期，量多色淡，或淋漓不止等。

【方解】 用人参、黄芪甘温补气健脾，为方中主药；白术、甘草补脾益气，助主药以资气血生化之源；当归甘辛温，养肝而生心血；茯神、枣仁、龙眼肉甘平，养心安神，共为辅药；远志交通心肾而定志宁心，为佐药；木香理气醒脾，且防止益气补血等药物滋腻滞气，为使药，诸药并用，共奏气血双补，心脾同治之功。

【按语】

（1）胃及十二指肠溃疡出血、功能性子宫出血、再生障碍性贫血、血小板减少性紫癜、神经衰弱、心脏病等，属于心脾两虚及脾不统血等，均可应用本方加减治疗。

（2）邪热内伏，或阴虚脉数者，不宜使用本方。

（3）临床亦可作汤剂水煎服，用党参12g　炙黄芪15g　白术　茯苓　当归　枣仁　龙眼肉各9g　远志6g　木香3g　炙甘草5g　生姜2片　大枣3枚。

炙甘草汤（复脉汤）
《伤寒论》

【组成】 炙甘草12g　生姜9g　桂枝9g　人参6g　生地30g　阿胶6g　麦冬10g　麻仁10g　大枣10g

【用法】 除阿胶外，它药水煎，取汁倒出，加清酒（可用黄酒）10ml，另将阿胶烊化，分2次入药汁和匀服用。

【功效】 益气养血，滋阴复脉。

【主治】 阴血不足，阳气虚弱。脉结代，心动悸，虚羸少气，舌光少苔而干；虚劳咳嗽。咳嗽，痰中带血，短气，虚烦眠少，形体消瘦，自汗盗汗，咽干舌燥，脉虚数。

【方解】 用炙甘草"通经脉，利气血"甘温益气，为方中主药；人参、大枣益气补脾生脉；生地、阿胶、麦冬、麻仁滋阴补血，养血复脉为辅药；佐以桂枝、生姜、清酒辛温走散，行阳气而复脉，诸药配伍，共奏滋阴养血、益气复脉之功。

【按语】

（1）功能性心律不齐、期外收缩、冠心病、风湿性心脏病、病毒性心肌炎、甲状腺功能亢进者等属阴血不足、心气虚弱者，均可用本方治疗。

（2）胃肠虚弱、或腹泻下利者，不宜应用本方。

【附方】

加减复脉汤《温病条辨》 炙甘草 18g 干地黄 18g 生白芍 18g 麦冬 15g 阿胶 9g 麻仁 9g。功用养血滋阴，生津润燥。用治温病后期，邪热久留不去，阴液亏虚。手足心热，口干舌燥，脉虚大。

10.3 气血双补

气血双补的方剂，适用于气血两虚而出现的气短乏力，心悸失眠，舌淡脉虚无力等证。

八 珍 汤
《正体类要》

【组成】 人参 白术 茯苓 当归 川芎 熟地 白芍各 9g 炙甘草 4.5g
【用法】 加生姜 3 片、大枣 2 枚水煎服。
【功效】 补益气血。
【主治】 气血两虚。面色苍白或萎黄，头晕目眩、倦怠乏力、气短懒言、心悸怔忡、饮食减少、脉细弱。
【方解】 本方即四君子汤和四物汤之合方。方中用人参、熟地甘温益气养血，共为方中主药；白术、茯苓健脾渗湿，协人参益气补脾；当归、白芍养血和营，助熟地补益阴血，均为辅药；佐以川芎活血行气，补而不滞；炙甘草益气和中，调和诸药，为使药。诸药配伍，共奏气血双补之功。
【按语】
病后虚弱、贫血及各种慢性病，妇女月经不调、胎产崩漏，外科疮疡久不收口等属于气血两虚者，均可使用。
【附方】
(1) 十全大补汤《太平惠民和剂局方》 即八珍汤加黄芪、肉桂。功能温补气血。用治气血不足、虚劳咳嗽、腰膝无力，食少遗精、疮疡不敛、妇女崩漏等证。
(2) 毓麟珠《景岳全书》 人参 60g、炒白术 60g、茯苓 60g、当归 120g、熟地 120g、川芎 30g、炙甘草 30g、菟丝子 120g、酒炒杜仲 60g、鹿角霜 60g、川椒 60g，共为细末，炼蜜为丸、每服 6g，温开水送下。功能补益气血，滋养肝肾，强固冲任，调经助孕。用治妇人气血不足，肝肾两虚，月经不调，或后错色淡，或量少腹痛，或淋漓不断、腰膝酸软，小腹冷痛、性欲减退、久不受孕等症。

10.4 补阴

补阴的方剂，适用于阴虚所致的腰膝酸软，潮热盗汗，舌红少苔，脉细数等证。

六味地黄丸
《小儿药证直诀》

【组成】 熟地 24g 山萸肉 山药各 12g 泽泻 丹皮 茯苓各 9g
【用法】 以上 6 味药共为细末，炼蜜为丸，每丸 15g，每服 1 丸，每日 3 次，温开水送服。亦可作汤剂，水煎服。

【功效】 滋补肝肾。

【主治】 肝肾阴虚，腰膝酸软、头晕目眩，耳鸣耳聋，潮热盗汗，五心烦热、消渴遗尿，舌燥咽痛，舌红少苔，脉细数。

【方解】 用熟地甘温滋阴补肾，填精益髓，为主药；山萸肉补养肝肾，涩精秘气，山药甘平补益脾阴、固精，为辅药（此三药相伍，滋补肝脾肾，三阴并补，但以补肾为主）；用泽泻泄浊利湿，并防熟地之滋腻，丹皮清肝凉血散血，且制山茱萸之温，茯苓淡渗利湿，以助山药强健脾运，为佐使药。诸药相伍，共奏滋阴补肝肾之功。

【按语】

(1) 慢性肾炎、高血压、糖尿病、肺结核、肾结核、甲状腺机能亢进、中心性视网膜炎、更年期综合征、闭经、经少、小儿发育不良等，系肝肾阴虚者，均可用本方加减治疗。

(2) 脾虚运化无力者慎用。

(3) 本方方中药物配伍有"三补（补益）三泻（防止滋补药产生滞腻之弊）"之说，即熟地（补肾）填精益髓，泽泻（泻肾）利湿降浊；山茱萸（补肝）涩精秘气，丹皮（泻肝）凉血散血；山药（补脾）益阴固精，茯苓（泻脾）淡渗利湿。可参。

左 归 丸
《景岳全书》

【组成】 熟地24g 山药（炒）12g 枸杞12g 山萸肉12g 菟丝子12g 鹿角胶12g 龟板胶12g 牛膝9g

【用法】 炼蜜为丸，每丸9g。早晚空腹各服1丸，淡盐汤送下。

【功效】 滋阴补肾。

【主治】 真阴不足，头目眩晕，腰酸腿软，遗精滑泄，自汗盗汗，口燥舌干，舌红少苔，脉细或细数。

【方解】 用熟地甘温滋肾益精，以填真阴，为方中主药；山药补脾益阴，滋肾固精，枸杞子补肾益精，养肝明目，山萸肉养肝滋肾，涩精敛汗，龟板胶、鹿角胶，为血肉有情之品，鹿角胶偏于补阳，龟板胶偏于补阴，二胶合用，"阳中求阴"，益精填髓，为辅药；菟丝子、牛膝益肝肾，强腰膝、健筋骨，俱为佐使药。诸药配伍，共奏滋肾填阴之功。

【按语】

(1) 慢性疾患、年老体衰，热病恢复期等，见真阴不足证者，均可用本方治疗。

(2) 本方常服久服，每易滞脾碍胃，运用时宜加陈皮、砂仁等理气醒脾之品。脾虚泄泻者慎用。

一 贯 煎
《柳洲医话》

【组成】 生地30g 枸杞子15g 沙参9g 麦冬9g 当归9g 川楝子5g

【用法】 水煎服。

【功效】 滋阴疏肝。

【主治】 肝阴不足，血燥气郁，胸脘胁痛，或呕吐酸水苦水，咽喉干燥，舌红少津，脉细弱。

【方解】 用生地甘寒、枸杞子甘平，滋养肝阴，为方中主药；用沙参、麦冬、当归等补血养液柔肝为辅药；川楝子疏肝利气，虽苦寒，但配伍在滋阴养血药中，无伤阴之弊，为佐使药。诸药配伍，共奏滋阴疏肝之功。

【按语】

慢性肝炎，早期肝硬变及慢性胃炎属阴虚气滞者，可用本方加减治疗。

10.5 补阳

补阳的方剂，适用于肾阳虚弱而出现的腰痛脚软，小便不利或反多，脉虚弱而尺部沉细等证。

肾 气 丸
《金匮要略》

【组成】 干地黄24g 山药 山茱萸各12g 泽泻 茯苓 丹皮各9g 桂枝3g 附子3g

【用法】 共为细末，炼蜜为丸，每丸9g，每日2次，温开水送服。亦可用作汤剂，水煎服。

【功效】 温补肾阳。

【主治】 肾阳不足，腰酸腿软，下半身常有冷感，少腹拘急，小便不利或反多，舌淡而胖，尺脉沉细。以及痰饮、水肿、消渴、脚气等。

【方解】 用干地黄甘温补肾滋阴，为方中主药；山茱萸、山药补肝脾而益精血；以少量附子、桂枝微微生长少火以生肾气，温化肾阳为辅药；配用泽泻、丹皮、茯苓共泻湿浊，为佐使药。诸药配伍，阴中求阳，共奏温阳益肾之功。

【按语】

(1) 慢性肾炎、糖尿病、甲状腺功能低下、醛固酮增多症、性神经衰弱、肾上腺皮质功能减退、慢性支气管哮喘、更年期综合征等属于肾阳不足者，均可用本方加减治疗。

(2) 肾阴不足、虚火上炎者、或燥热伤津之病证，不宜使用。

右 归 丸
《景岳全书》

【组成】 熟地24g 山药（炒）12g 山茱萸9g 枸杞子12g 菟丝子12g 鹿角胶12g 杜仲12g 肉桂6g 当归9g 制附子6g

【用法】 作蜜丸，每丸9g，每日2次，白开水送下，或作汤剂水煎服。

【功效】 温补肾阳，填补精血。

【主治】 肾阳不足，命门火衰，年老或久病气衰神疲，畏寒肢冷，腰膝酸软，阳痿遗精，或阳衰无子；或饮食减少，或小便自遗，或腰肢软弱，下肢浮肿等。

【方解】 方中附子、肉桂辛热，鹿角胶甘咸温培补肾中之元阳，温里祛寒为方中主药；熟地、山萸肉、枸杞子、山药滋阴益肾，养肝补脾，填精补髓。为辅药；佐以菟丝子、杜仲补肝肾、健腰膝；当归养血和血，为使药，诸药配伍，温阳益肾，填精补血，而收培补肾中之阳之功。

【按语】

（1）肾病综合征、老年骨质疏松症、精少不育症、贫血、白细胞减少症等属于肾阳不足者，均可加减运用。

（2）肾虚而湿浊者，不宜使用。

小结

补益剂共选主方14首，按其功用分为补气、补血、气血双补、补阴、补阳等5类。

（1）补气　四君子汤、参苓白术散、补中益气汤、生脉散均有补气作用，适用于气虚诸证。四君子汤益气健脾为主，适用于脾胃气虚证，是补气的基础方剂。参苓白术散益气健脾，兼具和胃化湿之功，适用于脾虚湿停证。补中益气汤以益气升阳为主，适用于劳倦伤脾，气虚发热，以及气虚下陷诸证。生脉散益气生津为主，适用于热盛灼津，耗气伤阴所致气阴两伤之证。

（2）补血　四物汤、当归补血汤、归脾汤、炙甘草汤均有补血作用。四物汤以补血调血为主，为治疗血虚证的基础方。当归补血汤以补气生血为主，适用于劳倦内伤，气不生血，血虚发热之证。归脾汤益气补血，健脾养心为主，适用于心脾两虚诸证。炙甘草汤以益气滋阴、养血补阴为主，适用于气血不足，脉结代，心动悸以及虚劳肺痿等证。

（3）气血双补　八珍汤是气血双补的代表方剂，适用于失血过多或气血两虚诸证。

（4）补阴　六味地黄丸、左归丸、一贯煎，均能滋补肝肾之阴，治疗阴虚证。六味地黄丸是滋肾补阴的代表方剂，具有壮水制火的作用，适用于肾阴不足、虚火上炎证；左归丸则侧重于滋肾补阴，填精补髓，主要用于治疗真阴精髓内亏诸症，以方中有血肉有情之品，其滋补肝肾精血之力，较六味地黄丸大；一贯煎具有滋阴疏肝作用，长于滋养阴血而柔肝，用治肝肾阴血不足，肝气不舒者。

（5）补阳　肾气丸、右归丸均有温补肾阳作用，适用于肾阳不足诸证，肾气丸温补肾阳，以生少火；右归丸温补肾阳，填补精血，其填精补髓之功大于肾气丸。

复习思考题

（1）请按补益剂分类列出各自主要方剂及适应证。

（2）归脾汤用治心悸怔忡、健忘等证，为什么又能用治妇女崩漏？

（3）为什么在阳虚补阳时，辅以补阴之品？在阴虚补阴时，辅以补阳之品？并举例说明。

（4）当归补血汤为什么重用黄芪，其用量是当归的5倍？

（5）左归丸、右归丸、六味地黄丸、肾气丸在药物配伍上有什么不同？功用有何不同？

11 治风剂

凡是以辛散祛风或熄风止痉的药物为主组成,具有疏散外风或平熄内风的作用,用于治疗风病的方剂,统称为治风剂。

风病可分为外风和内风两大类。外风治宜疏散,内风治宜平熄。因此治风剂可分为疏散外风和平熄内风两类。

11.1 疏散外风

疏散外风的方剂,运用于感受外风出现的头痛恶风、肢体麻木等证。

川芎茶调饮
《太平惠民和剂局方》

【组成】 川芎 荆芥各120g 白芷 羌活 炙甘草各60g 细辛30g 防风45g 薄荷240g

【用法】 共为细末,每服6g,食后清茶送下。亦可作汤剂,水煎服,用量按原方酌减。

【功效】 疏风止痛。

【主治】 外感风邪头痛。偏正头痛或巅顶作痛,恶寒发热,目眩鼻塞,舌苔薄白,脉浮。

【方解】 用川芎、白芷、羌活辛温疏风止痛,共为方中主药,其中川芎善治少阳经、厥阴经头痛(头顶痛和两侧头痛),羌活善治太阳经头痛(后头痛),白芷善治阳明经头痛(前额部);细辛散寒止痛,并长于治少阴经头痛;薄荷能清利头目,搜风散邪;荆芥、防风疏散上部风邪,共为辅药;甘草和中益气、调和诸药;用清茶调服,可上清头目,又能制约辛散疏风药的过于温燥和升散,为佐使药。诸药配伍,共奏疏风止痛之功。

【按语】
(1)感冒、偏头痛、神经性头痛、慢性鼻炎引起的头痛,属外感风邪头痛者,均可用本方加减治疗。
(2)气虚、血虚或因肝阳上亢、肝肾阴亏,肝风内动引起的头痛,不宜使用。

牵 正 散
《杨氏家藏方》

【组成】 白附子 僵蚕 全蝎各等分

【用法】 共为细末,每服3g,热酒或温开水调下。亦可水煎服。

【功效】 祛风化痰止痉

【主治】 中风面瘫,口眼㖞斜。

【方解】 用白附子辛甘温祛风化痰,并长于治头面之风,为方中主药;用僵蚕、全蝎咸辛平祛风止痉，且僵蚕有化痰作用，全蝎善于通络，共为辅药；用热酒调服，可以宣通血脉，并能引药入络，直达病所。诸药配伍，共奏祛风化痰止痉之功。

【按语】

（1）颜面神经麻痹、三叉神经痛、偏头痛等属风痰痹阻经络者，均可使用本方加减治疗。

（2）气虚血瘀或肝风内动引起的口角㖞斜或半身不遂者，不宜单用本方。

（3）本方水煎服参考用量：白附子3～5g　全蝎、僵蚕各9g。

消 风 散
《外科正宗》

【组成】　当归　生地　防风　蝉蜕　知母　苦参　胡麻仁　荆芥　苍术　牛蒡子　石膏各9g，木通　甘草各4.5g

【用法】　水煎，空腹服。

【功效】　疏风养血，清热除湿。

【主治】　风疹、湿疹。皮肤疹出色红，或遍体云片斑点，瘙痒，抓破后渗出津水，苔白或黄，脉浮数。

【方解】　用荆芥、防风辛微温，牛蒡子辛苦寒，蝉蜕甘寒疏风透表，以去除在表之风邪，为方中主药；用苍术散风除湿，苦参清热燥湿，木通渗利湿热，石膏、知母清热泻火，共为辅药；当归、生地、胡麻仁以养血活血，滋阴润燥，为佐药；生甘草清热解毒，调和诸药，为使药。诸药配伍，共奏疏风养血、清热除湿之功。

【按语】

（1）过敏性皮炎、神经性皮炎、药物性皮炎、荨麻疹等属风热为患者，均可用本方加减治疗。

（2）服药期间，不宜食辛辣、鱼腥、烟酒、浓茶等，以免影响疗效。

11.2　平熄内风

平熄内风的方剂，适用于内风病证。阳邪亢盛，热极动风而出现的高热不退，四肢抽搐等证；或肝阳偏亢、肝风内动而出现的眩晕、头部热痛，甚则卒然昏倒，半身不遂等症，均属内风之实证，治宜平肝熄风；对温病邪热伤阴，阴虚生风，虚风内动而出现的筋脉拘挛、四肢蠕动等症，或下元虚衰，虚阳浮越，痰浊上泛，发为暗痱等，属内风之虚证，治宜滋养熄风。

羚角钩藤汤
《通俗伤寒论》

【组成】　羚羊角4.5g（先煎）　双钩藤9g（后下）　桑叶6g　菊花9g　鲜生地15g　白芍9g　川贝12g　竹茹（鲜制，与羚羊角先煎代水）15g　茯神木9g　生甘草3g

【用法】　水煎服。

【功效】　凉肝熄风，增液舒筋。

【主治】　肝热生风。高热不退，烦闷躁扰，手足搐搦，发为痉厥，甚则神昏，舌绛而干，或舌焦起刺，脉弦而数。

【方解】 用羚羊角咸寒凉肝熄风，钩藤甘寒清热解痉，共为方中主药；桑叶、菊花辛凉疏泄、清热平肝熄风，以加强凉肝熄风之效，为辅药；鲜生地、白芍、生甘草增液滋阴、柔肝舒筋，与羚羊角、钩藤等同用，有标本兼顾之义；贝母、竹茹清热化痰，茯神木平肝宁心安神，均为佐药；生甘草调和诸药，为使药。诸药配伍，共奏凉肝熄风，清热镇痉，增液舒筋之功。

【按语】

(1) 本方是治疗热极动风的代表方剂。高血压、植物神经失调、脑血管意外、甲状腺机能亢进、妊娠子痫、流行性乙型脑炎引起的头痛、眩晕、抽搐属肝热风动者，均可用本方加减治疗。

(2) 热病后期，阴虚风动而出现筋脉拘急、手足蠕动者，不宜应用。

(3) 羚羊角现今多研末冲服，每次 0.3～0.6g。

镇肝熄风汤
《医学衷中参西录》

【组成】 怀牛膝 30g　生赭石（研细）30g　生龙骨（捣碎）15g　生牡蛎 15g　生龟板（捣碎）15g　生杭芍 15g　玄参 15g　天冬 15g　川楝子（捣碎）6g　生麦芽 6g　茵陈 6g　甘草 4.5g

【用法】 水煎服。

【功效】 镇肝熄风，滋阴潜阳。

【主治】 阳亢风动。头目眩晕，目胀耳鸣，脑部热痛，面色如醉，心中烦热、或时常噫气，或肢体渐觉不利，口角渐渐歪斜，甚或眩晕颠扑、昏不知人，移时始醒，或醒后不能复原，脉弦有力。

【方解】 用淮牛膝苦酸引血下行，补益肝肾，为方中主药；赭石、龙骨、牡蛎镇逆潜阳、镇肝熄风，共为辅药；龟板、玄参、天冬、白芍滋养阴液以制阳亢。茵陈、川楝子、生麦芽疏肝清热、条达肝气；甘草与麦芽相配，和胃调中，防止金石类药物碍胃之弊，且调和诸药，均为佐使药。诸药配伍，共奏镇肝熄风、滋阴潜阳之功。

【按语】

高血压、脑血管意外、高血压性脑病等属肝肾阴虚、肝阳上亢、气血逆乱者均可用本方加减治疗。

天麻钩藤饮
《杂病证治新义》

【组成】 天麻 9g　钩藤（后下）12g　石决明（先煎）18g　栀子 9g　黄芩 9g　川牛膝 12g　杜仲、益母草、桑寄生、夜交藤、茯神各 9g

【用法】 水煎服。

【功效】 平肝熄风、清热活血、补益肝肾。

【主治】 肝阳化风。头痛、眩晕、失眠、耳鸣眼花，手足震颤、甚或半身不遂、舌红苔黄脉弦数。

【方解】 用天麻甘平、钩藤甘寒、石决明咸寒平肝熄风，为方中主药；栀子、黄芩苦寒清热泻火，以清肝经之热，为辅药；益母草活血利水，牛膝引血下行，杜仲、桑寄生补益肝肾，夜交藤、茯神安神定志，俱为佐使药。诸药配伍，共奏平肝熄风，清热活血，补益肝肾之功。

【按语】

高血压、脑血管意外、甲状腺机能亢进、植物神经功能失调、癫痫、眩晕等，属肝阳化风者，均可用本方加减治疗。

大 定 风 珠
《温病条辨》

【组成】 白芍 18g 阿胶 9g 龟板 12g 生地 18g 麻仁 6g 五味子 6g 生牡蛎 12g 麦门冬 18g 炙甘草 12g 鸡子黄（生）2 个 鳖甲 12g

【用法】 水煎去滓，入阿胶烊化，再入鸡子黄搅匀，温服。

【功效】 滋阴熄风。

【主治】 阴虚动风。温病后期，热邪久羁，神倦瘛疭，脉气虚弱，舌绛苔少，有时时欲脱之势。

【方解】 用鸡子黄、阿胶甘平滋阴养液以熄内风，为方中主药；用白芍、地黄、麦冬滋阴柔肝、壮水涵木；龟板、鳖甲滋阴潜阳，共为辅药；麻仁养阴润燥，牡蛎平肝潜阳，五味子、炙甘草酸甘化阴，均可加强滋阴熄风之功，俱为佐使药。诸药配伍，共奏滋养阴液，柔肝熄风之功。

【按语】

(1) 流脑、乙脑后期的心悸、失眠、眩晕、肢体震颤属于阴虚风动或血不养心者，均可用本方加减。

(2) 阴液虽亏而邪热犹炽者，不宜用本方。

地 黄 饮 子
《宣明论方》

【组成】 熟地 15～30g 肉苁蓉 10～15g 巴戟天 10g 山茱萸 10g 石斛 10g 麦冬 10g 茯苓 10g 炮附子 4.5～10g 肉桂 3～6g 石菖蒲 4.5～6g 五味子 6g 远志 6g 薄荷 1.5g 生姜 3 片 大枣 4 枚

【用法】 水煎 2 次分服。

【功效】 滋肾阴，温肾阳，开窍化痰。

【主治】 中风喑痱证。肾之虚衰，语声不出，下肢痿弱或瘫痪，或手足皆不能运转，但不知痛处，脉象微弱。

【方解】 用熟地甘温、山茱萸酸温滋补肾阴，用巴戟、肉苁蓉、附子、肉桂辛温甘咸，温补肾阳，共为方中主药；用石斛、麦冬、五味子滋阴敛液，使阴阳相配，共为辅药；菖蒲、远志、茯苓交通心肾，开窍化痰，为佐药；姜、枣、薄荷为引，调和营卫，为使药。诸药配伍，共奏滋肾阴，补肾阳，开窍化痰之功。

【按语】

（1）脊髓炎、侧索硬化、脊髓空洞症、慢性进行性延髓麻痹等病出现中风、喑痱证候者可用本方加减治疗。

（2）本方适用于虚极之"语声不出，足废不用，中风瘫痪"，故肝阳偏亢之人不宜使用。

（3）原方各药等份，为末，每服 9g，加生姜 5 片、大枣 1 枚、薄荷 5～7 叶，水煎服。

小结

治风剂选主方 8 首，按其功效分为疏散外风和平熄内风两类。

（1）疏散外风　川芎茶调散长于疏散上部风邪，适用于风邪上犯头目的偏正头痛。牵正散善于祛风化痰，适用于风痰阻滞经络所致的口眼㖞斜。消风散疏风养血，清热除湿，是治疗风疹、湿疹的常用方剂。

（2）平熄内风　羚角钩藤汤、镇肝熄风汤、天麻钩藤饮都能平肝熄风。羚角钩藤汤凉肝清热镇痉之力强，适用于肝经热盛，热极动风证。镇肝熄风汤潜阳镇肝熄风之力大，适用于肝阳上亢，肝风内动证。天麻钩藤饮兼有清热活血安神作用，适用于肝阳偏亢，肝风上扰所致头痛、眩晕、失眠。大定风珠为滋阴熄风之剂，适用于热灼真阴，虚风内动之症。地黄饮子长于滋肾阴，补肾阳，开窍化痰，适用于下元虚弱，痰浊上逆的喑痱证。

复习思考题

（1）试述川芎茶调散和消风散的组成意义及主治病证。

（2）羚角钩藤汤与镇肝熄风汤均能平熄内风而治肝风内动之证，其主治和治法有什么不同？

（3）试述天麻钩藤饮的组成意义和主治病证。

（4）试述大定风珠与羚角钩藤汤在组成、功用、主治上的异同。

（5）地黄饮子为什么能治喑痱证？其用药有何特点？

12 治燥剂

凡以轻宣辛散或甘凉滋润的药物为主组成，具有轻宣润燥或滋阴润燥作用，用于治疗燥证的方剂，统称治燥剂。

根据燥证有内燥、外燥之分，治燥剂分为轻宣润燥和滋阴润燥两类。

治燥剂的适应证，是用于外感或内伤所致的燥证，故素体多湿者忌用。脾虚便溏以及气滞、痰盛者慎用。

12.1 轻宣润燥

轻宣润燥的方剂，适应于外感凉燥证。

杏 苏 散
《温病条辨》

【组成】 苏叶9g 杏仁9g 半夏9g 茯苓9g 前胡9g 苦桔梗6g 橘皮6g 枳壳6g 甘草3g 生姜3片 大枣3枚

【用法】 水煎服。

【功效】 轻宣凉燥、宣肺化痰。

【主治】 外感凉燥证。头微痛，恶寒无汗，咳嗽痰稀，鼻塞咽干，苔白，脉弦。

【方解】 用苏叶辛温解肌发汗，开宣肺气，使凉燥从表而解；杏仁苦微温宣肺止咳化痰，为方中主药；前胡疏风降气化痰，桔梗、枳壳宣降肺气为辅药；半夏、橘皮、茯苓理气化痰为佐药；生姜、大枣、甘草调营卫和诸药，为使药。诸药配伍，共奏发表宣肺、理气化痰之功。

【按语】

(1) 流行性感冒、支气管炎、肺气肿等表现为外感凉燥证者，均可用本方。

(2) 本方不宜用于温燥之证。

桑 杏 汤
《温病条辨》

【组成】 桑叶6g 杏仁9g 沙参12g 浙贝6g 淡豆豉6g 栀子皮6g 梨皮6g

【用法】 水煎服。

【功效】 轻宣温燥、润肺止咳。

【主治】 外感温燥证。头痛、身热、口渴咽干鼻燥，干咳无痰，或痰少而粘，舌红，苔薄白而干，脉浮数。

【方解】 用桑叶苦甘寒轻宣燥热，杏仁宣肺利气，润燥止咳，为方中主药；豆豉辛凉解表，助桑叶轻宣透热；贝母清热化痰，助杏仁止咳化痰；沙参润肺止咳生津，为辅药；栀子皮质轻而入上焦，清泄肺热；梨皮清热润燥，止咳化痰，共为佐使药。诸药配伍，共奏轻宣燥热，润肺止咳之功。

【按语】

本方是治疗外感温燥轻证的代表方剂。上呼吸道感染、急性支气管炎、支气管扩张咯血、百日咳等，属外感温燥而邪气较轻者，可用本方加减治疗。

清燥救肺汤
《医门法律》

【组成】 冬桑叶 9g 石膏 8g 甘草 3g 人参 2g 胡麻仁（炒研）3g 阿胶 3g 麦门冬 4g 杏仁（去皮尖、炒黄）2g 枇杷叶（刷去毛、蜜涂炙黄）3g

【用法】 水煎服。

【功效】 清燥润肺。

【主治】 温燥伤肺证。头痛身热，干咳无痰，气逆而喘，咽喉干燥，口渴鼻燥，胸膈满闷，舌干少苔，脉虚大而数。

【方解】 用桑叶苦甘寒清透肺中燥热之邪，为方中主药；石膏甘寒清泄肺热；麦冬养阴润肺，共为辅药；人参、甘草益气和中，培土生金，麻仁、阿胶养阴润肺；杏仁、杷叶降泄肺气，均为佐药。诸药配伍，共奏清燥热、养气阴之功。

【按语】

肺炎、支气管哮喘、急慢性支气管炎、肺气肿、肺癌，以及肺结核早期咳嗽痰少，属燥热伤肺、气阴两伤者，均可用本方加减治疗。

【附方】

翘荷汤《温病条辨》 薄荷 5g 连翘 5g 生甘草 3g 黑栀子 5g 桔梗 9g 绿豆皮 6g。功能轻清宣透，清解上焦气分燥热。用治上焦气分燥热证。耳鸣、目赤、龈肿、咽痛，苔薄黄而干，脉数。

12.2　滋阴润燥

滋阴润燥的方剂，适用于脏腑津伤液耗的内燥证。

养阴清肺汤
《重楼玉钥》

【组成】 大生地 12g 麦冬 9g 生甘草 3g 玄参 9g 贝母（去心）5g 丹皮 5g 薄荷 3g 炒白芍 5g

【用法】 水煎服。

【功效】 养阴清肺，解毒利咽。

【主治】 白喉。喉间起白膜如腐，不易拭去，咽喉肿痛，初起可发热或不发热，鼻干唇燥，或咳或不咳，呼吸不利，似喘非喘，脉数无力或细数。

【方解】 用生地甘苦寒养阴清热，为方中主药；玄参苦甘咸寒养阴生津，泻火解毒；麦冬甘寒养阴清肺，共为辅药；丹皮清热凉血消肿，白芍益阴养血；贝母润肺化痰，清热散结为佐药；加少量薄荷疏表利咽。生甘草泻火解毒，调和诸药，为使药。诸药配伍，共奏滋养肝肾，消肿利咽，微散表邪之功。

【按语】

急性扁桃体炎、急性咽喉炎、鼻咽癌。以及慢性支气管炎等，属阴虚燥热者，均可用本方加减治疗。

麦门冬汤
《金匮要略》

【组成】　麦门冬 60g　半夏 9g　人参 6g　甘草 4g　粳米 6g　大枣 3 枚

【用法】　水煎服。

【功效】　滋养肺胃，降逆下气。

【主治】　肺痿证。咳唾涎沫，短气喘促，咽喉干燥，舌干红少苔，脉虚数。

【方解】　重用麦门冬甘寒滋养肺胃之阴，为方中主药；人参、甘草、粳米、大枣甘温益气，补益后天化源以生津液，为辅药；半夏降逆下气，与麦门冬配伍，使其滋阴而不腻，为佐使药。诸药配伍，共奏滋肺胃、降逆气之功。

【按语】

(1) 慢性支气管炎、支气管扩张、慢性咽喉炎、矽肺、肺结核等，属肺阴虚，气火上逆者。以及胃、十二指肠溃疡、萎缩性胃炎，属胃阴不足，气逆呕吐者，均可用本方治疗。

(2) 肺痿属于虚寒者，不宜使用。

小结

治燥剂选主方 5 首，按其功效分为轻宣外燥和滋阴润燥两类。

(1) 轻宣外燥　杏苏散、桑杏汤、清燥救肺汤均能轻宣外燥，而杏苏散轻宣凉燥，是治疗凉燥袭肺的代表剂。桑杏汤、清燥救肺汤均具轻宣温燥之功，治疗燥热伤肺证。桑杏汤清热之力较弱，适用于外感温燥之轻证，而清燥救肺汤清热滋阴之功较强，适用于外感燥热之重证。

(2) 滋阴润燥　养阴清肺汤、麦门冬汤均有滋阴润燥作用，养阴清肺汤滋养肺胃，兼能疏散外邪，是治疗白喉的有效方剂，且可用于阴虚喉痛。而麦门冬汤滋养肺胃，兼降逆气，主治肺阴虚的咳逆上气、胃阴虚的气逆呕吐。

复习思考题

(1) 治燥剂分几类？各用于治疗何种病证？

(2) 试述桑杏汤、杏苏散药物组成、功效、主治的异同。

(3) 麦门冬汤出于何书？试述其组成、功用、主治及方义。

13 安神剂

凡以重镇安神或滋养心神的药物为主要组成，具有安神作用，用于治疗神志不安疾患的方剂，统称为安神剂。

根据神志不安有实证和虚证之分，将安神剂分为重镇安神和滋养安神两类。由于临床上神志不安的原因较多，又常虚实夹杂，互为因果，治疗方法上也非只一途，临床使用时，往往重镇与滋养药合用。重镇安神类多由金石碍胃的药物组成，不宜久服，对脾胃虚弱患者尤应注意。

13.1 重镇安神

重镇安神的方剂。多用于心阳偏亢证，临床多见心烦、失眠、惊悸、怔忡等症状。

朱砂安神丸（又名安神丸）
《医学发明》

【组成】 朱砂 1.5g 黄连 18g 炙甘草 16g 生地黄 8g 当归 8g

【用法】 上药为丸，每次服 6~9g，睡前开水送下；也可水煎服，用量按原方比例酌情增减，朱砂研细末水飞，以药汤送服。

【功效】 镇心安神，清热养血。

【主治】 心火上炎，灼伤阴血所致的心神烦乱，失眠多梦，惊悸怔忡，甚则欲吐不果，胸中气乱而热，舌红，脉细数。

【方解】 用朱砂微寒重镇，安心神，清心火，用黄连苦寒，清心除烦安神，共为方中主药；当归、生地养血滋阴，为辅药；用甘草和中调药，为佐使药。诸药配伍，标本兼顾，共奏镇心安神，泻火养阴之功。

【按语】

(1) 神经衰弱失眠、健忘，心悸或精神抑郁证神志恍惚属心火偏盛者，均可使用本方治疗。

(2) 本方水煎服，朱砂用水飞末，以汤送服 0.3~1g，且不宜多服久服。

13.2 滋养安神

滋养安神的方剂，适用于阴血不足，虚阳偏亢病证，症见虚烦失眠，心悸盗汗，梦遗健忘，舌红苔少等。

酸枣仁汤
《金匮要略》

【组成】 酸枣仁 18g 甘草 3g 知母 10g 茯苓 10g 川芎 5g

【用法】 水煎服。

【功效】 养血安神，清热除烦。

【主治】　虚劳虚烦不得眠，心悸盗汗，头目眩晕，咽干口燥，脉细弦。

【方解】　用酸枣仁甘平，养肝血，安心神，为方中主药；用川芎调养肝血，茯苓宁心安神为辅药；用知母清热除烦为佐药；甘草清热调和为使药。诸药配伍，滋清兼备，共奏养血安神，清热除烦之功。

【按语】

神经衰弱及更年期综合征具有烦躁失眠，心悸，盗汗等症，属肝血不足，阴虚内热者，均可使用本方治疗。

天王补心丹
《摄生秘剖》

【组成】　生地黄 120g　人参、丹参、元参、茯苓、五味子、远志、桔梗各 15g　当归、天门冬、麦门冬、柏子仁、酸枣仁各 60g

【用法】　上药为末，炼蜜为丸，朱砂为衣，每服 9g，温开水送下。亦可水煎服，用量按原方比例酌减。

【功效】　滋阴清热，补心安神。

【主治】　阴亏血少，虚烦心悸，失眠健忘，口舌生疮，大便干燥，舌红少苔，脉细数。

【方解】　用生地甘苦寒，滋肾水，清虚热，为方中主药；用玄参、天冬、麦冬甘咸寒，助主药滋阴清热，当归、丹参补血养血，共为辅药；人参、茯苓益气宁心，酸枣仁、五味子收敛心气而安神，柏子仁、远志、朱砂养心安神为佐药；桔梗宣肺以通心气，并载药上行，为使药。诸药配伍，标本并图，共奏滋阴清热，补心安神之功。

【按语】

神经衰弱的失眠多梦，某些心脏病属于阴血亏虚者，用本方治疗。

小结

安神剂选主方 3 首，按功用分为重镇安神和滋阴安神两类。

（1）重镇安神　朱砂安神丸具有镇心安神、清热养血之功，适用于心火亢盛，灼伤阴血的烦乱不眠、心悸、多梦等症状。

（2）滋养安神　酸枣仁汤、天王补心丹同有滋阴养血、补心安神的功效，酸枣仁汤长于养肝血，平虚阳，适用于肝血不足，阴虚阳亢的心悸失眠；而天王补心丹侧重于滋阴养血，补心安神，适用于阴血不足的虚烦不寐，失眠健忘。

复习思考题

（1）试述朱砂安神丸的组成、功用、主治及方义。

（2）酸枣仁汤和天王补心丹在功效、主治上有何异同？

14 开窍剂

凡以芳香开窍药物为主组成，具有开窍醒神作用，用于治疗窍闭神昏证的方剂，统称为开窍剂。

窍闭神昏之证，有虚实之分。属实证者，称为闭证。根据其证候有热闭与寒闭的不同，把开窍剂分为凉开与温开两类。

开窍剂只适用于邪盛气实的闭证，对于大汗肢冷，气微遗尿，口开目闭的脱证，即使有神志昏迷，也不能使用。阳明腑实证，邪热熏蒸，而见神昏谵语者，治宜寒下，不可误用开窍剂。

开窍剂方药大都气味芳香，善于辛散走窜，宜制成丸、散剂，温开水冲服，不宜加热煎煮，而且只可暂用，不可久服，中病即止。

14.1 凉开

凉开法，适用于温邪热毒内陷心包的热闭证以及中风、痰厥及感触秽浊之气，卒然昏倒，不省人事而有热象者。

安宫牛黄丸
《温病条辨》

【组成】 牛黄 郁金 犀角（水牛角代） 黄连 黄芩 山栀 朱砂 雄黄各30g 冰片 麝香各7.5g 珍珠15g 金箔衣

【用法】 为极细末，炼蜜为丸，每丸3g，每服1丸，小儿减量。

【功效】 清热开窍，豁痰解毒。

【主治】 温热病，热陷心包，痰热闭窍。高热，神昏谵语，以及中风昏迷，小儿惊厥属邪热内闭者。

【方解】 用牛黄、麝香苦凉芳香，清热解毒，豁痰开窍，为方中主药；用水牛角咸寒，清心凉血解毒，黄芩、黄连、山栀苦寒，清热泻火解毒，冰片、郁金芳香辟秽，通窍开闭，共为辅药；朱砂、珍珠镇心安神，雄黄豁痰解毒，为佐药；蜂蜜和胃调中为使药。金箔为衣，取其重镇安神之效。诸药配伍，共奏清热解毒，豁痰开窍之功。

【按语】

(1) 乙脑、流脑等急性传染病高热、昏迷以及脑血管意外的昏迷、肝昏迷属于热毒炽盛者，均可以使用本方。

(2) 方中犀角用水牛角代替，用量可增大5～10倍。

至 宝 丹
《太平惠民和剂局方》

【组成】 生乌犀屑（研）（水牛角代） 生玳瑁屑（研） 琥珀（研） 朱砂（研飞） 雄黄（研飞）各30g 龙脑（研） 麝香（研）各7.5g 牛黄（研）15g 安息

香 45g　金箔（半入药，半为衣）　银箔（研）各 50 片

【用法】　水牛角、玳瑁、安息香、琥珀分别粉碎成细粉；朱砂、雄黄分别水飞或粉碎成极细粉；将牛黄、麝香、冰片研细，与上述粉末配研，过筛，混匀，加适量炼蜜制成大蜜丸，每丸重 3g。口服，每次 1 丸，1 日 1 次。小儿减量。

【功效】　化浊开窍，清热解毒。

【主治】　中暑、中恶、中风及温病因于痰浊内闭所致神昏谵语，痰盛气粗，身热烦躁，舌红，苔黄垢腻，脉滑数，以及小儿惊厥属于痰热内闭者。

【方解】　用麝香、冰片、安息香芳香开窍，辟秽化浊；水牛角、牛黄、玳瑁清热解毒，为方中主药；用朱砂、琥珀镇心安神，雄黄豁痰解毒，共为辅药；金箔、银箔与朱砂、琥珀同用，意在加强重镇安神之效，现在成方均已不用。诸药配伍，共奏清热解毒，化痰开窍之功。

【按语】

(1) 脑血管意外、肝昏迷，乙脑、癫痫等属于痰迷心窍而见昏厥者，均可使用本方治疗。

(2) 本方芳香辛燥之药较多，虽善于开窍，但有耗阴劫液之弊，故凡中风昏厥因于肝阳上亢所致的不宜用。

紫 雪 散
《外台秘要》

【组成】　石膏　寒水石　磁石　滑石各 1.5kg　犀角屑（水牛角代）　羚羊角屑各 150g　青木香　沉香各 150g　玄参　升麻各 500g　甘草 240g　朴硝 5kg　硝石（精制）96g　麝香 1.5g　朱砂 90g　黄金（原方 100 两）　丁香 30g

【用法】　制成散剂。口服，1 次 1.5~3g，1 日 2 次。小儿酌量。

【功效】　清热解毒，镇痉开窍。

【主治】　温热病，邪热内陷心包而致的高热烦躁，神昏谵语，痉厥，口渴唇燥，尿赤便闭，以及小儿热盛惊厥。

【方解】　用石膏、滑石、寒水石甘寒清热；用水牛角清心解毒；麝香、青木香、丁香行气开窍；玄参、升麻、甘草清热解毒，玄参并能养阴生津，甘草兼能和胃安中。以上清热与开窍二组药物是方中的重要部分。用羚羊角咸寒，清肝息风以解痉厥；朱砂、磁石、黄金重镇安神；更用朴硝、硝石泄热散结，以上药物均为方中辅助部分。诸药合用，共奏清热开窍，息风镇痉之功。

【按语】

(1) 流脑、乙脑、猩红热等急性热病，见高热神昏，抽搐痉厥，口渴唇燥等症状及小儿高热惊厥属热盛风动者均可使用。

(2) 小儿麻疹、热毒内盛，疹色紫红，或透发不畅，见高热、喘促、昏迷、指纹紫红者，也可使用。

(3) 现在成方不用黄金。

14.2 温开

温开法，适用于中风、中寒、痰厥等属于寒闭之证，症见突然昏倒，牙关紧闭，神昏不语，苔白脉迟等。

苏 合 香 丸
《太平惠民和剂局方》

【组成】 白术　青木香　乌犀屑（水牛角代）　香附　朱砂　诃子　白檀香　安息香　沉香　麝香　丁香　荜茇各60g　龙脑（研）　苏合香油（入安息香膏内）　乳香各30g

【用法】 炼蜜制成药丸（每丸重3g）。口服，1次1丸，1日1～2次，小儿用量酌减。

【功效】 芳香开窍，行气止痛。

【主治】 中风或感受时行瘴疠之气，突然昏倒，牙关紧闭，不省人事。或中寒气闭，心腹卒痛，甚则昏厥。或痰壅气阻，突然昏倒。

【方解】 用苏合香、麝香、冰片、安息香芳香开窍，为方中主药；用青木香、白檀香、沉香、乳香、丁香、香附行气解郁，散寒化浊，解除脏腑气血之郁滞，为辅药；荜茇配合诸香药，增强散寒、止痛、开郁的作用；用水牛角解毒，朱砂镇心安神，白术补气健脾，燥湿化浊；煨诃子温涩敛气，以防诸香药辛香太过，耗散正气，共为佐使药。诸药配伍，共奏芳香开窍，行气止痛之功。

【按语】

(1) 冠心病、心绞痛以及胸腹诸痛属气滞寒凝者，均可用本方治疗。

(2) 本方香窜走泄，有损胎气，孕妇慎服。对于脱证，非本方所宜。

小结

开窍剂选方4首，根据功用分为凉开与温开两类。

(1) 凉开　安宫牛黄丸、至宝丹、紫雪散是凉开代表方剂，均有清热解毒，开窍醒神之功，治疗热闭证。而安宫牛黄丸长于清热解毒，适用于热陷心包，神昏谵语之证。而至宝丹长于芳香辟秽化浊，适用于一切痰热内闭的神昏；紫雪散则优于息风止痉，适用于热陷心包，神昏痉厥并见者。

(2) 温开　苏合香丸是温开的代表方剂，治疗寒闭证，因长于行气止痛，适用于气滞寒凝的心腹疼痛。

复习思考题

(1) 凉开剂的组方要点是什么？试述其代表方剂在功效、主治方面的异同。

(2) 苏合香丸的配伍特点是什么？试述其功效、主治。

15　固涩剂

凡以固涩药为主组成，具有收敛固涩的作用，用于治疗气、血、精、津液耗散滑脱之证的方剂，统称为固涩剂。

根据病因和发病部位的不同，耗散滑脱之证可分为固表止汗、敛肺止咳、涩肠固脱、涩精止遗、固崩止带 5 类。

固涩剂的适应证是正气内虚、耗散滑脱证。在使用时，应根据患者气、血、精、津液耗伤程度的不同，配伍相应的补益药，使之标本兼顾。外邪未去，不可用固涩，恐有"闭门留寇"之弊，转生他变。对于由实邪所致的热病多汗，火扰遗精，热痢初起，食滞泄泻，实热崩带等，均非本类方剂所宜。

15.1　固表止汗

固表止汗的方剂，适用于体虚卫外不固，阴液不能内守而出现的自汗、盗汗等证。

玉屏风散
《丹溪心法》

【组成】　防风 30g　黄芪 30g　白术 60g

【用法】　共研细末，每日 2 次，每次 6～9g，温开水送服。亦可作汤剂，用量按原方比例酌减。

【功效】　益气固表止汗。

【主治】　表虚卫阳不固，易感风邪。自汗，多汗，恶风，面色㿠白，舌淡苔白，脉浮虚软。

【方解】　用黄芪甘温益气固表，为方中主药；白术苦甘温健脾益气，以助黄芪益气固表之功，为辅药；二药合用，则气旺表实，汗不能外泄，邪不能内侵；防风走表祛风，为佐使药。且黄芪得防风之散，固表而不留邪；防风得黄芪之补，祛邪而不伤卫，实属补中有散，散中有补，相得益彰。三药配伍，共奏益气固表止汗之功。

【按语】

（1）多汗证、过敏性鼻炎、慢性鼻炎、上呼吸道感染，易感风邪表现为表虚卫阳不固者，均可用本方加减治疗。

（2）外感自汗，阴虚盗汗者不宜使用。

牡蛎散
《太平惠民和剂局方》

【组成】　黄芪　麻黄根　牡蛎各 30g

【用法】　共为粗末，每服 9g，与浮小麦 30g 同煎，去渣热服，日 2 服。或作汤剂，水煎服。

【功效】　益气固表，敛阴止汗。

【主治】 自汗、盗汗。身常自汗，夜卧尤甚，心悸惊惕，短气烦倦，舌淡红，脉细弱。

【方解】 用牡蛎咸寒，敛阴潜阳，固涩止汗，为方中主药；黄芪益气实卫，固表止汗，为辅药；麻黄根走表，固卫专于止汗，为佐药；浮小麦养心气，除烦热止虚汗，为使药。四药配伍，共奏养气阴，固肌表，止汗出之功。

【按语】

(1) 多汗证、植物神经功能失调、术后及产后自汗、盗汗属卫外不固、阴液外泄者，可用本方治疗。

(2) 阴虚火旺而致的盗汗，不宜用本方。

(3) 原方牡蛎要求"米泔浸，刷去土，火烧通红"。

15.2　敛肺止咳

敛肺止咳的方剂，适用于久咳肺虚，气阴耗伤而出现的咳嗽、气喘、自汗，脉虚数等证。

九　仙　散
《医学正传》

【组成】 人参（另炖）　款冬花　桑白皮　桔梗　五味子　阿胶　乌梅　贝母各2g　罂粟壳（蜜炙）6g　乌梅6g

【用法】 共为细末，加生姜1片，枣1枚，水煎温服。

【功效】 敛肺止咳，益气养阴。

【主治】 久咳肺虚证。久咳不已，咳甚则自汗气喘，痰少而粘，脉虚数。

【方解】 用罂粟壳酸涩敛肺止咳，人参补气益肺，为方中主药；阿胶养阴益肺，五味子、乌梅收敛肺气止咳，为辅药；款冬花、桑白皮降气化痰，止咳平喘，贝母化痰止咳，共为佐药；桔梗宣肺祛痰，载药上行，为使药。诸药配伍，共奏敛肺止咳，益气养阴之功。

【按语】

(1) 慢性气管炎、肺气肿属于久咳肺虚、气阴两虚者，可用本方加减治疗。

(2) 久咳不止，但内多痰涎，或外有表邪者不宜使用。

(3) 方中罂粟壳不宜多服、久服。

15.3　涩肠固脱

涩肠固脱的方剂，适用于脾肾虚寒，固摄无权而出现的久泻久痢，大便滑脱不禁等证。

真人养脏汤
《太平惠民和剂局方》

【组成】 人参6g　当归9g　白术12g　肉豆蔻12g　肉桂3g　炙甘草6g　白芍15g　木香9g　诃子12g　罂粟壳20g

【用法】 水煎服。

【功效】 温补脾胃，涩肠止泻。

【主治】 脾肾虚寒之久泻久痢。泻痢日久，滑脱不禁，或脱肛坠下，腹痛喜温、喜按，不思饮食，舌淡苔白，脉沉迟。

【方解】 用罂粟壳酸涩，涩肠止泻，肉桂辛热，温补脾肾，为方中主药；肉豆蔻暖脾温中，涩肠止泻，为辅药；人参、白术益气健脾，当归、白芍养血和血止痛，木香理气，为佐药；炙甘草调和诸药，为使药，诸药配伍，共奏温补脾肾，涩肠止泻之功。

【按语】

（1）慢性肠炎、肠结核、慢性痢疾、脱肛等属脾肾虚寒者，均可用本方加减治疗。

（2）泻痢初起，湿热积滞未去者，忌用。

四 神 丸
《证治准绳》

【组成】 肉豆蔻 60g　补骨脂 120g　五味子 60g　吴茱萸 30g

【用法】 共为细末，生姜 240g　红枣 100 枚，用水煮姜、枣，取枣肉与药末为丸，如桐子大，每服 6～9g，空腹食前服。或按原方比例酌减，水煎服。

【功效】 温肾暖脾，涩肠止泻。

【主治】 脾肾虚寒。五更泄泻，不思饮食，食不消化，或久泻不愈，或腹痛肢冷，神疲乏力，舌淡苔薄白，脉沉迟无力。

【方解】 用补骨脂辛苦大温，补命门之火，温补肾阳，为主药；肉豆蔻温脾暖胃，涩肠止泻，为辅药；五味子收敛止泻，吴茱萸辛热暖脾胃散阴寒止腹痛，共为佐药；生姜温胃散寒，大枣补脾养胃，为使药。诸药配伍，共奏温肾暖脾，涩肠止泻之功。

【按语】

（1）慢性结肠炎、过敏性结肠炎、慢性痢疾、肠结核的久泻证属脾肾虚寒者，均可用本方加减治疗。

（2）食滞不化或肠胃湿热蕴结所致的泄泻，不宜使用本方。

赤石脂禹余粮丸
《伤寒论》

【组成】 赤石脂（碎）30g　禹余粮（碎）30g

【用法】 水煎服。

【功效】 涩肠止泻。

【主治】 泻痢日久，滑脱不禁。

【方解】 用赤石脂甘酸温涩，收敛止泻固脱，为方中主药；禹余粮甘涩固涩收敛，为辅佐药。二药配伍，共奏涩肠止泻之功。

【按语】

本方属于泻痢日久，滑脱不禁治标之剂，慢性结肠炎、脱肛等可用本方加减治疗。

15.4 涩精止遗

涩精止遗剂，适用于肾虚失藏、精关不固而出现的遗精滑泄，或肾虚不摄，膀胱失约而出现的遗尿、尿频证。

桑 螵 蛸 散
《本草衍义》

【组成】 桑螵蛸 远志 菖蒲 龙骨 人参 茯神 当归 龟甲（炙）各30g

【用法】 研末，睡前人参汤调下6g。亦可按本方比例酌减，水煎服。

【功效】 调补心肾，固精止遗。

【主治】 心肾两虚证。小便频数或遗尿遗精，心神恍惚，健忘多梦，舌淡苔白，脉细弱。

【方解】 用桑螵蛸甘咸，补肾益精，固涩止遗，为方中主药；龙骨敛心神而涩精气，龟甲益阴气而补心肾，为辅药；人参补中气，当归养心血，茯神安心神，为佐药；远志、菖蒲安神定志，交通心肾，为佐使药。诸药配伍，共奏调补心肾，固精止遗之功。

【按语】

（1）神经衰弱、糖尿病及小儿遗尿证等属心肾不交者，可用本方治疗。

（2）下焦火盛，或湿热困扰所致的尿频失禁，不宜使用。

缩 泉 丸
《妇人良方》

【组成】 乌药 益智仁等份

【用法】 上为末，酒煎山药末为糊，如绿豆大。每服6~9g，每日1~2次，开水送下，亦可用原方比例酌定，水煎服。

【功效】 温肾祛寒，缩尿止遗。

【主治】 下元虚冷。小便频数或遗尿不止，舌淡，脉沉弱。

【方解】 用益智仁辛温，温补脾肾，固精气，缩小便，为方中主药；乌药辛温调气散寒，能除膀胱肾间冷气，止小便频数，固涩精气，为辅药；山药健脾补肾涩精气，为佐使药。三药配伍，温而不燥，共奏温肾祛寒，缩尿止遗之功。

【按语】

神经性尿频、尿崩证等属脾肾虚寒者，或多涕证属脾肾虚寒者，均可用本方治疗。

秘 元 煎
《景岳全书》

【组成】 远志（炒）2.5g 山药（炒）6g 芡实6g 酸枣仁（炒）6g 金樱子6g 白术（炒）4.5g 茯苓4.5g 炙甘草3g 人参3~6g 五味子14粒

【用法】 水煎服。

【功效】 收涩固精，健脾益肾，交通心肾。

【主治】 无火滑精。梦遗日久，下焦已无火邪而频频滑精，腰膝酸软，脉沉细。

【方解】 用远志辛苦微温，五味子酸温，酸枣仁甘平收敛心神，交通心肾，为方中主药；用金樱子酸涩补肾涩精，以固滑泄，为辅药；用四君子（参、苓、术、草）汤健脾益气。加山药、芡实健脾兼能收涩下焦精气，为佐使药。诸药配伍，共奏收涩固精，健脾益肾，交通心肾之功。

【按语】

(1) 神经衰弱、睾丸炎及阴囊炎等属心肾不交者，均可用本方加减治疗。

(2) 下焦有湿热者，禁用本方。畏酸者，亦非所宜。

(3) 如尚有火，觉热者加苦参 3~6g；气虚甚加黄芪 3~9g。

15.5 固崩止带

固崩止带的方剂，适用于妇人的崩中漏下，或带下日久不止等证。

固 经 丸
《丹溪心法》

【组成】 黄芩 白芍 龟板各 30g 椿根皮 21g 黄柏 9g 香附 7.5g

【用法】 共为末，酒糊丸，每服 9g，空腹温酒或温开水送下。亦可按原方用量比例酌定，水煎服。

【功效】 滋阴清热，止血固经。

【主治】 阴虚内热崩漏。经行不止，崩中漏下，血色深红，或夹紫黑瘀块，心胸烦热，腹痛溲赤，舌红，脉弦数。

【方解】 用龟板甘咸寒，益肾滋阴而降火，白芍苦酸微寒，敛阴益血而养肝，为方中主药；黄芩清热止血，黄柏泻火坚阴，共为辅药；佐以椿根皮固经止血，香附调气活血。诸药配伍，共奏养阴清热疏肝、固经止崩之功。

【按语】

功能性子宫出血或慢性附件炎而致的经行量多，淋漓不止属阴虚血热者，均可用本方加减治疗。

完 带 汤
《傅青主女科》

【组成】 白术 30g 山药 30g 人参 6g 白芍（炒）15g 车前子（炒）9g 苍术 9g 甘草 3g 陈皮 2g 黑芥穗 2g 柴胡 2g

【用法】 水煎服。

【功效】 补中健脾疏肝，化湿止带。

【主治】 脾虚带下。带下色白或淡黄，清稀无臭，倦怠便溏，面色㿠白，舌淡苔白，脉濡缓或濡弱。

【方解】 用人参、白术、山药甘苦温，补气健脾燥湿，为方中主药；苍术、陈皮燥湿运脾，芳香行气，使主药补而不滞，气行湿自去，车前子淡渗利湿，使水湿从小便而去，共为辅药；白芍疏肝扶脾，柴胡升阳，使湿气不致下流入里，芥穗入血分祛风胜湿以止带，共为佐药；甘草调合诸药，为使药。诸药配伍，共奏健脾疏肝，化湿止带之功。

【按语】

（1）慢性宫颈炎、盆腔炎等引起的白带过多属脾虚湿盛者，可用本方治疗。

（2）湿热下注所致的带下色黄，或带下赤白等证，不宜使用。

小结

固涩剂选方 11 首，按其功用不同，分为固表止汗、敛肺止咳、涩肠固脱、涩精止遗和固崩止带 5 类。

（1）固表止汗　玉屏风散、牡蛎散均能固表止汗。玉屏风散益气固表之力较大，适用于表虚自汗，易感风邪者；牡蛎散敛汗之力较强，兼能益阴潜阳，适用于气阴不足的汗出，夜卧尤甚者。

（2）敛肺止咳　九仙散补气益肺，敛肺止咳，适用于治疗肺虚气弱的久咳不止，短气自汗。

（3）涩肠固脱　真人养脏汤、四神丸均能温阳补肾，涩肠固脱，适用于脾肾虚寒，久泻久痢之证，为治本之剂。真人养脏汤长于益气健脾，固涩之力较大；四神丸则偏于温肾暖脾而固肠止泻。赤石脂禹余粮丸则以涩肠止泻为主，属于泻痢日久，滑脱不禁治标之剂。

（4）涩精止遗　桑螵蛸散、缩泉丸、秘元煎都能涩精止遗，适用于遗精、遗尿诸证。桑螵蛸散长于调补心肾，固精止遗，主要用于心肾两虚的尿频、色如米泔而神志恍惚谵妄者；缩泉丸专于固肾缩泉，主治肾虚遗尿；秘元煎则收涩固精，健脾益肾，标本兼治，适用于无火之滑精证。

（5）固崩止带　固经丸长于滋阴清热，固经止血，适用于阴虚内热的崩漏。而完带汤补气健脾，祛湿止带，适用于脾虚肝郁湿盛之带下证。

复习思考题

（1）固涩剂的适用范围是什么？请按固涩剂分类分述各类代表方剂。

（2）分析真人养脏汤的功用、主治及配伍特点，木香在方中的意义是什么？

（3）桑螵蛸散主治什么病证？简述其配伍意义。

16 理气剂

凡以理气药为主要组成，具有行气、降气的作用，用于治疗气滞、气逆病证的方剂，称为理气剂。

因于脏腑气机功能失调大多表现为气滞和气逆，气滞当采用行气方法治之，气逆当采用降气方法治之。使用理气剂要注意辨别病情的寒热虚实与兼证的有无，分别给予不同的配伍，使方证一致。另外，理气剂多属芳香辛燥之品，易伤津耗气，故应中病即止。单纯气虚及阴虚火旺者忌用，年老体弱、孕妇及有出血倾向者慎用。

16.1 行气

行气剂适用于脾胃气滞而出现的脘腹胀满，嗳气吞酸等证、或肝气郁滞而出现的胸胁胀痛、或疝气痛、或月经不调等证。

柴胡疏肝散
《景岳全书》

【组成】 陈皮（醋炒）6g 柴胡 6g 川芎 5g 香附 5g 枳壳 5g 芍药 5g 炙甘草 3g

【用法】 水煎服。

【功效】 疏肝解郁，行气止痛。

【主治】 肝郁气滞。胁肋疼痛，或寒热往来，嗳气叹息，脘腹胀满，脉弦。

【方解】 用柴胡苦辛微寒疏肝解郁，为方中主药；香附理气疏肝，川芎行气活血散瘀止痛，共为辅药；陈皮理气开胃，枳壳宽中消胀，芍药养血柔肝，均为佐药；甘草调合诸药，为使药。诸药配伍，共奏疏肝解郁，行气止痛之功。

【按语】

（1）慢性肝炎、慢性胃炎、肋间神经痛等属于肝郁气滞者，均可用本方加减治疗。

（2）肝火旺或肝胆湿热者不宜使用。

越 鞠 丸
《丹溪心法》

【组成】 香附 川芎 苍术 神曲 栀子各 6g

【用法】 共为细末，水丸如绿豆大，每服 6～9g。亦可作汤剂水煎服。

【功效】 行气解郁。

【主治】 气、血、痰、火、湿、食诸郁证。胸膈痞闷，脘腹胀痛，嗳腐吞酸，恶心呕吐，饮食不消，苔白腻，脉弦。

【方解】 用香附辛苦甘平，行气解郁以治气郁，为方中主药；川芎活血祛瘀以治血郁；山栀子清热泻火以治火郁，苍术燥湿健脾以治湿郁，胸痞痰多，神曲消食导滞以治食郁，俱为佐使药。诸药配伍，气畅郁舒，诸郁得解。

【按语】

（1）胃神经官能证、胃及十二指肠溃疡、慢性胃炎、胆石证、胆囊炎、肝炎、肋间神经痛、精神抑郁证、妇女痛经、月经不调等有六郁见证者，可加减使用。

（2）本方所治诸郁均为实证，虚证不宜使用。

瓜蒌薤白白酒汤
《金匮要略》

【组成】　全瓜蒌 30g　薤白 9g　白酒　适量

【用法】　水酒同煎，分温 2 服。

【功效】　通阳散结，行气祛痰。

【主治】　胸痹。胸中闷痛、甚痛彻背，喘息咳唾、短气。苔白腻，脉沉弦或紧。

【方解】　用瓜蒌甘寒涤痰散结，为方中主药；薤白辛温通阳散结，行气止痛，为辅药；白酒行气活血，可增强主辅药行气通阳之力，为佐使药。诸药配伍，共奏通阳散结，行气祛痰之功。

【按语】

（1）冠心病心绞痛、肋间神经痛、慢性支气管炎、非化脓性肋软骨炎等，有上述见证者，均可运用。

（2）本方属于温开之剂，如阴虚胸痛，肺热痰喘胸痛不宜使用。

（3）方中白酒，可用黄酒或绍兴酒 10～60ml 加水适量煎瓜蒌、薤白。

【附方】

（1）枳实薤白桂枝汤（《金匮要略》）　枳实 12g　厚朴 12g　薤白 9g　桂枝 3g　全瓜蒌 30g。功能通阳散结，祛痰下气。用治胸痹，胸满而痛，喘息咳唾，短气，气从胁下上逆至心，舌苔白腻，脉沉弦或紧。

（2）瓜蒌薤白半夏汤（《金匮要略》）　全瓜蒌 30g　薤白 6g　半夏 12g　白酒（黄酒）30～60ml。功能通阳散结，祛痰宽胸。用治胸痹，而痰浊较甚者。胸中满痛彻背，不能安卧。

16.2　降气

降气剂适用于肺胃气逆而出现的咳喘、或呃逆、呕吐等证。

苏子降气汤
《太平惠民和剂局方》

【组成】　苏子 9g　半夏 9g　当归 6g　甘草 6g　前胡 6g　厚朴 6g　肉桂 3g　生姜 3g　苏叶 2g　大枣 3 枚

【用法】　水煎服。

【功效】　降气平喘，祛痰止咳。

【主治】　上实下虚。痰涎壅盛，喘咳短气，胸膈满闷，腰痛脚软，肢体倦怠，舌苔白腻或滑。

【方解】　用苏子辛温降气祛痰，止咳平喘，为方中主药；半夏、厚朴、前胡祛痰止咳，降气平喘，共为辅药；肉桂温肾祛寒，纳气平喘，当归养血补肝，二药配伍，以温补下虚，又能治咳逆上气，加生姜、苏叶宣肺散寒，共为佐药；大枣、甘草和中而调药为使。诸药配伍，上实下虚兼顾，以治上实为主，气降痰消，喘咳自愈。

【按语】

(1) 本方是急则治其标之方，重在降气祛痰、辅以温肾纳气，主治上实下虚而以上实为主的咳喘证。慢性支气管炎、肺气肿、肺原性心脏病、支气管哮喘等，可用本方加减治疗。

(2) 肺肾阴虚的咳喘，或肺热痰喘，均不宜使用。

旋覆代赭汤
《伤寒论》

【组成】 旋覆花（包）9g 人参6g 生姜10g 代赭石9g 炙甘草6g 半夏9g 大枣4枚

【用法】 水煎服。

【功效】 降气化痰，益气和胃。

【主治】 胃虚气逆。心下痞硬，噫气不除，反胃呕吐，吐涎沫，苔白滑，脉弦而虚。

【方解】 用旋覆花苦辛咸，下气化痰，降逆止噫，为方中主药；代赭石降逆下气，助旋覆花降逆化痰而止呕噫，为辅药；半夏燥湿化痰，降逆和胃，生姜祛痰散结，降逆止呕，二药合用，可增强主、辅的降逆止呕之力，人参、大枣、甘草益气补中，以疗胃虚，且防金石之伤胃之弊，均为佐药。诸药配伍，共奏降气化痰，益气和胃止呕之功。

【按语】

胃神经官能证、慢性胃炎、胃下垂、胃扩张、胃及十二指肠溃疡、幽门不全梗阻、神经性呃逆等属胃虚气逆者，均可加减使用。

定 喘 汤
《摄生众妙方》

【组成】 白果9g 麻黄9g 苏子6g 甘草3g 款冬花9g 杏仁9g 半夏9g 桑白皮9g 黄芩6g

【用法】 水煎服。

【功效】 宣肺降气，清热化痰。

【主治】 风寒外束，痰热内蕴之哮喘证。哮喘咳嗽，痰多气急，痰稠色黄，或有恶寒发热，苔黄腻，脉滑数。

【方解】 用麻黄辛温宣肺散邪平喘，白果甘苦涩敛肺化痰定喘，二者一散一收，既可加强平喘之功，又可防麻黄耗散肺气，共为方中主药；苏子、杏仁、半夏、款冬花降气平喘，止咳祛痰，均为辅药；桑白皮、黄芩清泄肺热，止咳平喘，共为佐药；甘草调合诸药，为使药。诸药配伍，共奏宣降肺气，清痰平喘之功。

【按语】

(1) 慢性支气管炎、支气管哮喘等属于痰热蕴肺者，可用本方加减治疗。

（2）新感风寒，无汗而喘，内无痰热者及哮喘日久，气虚脉弱者，忌用。

四 磨 饮
《成方便读》

【组成】 人参 3g　槟榔 9g　沉香 3g　乌药 9g

【用法】 水煎服。

【功效】 行气降逆，宽胸散结。

【主治】 气滞气逆，胸膈烦闷，上气喘急，心下痞满，不思饮食。

【方解】 用乌药辛温行气疏肝以解郁，沉香辛苦温顺气降逆以平喘，槟榔行气化滞以除满，用人参益气扶正，使郁结之气散而不伤正气。四药配伍，降中有升，泻中带补，疏肝气，和肺胃，诸证自愈。

【按语】

（1）支气管哮喘、肺气肿属气滞兼有气逆者，可用本方加减治疗。

（2）方中人参亦可用党参 6g。

参赭镇气汤
《医学衷中参西录》

【组成】 党参 12g　生赭石（轧细）18g　生芡实 15g　生山药 15g　萸肉 18g　生龙骨　生牡蛎各 18g　杭芍 12g　苏子 6g

【用法】 水煎服。

【功效】 补气摄纳，镇逆定喘。

【主治】 阴阳两虚，喘逆迫促，有将脱之势，或肾虚不摄，冲气上干，胃气上逆而满闷，脉浮大，按之空豁无力。

【方解】 用党参甘温补中益气，赭石质重镇降平喘，为方中主药；山药、山萸肉、白芍、芡实滋补肝肾，以收摄肾气，龙骨、牡蛎潜镇浮阳，收敛固脱，为辅药；苏子消痰降气，以平喘息，为佐药。诸药配伍，共奏补气摄纳，镇逆定喘之功。

【按语】

慢性支气管炎、肺扩张、胃及十二指肠溃疡等有上述见证者，可用本方加减治疗。

小结

理气剂选主方 8 首，按其功效分为行气和降气两大类。

（1）行气　本类方剂都有行气作用，适用于气机郁滞之证。柴胡疏肝散长于疏肝解郁，适用于肝气郁滞所致疼痛胀满之证。越鞠丸行气解郁，主治以气郁为主的诸郁证。瓜蒌薤白白酒汤行气止痛，通阳祛痰散结，适用于胸阳不振，痰湿内阻的胸痹证。

（2）降气　本类方剂都有降气作用，适用于气逆诸证。苏子降气汤、定喘汤长于降肺气、定喘逆。而苏子降气汤兼具温化寒痰之功，适用于上实下虚的寒湿痰喘证。定喘汤则兼具宣肺除痰之功，多用于风寒外束，痰热内蕴的哮喘证。四磨饮能降气行气，适用于气滞气逆证。旋覆代赭汤降逆化痰兼以补虚，适用于胃气虚弱，痰阻气逆的呕吐、嗳气等证。参赭镇气汤具有补气摄纳镇逆之功，适用于阴阳两虚，冲胃之气上逆证。

复习思考题

(1) 越鞠丸以何药为主药？为什么？

(2) 苏子降气汤、定喘汤均有降气平喘之功，二方组方意义有何不同？

(3) 试述旋覆代赭汤的组方意义及功效。

17 理血剂

凡以理血药为主组成，具有活血祛瘀或止血作用，以治疗血瘀或出血证的方剂，统称为理血剂。

血分病变范围广泛，有寒热虚实之分，故治疗方法也很多。本剂根据血瘀、血溢两证而分为活血祛瘀和止血的两类。

血证病情复杂，使用理血剂时，须探求其致病原因，分清标本缓急，做到急则治标，缓则治本，或标本兼顾，攻补兼施。应该注意逐瘀过猛，易于伤血，久用逐瘀亦易伤正，必要时可以酌情配伍益气养阴之品，使消瘀而不伤正。止血过急，易致留瘀，必要时可在止血剂中辅以少量活血祛瘀之品，或选用兼有活血祛瘀作用的止血药。此外，活血祛瘀之剂属于消法，只可暂用，不可久服，中病即止。且其性多破泄，易于动血、堕胎，故凡月经过多及孕妇均当慎用。

17.1 活血祛瘀

活血祛瘀剂，适用于蓄血及瘀血证。

失 笑 散
《太平惠民和剂局方》

【组成】 五灵脂、蒲黄各等分。

【用法】 原方为末，先用酽醋调2钱，熬成膏，入水1盏，煎7分，食前热服。现代用法：共为细末，每服6g，用黄酒或醋冲服；亦可每日用6～12g，包煎，作汤剂。

【功效】 活血祛瘀，散结止痛。

【主治】 瘀血停滞。心腹剧痛，或产后恶露不行，或月经不调，少腹急痛等。

【方解】 用五灵脂苦温甘，活血化瘀止痛，为方中主药；用蒲黄甘平，行血祛瘀止痛，为辅药；用醋或黄酒冲服，取其活血脉，行药力，化瘀血，以加强活血止痛作用。诸药配伍，共奏活血化瘀止痛之功。

【按语】

（1）本方为治疗血瘀作痛的常用方剂。冠心病心绞痛以及宫外孕等病属于瘀血停滞者，均可用本方加味治疗。

（2）方中五灵脂腥臊伤胃，胃气弱者慎用。孕妇忌服本方。

【附方】

手拈散（《奇效良方》） 延胡索 五灵脂 草果 没药各等分研末，每服6g，开水送下。功能活血祛瘀，行气止痛。用治气血凝滞之脘腹疼痛。

血府逐瘀汤
《医林改错》

【组成】 桃仁12g 红花9g 当归9g 生地黄9g 川芎5g 赤芍6g 牛膝9g 桔

梗 5g　柴胡 3g　枳壳 6g　甘草 3g

【用法】　水煎服。

【功效】　活血祛瘀，行气止痛。

【主治】　胸中血瘀，而致头痛。胸痛日久不愈，痛如针刺，且有定处，或呃逆干呕，或急躁易怒，或多梦失眠，或心悸怔忡，或入暮发热，舌质黯红，舌边有瘀斑瘀点，脉涩。

【方解】　用桃红四物汤活血化瘀而养血，四逆散行气和血而疏肝，桔梗开肺气，载药上行，合枳壳则升降上焦之气而宽胸，尤以牛膝通利血脉，引血下行，诸药配伍，共奏活血行气，化瘀止痛之功。

【按语】

(1) 冠心病心绞痛、风湿性心脏病、胸部挫伤与肋软骨炎之胸痛，以及脑震荡后遗症之头痛头晕，精神抑郁等证属于血瘀者，均可用本方加减治疗。

(2) 本方活血祛瘀之品较多，非确有瘀血之证者，不宜使用；孕妇忌用。

【附方】

(1) 通窍活血汤（《医林改错》）　赤芍 3g　川芎 3g　桃仁 9g　红花 9g　老葱 3g　红枣 5g　麝香五厘　黄酒 250g。功能活血通窍。用治血瘀头面的头痛昏晕，或耳聋年久，或头发脱落，面色青紫，或酒渣鼻，或白癜风，以及妇女干血痨，小儿疳积而见肌肉消瘦、腹大青筋、潮热等。

(2) 膈下逐瘀汤（《医林改错》）　五灵脂 9g　当归 9g　川芎 6g　桃仁 9g　丹皮 6g　赤芍 6g　乌药 6g　延胡索 3g　甘草 9g　香附 3g　红花 9g　枳壳 5g。功能活血祛瘀，行气止痛。用治瘀在膈下，形成积块；或小儿痞块，或肚腹疼痛，痛处不移；或卧则腹坠似有物者。

(3) 少腹逐瘀汤（《医林改错》）　小茴香 1.5g　干姜 3g　延胡索 3g　当归 9g　川芎 3g　官桂 3g　赤芍 6g　蒲黄 9g　五灵脂 6g。功能活血祛瘀，温经止痛。用治少腹瘀血积块疼痛或不痛，或痛无积块，或少腹胀满，或经期腰酸少腹胀，或月经1月见3、5次，连续不断，断而又来，其色或紫或黑，或有瘀块，或崩漏兼少腹疼痛等证。

补阳还五汤
《医林改错》

【组成】　黄芪 120g　当归 6g　赤芍 6g　地龙 3g　川芎 3g　红花 3g　桃仁 3g

【用法】　水煎服。

【功效】　补气、活血、通络。

【主治】　中风后遗症。半身不遂，口眼㖞斜，语言謇涩，口角流涎，下肢痿废，小便频数或遗尿不禁，苔白，脉缓。

【方解】　用生黄芪甘温补益元气，使气旺则血行，为方中主药；用当归活血，有祛瘀不伤血之妙，为辅药；赤芍、川芎、桃仁、红花助当归活血和营，地龙通经活络。诸药配伍，共奏补益元气，活血通络之功。

【按语】

(1) 本方主要用于治疗中风后半身不遂之证。以舌淡苔白，脉缓无力，为其辨证要点。脑血管意外后遗症、小儿麻痹后遗症引起的瘫痪，属气虚血瘀者，均可用本方加减治疗。

（2）原方黄芪用量120g，临床可根据病情少用，一般从30～60g开始。

生 化 汤
《傅青主女科》

【组成】 全当归25g 川芎9g 桃仁6g 干姜2g 甘草2g

【用法】 黄酒、童便各半煎服（现代用法：水煎服，或酌加黄酒同煎）。

【功效】 活血化瘀，温经止痛。

【主治】 产后血虚受寒，恶露不行，小腹冷痛。

【方解】 用当归甘辛温补血活血，化瘀生新，为方中主药；用川芎辛温活血行气；桃仁苦平活血化瘀，为辅药；炮姜入血散寒，温经止痛；黄酒温通血脉，以助药力，加入童便者，取其益阳化瘀，并有引败血下行之效，共为辅药。炙甘草调合诸药，为使药。诸药配伍，共奏活血化瘀，温经止痛之功。

【按语】

本方为产后常用方，但药性偏温，应以产后寒凝血瘀者为宜。胎盘残留，产后宫缩腹痛可用本方加减治疗。血热而有瘀滞者，不宜使用。

桃核承气汤
《伤寒论》

【组成】 桃仁12g 大黄12g 桂枝6g 甘草6g 芒硝6g

【用法】 水煎，去滓，冲入芒硝，温服。

【功效】 破血下瘀。

【主治】 下焦蓄血。少腹胀满，疼痛拒按，小便自利，谵语烦渴，至夜发热，其人如狂，脉沉。

【方解】 用桃仁苦平破血祛瘀，大黄苦寒下瘀泄热，二药合用，瘀热并泄，共为方中主药；桂枝通行血脉，助桃仁破血祛瘀，芒硝泄热软坚，助大黄下瘀泄热，共为辅药；炙甘草益气和中，并缓诸药峻烈之性，为佐使药。五味配伍，共奏破血下瘀之功。

【按语】

（1）对跌打损伤、瘀血停留，疼痛不能转侧，二便秘涩者、火旺而血郁于上，头痛头胀，目赤齿痛者、血热妄行而致鼻衄，或吐血紫黑者、以及妇人血瘀经闭，或产后恶露不下，少腹坚痛，喘胀欲死等证，均可用本方加减治疗。

（2）若兼有表证未解者，当先解表，而后再下瘀。

（3）本方破血下瘀之力较为峻猛，孕妇忌服。

温 经 汤
《金匮要略》

【组成】 吴茱萸9g 当归9g 芍药6g 川芎6g 人参6g 桂枝6g 阿胶9g 牡丹皮6g 生姜6g 甘草6g 半夏6g 麦冬9g

【用法】 水煎服。

【功效】 温经散寒，祛瘀养血。

【主治】 冲任虚寒，瘀血阻滞。漏下不止，月经不调，或前或后，或逾期不止，或1月再行，或经停不至，而见入暮发热，手心烦热，唇口干燥，少腹里急，腹满；亦治妇人久不受孕。

【方解】 用吴茱萸辛苦热、桂枝辛甘温，温经散寒，通利血脉，共为方中主药；当归、川芎、芍药、阿胶养血调经，祛瘀生新，为辅药；丹皮助桂枝、当归、川芎活血祛瘀，且能清血分郁热；人参、甘草、麦冬益胃气养胃阴，使中气充盛，以化生血液，半夏降胃安冲，生姜暖肝和胃，且解半夏之毒，均为佐药。甘草调合诸药，为使药。诸药配伍，共奏温经通脉，养血祛瘀之功。

【按语】

功能性子宫出血、慢性盆腔炎等，辨证属冲任虚寒、瘀血阻滞者，可用本方治疗。

17.2 止血

止血剂，适用于血液离经妄行而出现的吐血、衄血、咳血、便血、崩漏等各种出血证。

小蓟饮子
《济生方》

【组成】 生地黄 30g 小蓟 15g 滑石 15g 木通 9g 炒蒲黄 9g 藕节 9g 淡竹叶 9g 当归 6g 山栀子 9g 炙甘草 6g

【用法】 水煎服。

【功效】 凉血止血，利水通淋。

【主治】 下焦瘀热，血淋，小便频数，赤涩热痛或尿血，舌红，脉数者。

【方解】 用小蓟甘凉，凉血止血，祛瘀生新，生地甘苦寒，清热凉血，止血消瘀，为方中主药；用蒲黄、藕节甘平涩收敛止血，行血化瘀，共为辅药；用滑石、木通、淡竹叶，清热利水通淋，栀子清泄下焦之热，从小便而出，当归祛瘀生新，使清热利水而不伤阴血，为佐药；用炙甘草缓急止痛，调合诸药，为使药。诸药配伍，共奏凉血止血，利水通淋之功。

【按语】

(1) 急性泌尿系感染及泌尿系结石等病，可用本方加减治疗。

(2) 本方药物多属寒凉通利之品，只适宜于实证、热证，若血淋、尿血日久正气虚弱者，不宜使用原方。

胶艾汤
《金匮要略》

【组成】 川芎 6g 阿胶 9g 艾叶 9g 甘草 6g 当归 9g 芍药 12g 干地黄 18g

【用法】 以水 1/3，黄酒 2/3，同煎，去滓，加入阿胶烊化，温服。

【功效】 养血调经，安胎止漏。

【主治】 妇女冲任虚损。崩中漏下，月经过多，淋漓不止，或产后下血不绝，或妊娠下血，腹中疼痛者。

【方解】 用阿胶甘平补血，止血，用艾叶苦辛温，温经止血，共为方中主药；熟地、白芍、当归、川芎补血活血调经，共为辅佐药；甘草调合诸药，清酒助药力运行，共为使药。诸药配伍，共奏养血调经，安胎止漏之功。

【按语】

（1）功能性子宫出血、先兆流产、习惯性流产等所致的出血不止，辨证属冲任虚损，血虚有寒者，均可用本方治疗。

（2）血分有热而致的月经过多，崩中漏下，或妊娠下血，则不宜使用。

咳 血 方
《丹溪心法》

【组成】 青黛6g 瓜蒌仁9g 海石9g 山栀子9g 诃子6g

【用法】 水煎服。

【功效】 清火化痰，敛肺止咳。

【主治】 肝火犯肺。咳嗽痰稠带血，咯吐不爽，或心烦易怒，胸胁刺痛，颊赤，便秘，舌红苔黄，脉弦数。

【方解】 用青黛、栀子苦咸寒，清肝泻火凉血，为方中主药；瓜蒌仁、海石清热降火，润燥化痰，为辅药；诃子清敛降肺，止咳化痰，为佐使药。诸药配伍，共奏清肝宁肺之功。

【按语】

（1）支气管扩张咯血、肺结核咯血等病而见上证者，可用本方加减治疗。

（2）肝火灼肺所致咳血，阴分每亦亏损，需酌加清肺养阴之品。

槐 花 散
《本事方》

【组成】 炒槐花12g 炒柏叶12g 荆芥炭6g 炒枳壳6g

【用法】 为细末，每服6g，开水或米汤调下；亦可作汤剂，水煎服，用量按原方比例酌定。

【功效】 清肠止血，疏风行气。

【主治】 肠风脏毒下血。便前出血，或便后出血，或粪中带血，以及痔疮出血，血色鲜红或晦暗。

【方解】 用槐花苦微寒，清大肠湿热，凉血止血，为方中主药；侧柏叶助槐花凉血止血，荆芥炒炭，疏风并入血分而止血，共为辅药；枳壳下气宽肠，为佐使药。诸药配伍，共奏凉血止血，清肠疏风之功。

【按语】

（1）本方为治肠风、脏毒下血的常用方剂，亦可用治痔疮出血。

（2）本方药性寒凉，不宜久服。如便血日久，见有气虚或阴虚者，不宜使用。

小结

理血剂共选主方 10 首，按其功用分为活血祛瘀和止血两类。

（1）活血祛瘀　本类方剂都具有活血祛瘀的作用，适宜于血行不畅或瘀血内结之证。其中血府逐瘀汤能活血化瘀，行气止痛，兼治胸中瘀血所致的各种痛证；而桃核承气汤能破血下瘀，荡涤瘀热，适宜于血热互结下焦的蓄血证；补阳还五汤长于补气活血通络，常用于治疗气虚血瘀，脉络瘀阻所致的半身不遂等证。失笑散、温经汤、生化汤均为妇科常用方剂。失笑散侧重于活血化瘀止痛，主要用于月经不调，或产后恶露不下的少腹急痛之证；而温经汤则长于温经散寒，养血行瘀，是治疗冲任虚寒，瘀血内阻的月经不调或不孕的常用方剂；生化汤具活血化瘀，温经止痛之功，多用于治疗产后恶露不下，少腹疼痛而有寒之证。

（2）止血　本类方剂具有止血作用，适用于出血证。小蓟饮子、咳血方、槐花散均为凉血止血之剂，主治血热妄行出血证。而小蓟饮子兼具利水通淋之功，主要用于血淋、尿血；咳血方兼具清火化痰之功，适用于肝火犯肺的咳血；槐花散善于清肠疏风，主要用于肠风便血证；胶艾汤则属温补止血之剂，能补血调经安胎，适用于妇人冲任虚损所致的月经过多，崩漏胎漏等。

复习思考题

（1）活血祛瘀剂为什么常配伍行气药或补益药？止血药为什么常配伍祛瘀药？

（2）试述血府逐瘀汤的组方、配伍意义及主治病证。

（3）补阳还五汤的配伍特点是什么？并试述其功效、主治。

（4）温经汤和生化汤均为治疗妇科常用方剂，二者如何区别使用？

（5）咳血方主治哪种咳血？为什么不用止血药而能使血自止？

18 消导化积剂

凡以消导药为主组成，具有消食导滞，化积消癥作用，治疗食积痞块、癥瘕积聚的方剂，统称为消导化积剂。

消导化积剂多属渐消缓散之剂，适用于食停中脘与逐渐形成的癥瘕积聚。故将本剂分为消食导滞和消痞化积两类。

消导化积剂属克伐之品，对于纯虚无积之证，应当禁用。若脾胃素虚，或积滞日久，耗损正气者，须适当配伍扶正健脾之药，消补兼施，以期消积不伤正，扶正以祛邪。使用本类方剂，应当掌握适当的剂量，中病即止。

另外，积滞内停，每使气机运化不畅，故消导化积剂中又常配伍理气药，使气利而积消。

18.1 消食导滞

消食导滞剂，适用于食积为病。

保 和 丸
《丹溪心法》

【组成】 山楂 180g 神曲 60g 半夏 茯苓各 90g 陈皮 连翘 萝卜子各 30g

【用法】 共为末，水泛为丸，每服 6～9g，温开水或炒麦芽汤送下。亦可作汤剂，水煎服，用量按原方比例酌减。

【功效】 消食和胃。

【主治】 一切食积。脘腹痞满胀痛，嗳腐吞酸，恶食呕逆，或大便泄泻，舌苔厚腻，脉滑。

【方解】 用山楂酸甘微温，消肉食油腻之积，为方中主药；用神曲甘平而温，消食和胃，化酒食陈腐之积；萝卜子辛甘下气，消面食之积，宽胸畅膈除满，为辅药；用半夏辛温，燥湿祛痰，下气散结；陈皮辛苦温，燥湿化痰，理气和中；茯苓甘平，健脾和中，化痰利湿；食积停滞，易郁而化热，又用连翘苦寒芳香，散结清热。诸药配伍，共奏消食和胃之功。

【按语】

本方为消食化积之剂，宜于食停中脘而正气未虚者。急性肠胃炎、小儿消化不良症，辨证属食积停滞者，可用本方治疗。

枳 术 丸
《脾胃论》

【组成】 枳实 30g 白术 60g

【用法】 丸剂，每服 6～9g，荷叶煎汤或温开水送下。亦可作汤剂，用量按原方比例酌减，加荷叶水煎服。

【功效】 健脾胃消痞满。

【主治】 脾胃气滞，饮食停聚。胸脘痞满，不思饮食，大便或溏或不畅。

【方解】 用白术苦甘温，健脾祛湿，以助脾之运化，为方中主药；用枳实苦辛微寒，下气化滞，消痞除满，为辅药；用荷叶取其养脾胃而升清，为佐使。诸药配伍，共奏升清降浊，调气和胃，健脾化积除痞之功。

【按语】

胃下垂、胃肌无力、胃神经官能证、慢性胃炎等病，属脾虚气滞者，均可用本方治疗。

健 脾 丸
《证治准绳》

【组成】 白术75g 木香 黄连 甘草各22g 白茯苓60g 人参45g 神曲 陈皮 砂仁 麦芽 山楂 山药 肉豆蔻各30g

【用法】 糊丸或水泛小丸，每服6~9g，温开水送下，日2次，或作汤剂水煎服。

【功效】 健脾和胃，消食止泻。

【主治】 脾胃虚弱，饮食停滞。食少难消，脘腹痞闷，大便溏薄，苔腻微黄，脉象虚弱。

【方解】 用四君子汤补气健脾，渗湿止泻，为方中主药；用山药、肉豆蔻助其健脾止泻之力，山楂、神曲、麦芽消食化滞为辅药；木香、砂仁、陈皮理气和胃；黄连清热燥湿，为佐使药。诸药配伍，共奏健脾消积止泻之功。

【按语】

本方系攻补兼施之剂。慢性胃炎、功能性消化不良、慢性肝炎，证见脾胃虚弱，饮食内停，脘腹痞闷泄泻者，均可用本方治疗。

18.2 消痞化积

消痞化积剂，适用于癥积痞块证。

枳实消痞丸
《兰室秘藏》

【组成】 干生姜3g 炙甘草 麦芽曲 白茯苓 白术各6g 半夏曲 人参各9g 厚朴12g 枳实 黄连各15g

【用法】 为细末，水泛小丸或糊丸，每服6~9g，温开水送下，日2次，亦可水煎服。

【功效】 消积除满，健脾和胃。

【主治】 脾虚气滞，寒热互结。心下痞满，不思饮食，倦怠乏力，大便不调。

【方解】 用枳实苦辛微寒行气消痞，厚朴苦辛温行气除满，共为方中主药；用黄连清热燥湿而除痞，半夏曲辛温散结和胃，干姜温中祛寒，三味配伍，辛开苦降，共助枳、朴行气开痞之功，为辅药；人参、白术、茯苓、炙甘草补气健脾，麦芽消食和胃共为佐使。诸药配伍，消补并施，寒热并用，共奏消痞祛积，健脾和胃之功。

【按语】

(1) 慢性肝炎、早期肝硬化、慢性胃炎，有上述见证者，可用本方加减治疗。

(2) 食积实证和虚寒证不宜服用。

小结

消导化积剂共选方 4 首，按其功用分为消食导滞和消痞化积两类。

(1) 消食导滞　保和丸消食和胃，是消食化积的通用方，适用于一切食积证。枳术丸、健脾丸均为消补兼施之剂，枳术丸健脾行气，主治脾虚气滞停食证；而健脾丸则是健脾消食，适用于脾虚食滞证。

(2) 消痞化积　枳实消痞丸行气消痞，健脾和胃，消中有补，主治虚实相兼，寒热错杂，气壅湿聚的痞满证。

复习思考题

(1) 保和丸为消食和胃之剂，为什么方中配伍连翘？

(2) 为什么说枳术丸是消补结合以补为主的方剂？

(3) 健脾丸由哪些药物组成？主治何证？

(4) 枳实消痞丸的功效、主治病证是什么？

19 驱虫剂

凡以驱虫药为主组合成方，用以治疗人体寄生虫病的方剂，统称驱虫剂。

驱虫剂常以乌梅、川椒、槟榔、雷丸、使君子、苦楝根皮等药组成。由于寄生虫在人体内所致病证有寒热虚实不同，故应注意据证配伍。

服用驱虫剂应事先作粪便检查，发现虫卵，再结合辨证服药。并注意忌食油腻，空腹为宜。

乌 梅 丸
《伤寒论》

【组成】 乌梅 480g 细辛 180g 干姜 300g 黄连 480g 当归 120g 附子 180g 蜀椒 120g 桂枝 180g 人参 180g 黄柏 180g

【用法】 乌梅用 50% 醋浸 1 宿，去核打烂，和全药打匀，烘干或晒干，研末，加蜜制丸，每服 9g，每日 1～3 次，空腹温开水送下，亦可按原方比例酌减用量，水煎服。

【功效】 温脏安蛔。

【主治】 蛔厥。心烦呕吐，时发时止，食入吐蛔，手足厥冷，腹痛；又治久痢、久泻。

【方解】 用乌梅酸以治蛔，用黄连苦以下蛔，用川椒辛以杀虫驱蛔，共为方中主药。用细辛、桂枝、干姜、附子温脏祛寒，黄柏助黄连清热燥湿，人参、当归补养气血，扶助正气。诸药配伍，寒热并用，标本兼顾，共奏温脏安蛔之功。

【按语】

本方是治疗胆道蛔虫、肠道蛔虫的代表方剂。慢性结肠炎、慢性痢疾属于肠胃虚弱，寒热错杂者，可用本方治疗。

化 虫 丸
《太平惠民和剂局方》

【组成】 胡粉（铅粉）1500g 鹤虱 1500g 槟榔 1500g 苦楝根皮 1500g 白矾 370g

【用法】 上药碾细筛净，水泛为丸，每丸如麻子大，1 岁儿服 5 丸，空腹时米汤送服。

【功效】 驱杀肠中诸虫。

【主治】 肠中诸虫。发作时腹中疼痛，往来上下，痛甚呕吐清水，或吐蛔虫。

【方解】 用鹤虱苦辛平，有小毒，驱杀蛔虫；苦楝根皮苦寒有毒，杀虫且缓解腹痛；槟榔驱虫排虫，白矾解毒化虫，铅粉有毒，性能化浊。诸药配伍，效专力雄，驱杀诸虫。

【按语】

（1）本方可用治驱杀蛔虫、蛲虫、绦虫、囊虫、姜片虫等。

（2）药性有毒，使用要适可而止。驱虫后当调补脾胃，恢复正气。若作汤剂减去铅粉。

小结

驱虫剂选方2首。乌梅丸有温脏、补虚、清热、安蛔之功，适用于上热下寒，寒热错杂的蛔厥证。化虫丸驱虫杀虫之力较强，是治疗各种肠寄生虫病的通剂。

复习思考题

试述乌梅丸组成、功用、主治及方义。

20 痈疡剂

凡主要由清热解毒、托毒排脓或温阳散结药物组成，具有解毒消痈作用，治疗痈、疽、疔、疖等的方剂，称为痈疡剂。

痈疡剂的范围很广，可概括为内、外两大类。故痈疡剂可分为外痈剂、内痈剂。

20.1 外痈

外痈剂，适用于体表痈疡。

仙方活命饮
《校注妇人良方》

【组成】 白芷 贝母 防风 赤芍药 当归尾 甘草节 皂角刺 炙穿山甲 天花粉 乳香 没药各3g 金银花 陈皮各9g

【用法】 水煎服。或水、酒各半煎服。

【功效】 清热解毒，消肿溃坚，活血止痛。

【主治】 痈疡肿毒初起，热毒壅聚，气滞血瘀。红肿焮痛，或身热凛寒，苔薄白或黄，脉数有力。

【方解】 用金银花甘凉清热解毒，消散疮痈，为方中主药；防风、白芷祛风排脓消肿，归尾、赤芍活血通络，乳香、没药散瘀止痛，陈皮理气化滞，共为辅药；贝母、花粉清热散结消肿，甘草泻火解毒，共为佐药；穿山甲、皂角刺消肿溃坚，酒能活血通络以助药势之行，共为使药。诸药配伍，共奏清热解毒，消肿溃坚，活血止痛之功。

【按语】

(1) 本方为治疗阳证痈肿的常用方，疖肿、蜂窝组织炎、乳腺炎以及多种化脓性炎症而未溃破者，均可用本方治疗。

(2) 疮疡已溃者，不宜使用。阴性疮疽禁用。脾胃本虚，气血不足者慎用。

四妙勇安汤
《验方新编》

【组成】 金银花 玄参各90g 当归30g 甘草15g

【用法】 水煎服。一连10剂……药味不可少，减则不效。

【功效】 清热解毒，活血止痛。

【主治】 脱疽。热毒炽盛，患肢黯红微肿灼热，溃烂腐臭，疼痛剧烈，或见发热口渴，舌红，脉数。

【方解】 用金银花甘凉清热解毒，为方中主药；玄参泻火解毒，当归活血散瘀，甘草配金银花加强清热解毒作用，共为辅佐药。诸药配伍，共奏清热解毒，活血通脉之功。

【按语】

（1）血栓闭塞性脉管炎或其他原因引起的血管栓塞病变，属阳证热毒火炽者可用本方治疗。

（2）阴寒型、气血两虚型的血管栓塞性病变，不宜用本方。

透 脓 散
《外科正宗》

【组成】　生黄芪 12g　当归 6g　穿山甲 3g　皂角刺 5g　川芎 9g

【用法】　水煎服。临服入酒 1 杯亦可。

【功效】　托毒溃脓。

【主治】　痈疡肿痛，正虚不能托毒。内已成脓，外不易溃，漫肿无头，或酸胀热痛。

【方解】　用生黄芪甘温益气托毒，为方中主药；用当归、川芎养血活血；山甲、皂角刺消散通透，软坚溃脓，为辅药；用酒少许，增强行血、活血作用，为佐使药。诸药配伍，共奏托毒溃脓之功。

【按语】

本方适用于痈肿不消，成脓不易，而又不宜切开者。

阳 和 汤
《外科全生集》

【组成】　熟地 30g　肉桂 3g　麻黄 2g　鹿角胶 9g　白芥子 6g　姜炭 2g　生甘草 3g

【用法】　水煎服。

【功效】　温阳补血，散寒通滞。

【主治】　阳虚寒凝阴疽。贴骨疽、脱疽、流注、痰核、鹤膝风等，患处漫肿无头，酸痛无热，皮色不变，口中不渴，舌苔淡白，脉沉细等。

【方解】　用熟地甘温，温补营血，为方中主药；用鹿角胶甘咸温，填补精髓，强壮筋骨，助熟地养血，炮姜、肉桂温阳散寒通血脉，共为辅药；麻黄、白芥子散寒凝，化瘀滞为佐药；生甘草解毒，并调合诸药为使药。诸药配伍，共奏温阳补血，散寒通滞之功。

【按语】

本方适用于一切慢性虚弱性阴疽证。骨结核、腹膜结核、淋巴结核、血栓闭塞性脉管炎、慢性深部脓肿等属虚寒证候者，均可用本方治疗。

小 金 丹
《外科全生集》

【组成】　白胶香　草乌　五灵脂　地龙　木鳖各 150g　乳香　没药　归身各 75g　麝香 30g　墨炭 12g

【用法】　以上 10 味，除麝香外，其余木鳖子等 9 味粉碎成细粉，将麝香研细，与上粉末配研，过筛。每 100g 粉末加淀粉 25g，混匀。另用淀粉 5g 制成稀糊泛丸，阴干或低温干燥即得。每服 2～5 丸，1 日 2 次，小儿酌减。

【功效】 化痰祛湿，祛瘀通络。

【主治】 寒湿痰瘀，阻滞凝结，如流注、痰核、瘰疬、乳岩、贴骨疽等病。初起皮色不变，肿硬作痛者。

【方解】 用草乌辛苦温，祛风湿，温经散寒，为方中主药；五灵脂、乳香、没药活血祛瘀，消肿定痛为辅药；当归和血，地龙通络，白胶香调气血，消痈疽，木鳖祛痰毒，消结肿，墨炭消肿化痰，麝香走窜通络，散结开壅，为佐使药。诸药配伍，共奏散寒通络，化湿祛痰，消瘀止痛之功。

【按语】

(1) 骨结核、肠系膜淋巴结核、寒性脓疡，可用本方治疗。

(2) 孕妇忌服。体虚者慎用。

犀 黄 丸
《外科全生集》

【组成】 犀黄（即上好牛黄）15g 麝香75g 乳香 没药各500g 黄米饭350g

【用法】 上药分别研细末，用黄米蒸熟烘干，为细粉与药相合，混匀，水泛为丸，阴干，每服9g，用陈黄酒送服。

【功效】 解毒消痈，化痰散结，活血祛瘀。

【主治】 乳癌、瘰疬、痰核、流注、肺痈、小肠痈等症。

【方解】 用犀黄苦凉清热解毒，化痰散结为方中主药；麝香辛温窜通消散，活血开壅为辅药；乳香、没药活血祛瘀，消肿定痛，为佐药；黄米饭调养胃气。酒送服，是用其活血行血以加速药效，为使药。诸药配伍，共奏解毒清热，活血祛瘀化痰散结之功。

【按语】

(1) 淋巴结炎、乳腺炎、乳腺癌、多发性脓肿、骨髓炎等有毒热结滞者，均可用本方治疗。对于食道癌、贲门癌亦可用本方加味治疗。

(2) 脓疡溃后脓水淋漓，气血皆虚者，阴虚火旺者禁用。

20.2 内痈

内痈剂，适用于内部脏腑痈疡。

苇 茎 汤
《备急千金要方》

【组成】 苇茎30g 薏苡仁30g 冬瓜子24g 桃仁9g

【用法】 水煎服。

【功效】 清肺化痰，逐瘀排脓。

【主治】 肺痈咳嗽，微热，甚则咳吐腥臭痰，胸中隐隐作痛，肌肤甲错，舌红苔黄腻，脉滑数。

【方解】 用苇茎甘寒，清肺泄热为方中主药；用薏苡仁甘淡微寒，清热利湿，化痰排脓，冬瓜子甘寒，清热化痰排脓，为辅药；桃仁润肺止咳，逐瘀行滞，为佐使药。诸药配伍，共奏清热化痰，逐瘀排脓之功。

【按语】

(1) 本方为治疗肺痈（肺脓疡）的常用方，不论肺痈之将成、已成，均可服用。支气管炎、肺炎、百日咳属痰热咳嗽者，亦可用本方加减治疗。

大黄牡丹皮汤
《金匮要略》

【组成】　大黄 12g　牡丹 9g　桃仁 12g　冬瓜子 30g　芒硝 9g

【用法】　水煎服。

【功效】　泻热破瘀，散结消肿。

【主治】　肠痈初起，右少腹疼痛拒按，甚则局部肿痞，小便自调，时时发热，自汗出复恶寒，或右足屈而不伸；舌苔薄腻而黄，脉迟紧有力。

【方解】　用大黄苦寒，泻肠中湿热瘀结之毒，用牡丹皮苦辛微寒，清热凉血散瘀，为方中主药；芒硝咸寒，泻热导滞，软坚散结，助大黄荡涤肠胃，推陈致新，桃仁性善破血，助牡丹皮活血散瘀，且润肠通便，二味共为辅药；冬瓜了排脓散结，为佐药。诸药配伍，共奏清热解毒，泻下逐瘀，散结消肿之功。

【按语】

(1) 急性阑尾炎、以及妇科盆腔、附件的急性炎症等，属于湿热瘀滞者可用本方治疗。

(2) 慢性复发性阑尾炎或急性化脓性坏疽性阑尾炎不宜使用。老人、孕妇、体虚者慎用。

薏苡附子败酱散
《金匮要略》

【组成】　薏苡仁 30g　附子 6g　败酱 15g

【用法】　水煎服。

【功效】　排脓消肿。

【主治】　肠痈内已成脓，身无热，肌肤甲错，腹皮急，如肿胀，按之濡软，脉数。

【方解】　用薏苡仁甘淡微寒，利湿消肿，为方中主药；用败酱草辛苦微寒，排脓破血，为辅药；少佐附子，辛热散结，振奋阳气。诸药配伍，共奏排脓消肿之功。

【按语】

慢性阑尾炎脓已成者，用本方治疗。

小结

疮疡剂共选方剂 9 首，根据疮痈有内、外之不同，分为外痈剂和内痈剂。

(1) 外痈剂　仙方活命饮、四妙勇安汤均能清热解毒。仙方活命饮兼有疏风透表，消肿溃坚，活血化瘀之功。适用于疮疡肿毒初期，属消法。四妙勇安汤兼具泻火散瘀之功，适用于热毒炽盛的脱疽。犀黄丸具有解毒化痰，散结消痈之功，是治疗痈疽、瘰疬、流注等病的主要成药。透脓散托毒溃脓，兼以扶正，适用于痈疡已成脓，外不易溃者，属托法。阳和汤和小金丹同治阴证或阴疽，阳和汤以温阳补血为主，兼以散寒通滞；而小金丹则以温化寒湿，祛痰通络为主。

（2）内痈剂　苇茎汤有清肺化痰排脓之功，用治肺痈；大黄牡丹皮汤、薏苡附子败酱散均能治疗肠痈，而二者的区别在于前者以泻热破瘀为主，后者以排脓消肿为主。

复习思考题

（1）痈疡剂中属于消法、托法的代表方剂是什么？请分述其组成功用，主治病证。

（2）简述苇茎汤、大黄牡丹皮汤的药物组成及主治。

（3）四妙勇安汤的药物用量与用法有何特点？

（4）阳和汤和仙方活命饮的用药法度有何不同？

附：方剂笔画索引

INTRODUCTION

A prescription is composed of herbs whose selection is based on the determination of treatment methods according to differentiation of syndromes, as well as subject to a certain principle of formulation. The science of prescriptions is one that studies and expounds the theories of prescriptions and their clinical applications.

Prescriptions of Traditional Chinese Medicine have a long history, dating far back to the period of slave society when our ancestors began to treat diseases with only one herb. It was in the course of practice that they came to realize that the curative effects of several herbs combined was better than that of a single herb, hence the formation of embryonic prescriptions. In 1979, a book entitled *Wu Shi Er Bing Fang* (Prescriptions for Fifty Two Kinds of Diseases) was discovered inside the Third *Han* Dynasty Tomb of "*Ma Wang Dui*" in *Changsha* City. The book was completed in the 3rd century B.C., probably the earliest formulary extant in China.

Huang Di Nei Jing (The Yellow Emperor's Classic of Internal Medicine) written from the Warring States period to the *Qin* and *Han* Dynasties, is the earliest extant classic on TCM theories. Though not specializing in prescriptions, the book discusses such fundamentals of prescriptions as principles and methods of treatment, selection of drugs and formulation of prescriptions, as well as compatibility and incompatibility of drugs, etc. Besides, it records 13 prescriptions and such forms of processed drugs as decoction, extract, pill and tincture, etc, thus lays a theoretical foundation for the formation and development of the science of prescriptions. *Shang Han Za Bing Lun* (Treatise on Cold-Induced and Miscellaneous Diseases) written by *Zhang Zhongjing* of the Eastern *Han* Dynasty covers 375 prescriptions with names and methods of administration, each of which being a combination of theories, treatment method, prescription and drugs. Owing to its well-knit and effective prescriptions, the book earns a reputation of "Forerunner of Prescription Books" from the later generations. The *Jin* and *Tang* dynasties witnessed further development in prescriptions, marked by the birth of *Qian Jin Yao Fang* (Prescriptions Worth a Thousand Gold for Emergencies) and *Qian Jin Yi Fang* (A Supplement to Prescriptions Worth a Thousand Gold for Emergencies) written by *Sun Simiao* and *Wai Tai Mi Yao* (The Medical Secrets of An Official) compiled by *Wang Tao*, which have a complete collection of the prescriptions before the *Tang* Dynasty. *Tai Ping Shen Hui Fang* (Peaceful Holy Benevolent Prescriptions) and *Sheng Ji Zong Lu* (General Collection for Holy Relief), famous formularies of the *Song* Dynasty, records respectively 16, 834 and nearly 20, 000 prescriptions. *Tai Ping Hui Min He Ji Ju Fang* (Prescriptions of Peaceful Benevolent Dispensary), a pharmacopoeia of patent medicines compiled by the government, is the first of its kind in the history of China and among one of the earliest formularies compiled by national pharmaceutic bureaus worldwide. *Shang Han Ming Li Lun* (Expoundings on the Treatise on Cold-Induced.Diseases) written by *Cheng Wuji* of the Song dynasty becomes the pioneer of prescription theories for its interpretation of 20 prescriptions. *Pu Ji Fang* (Prescriptions for Universal Relie) of the *Ming* dynasty is the most voluminous formulary that houses over 60, 000 prescriptions. *Yi Fang Kao* (Textual Criticism on Prescriptions) by *Wu Kun* is historically the first book devoting exclusively to the elaboration of prescriptions. Its birth signifies a breakthrough in the history of the development of prescriptions, namely, the switch from collection to interpretation. The boom of the school of epidemic febrile disease brought about numerous prescriptions for the treatment of epidemic febrile diseases, which contributed to the richness and perfection of the science of prescriptions.

After the founding of the People's Republic of China, a work was started on the extensive collection, annotation and correction on TCM formularies. Through clinical and experimental research, the mechanism of the effects of prescriptions is further explained, and large number of effective prescriptions is proved. The reformation of the preparation of Chinese drugs shows a bright future for the development of Chinese formularies.

In general, Chinese medical formulary is developed with the extensive practice by doctors of previous dynasties, and it is an important component part of the system of applying treatment based on differentiation of syndromes, and it is also the bases for all the clinical specialities. Therefore, studying of the prescriptions should be under the direction of the theories of traditional Chinese medicine. During the study, we should master the principles of forming prescriptions, i.e. setting up treatment principles according to clinical differentiation and choosing drugs to make a prescription based on the treatment principle. We should also pay attention to the explanation of prescriptions, and give careful consideration of the actions, indications of drugs so as to make a prescription which is in accordance with the treatment principle. While explaining a prescription, we should not only pay attention to the functions of the individual drugs but also the coordinate functions of combined drugs. In this way, we can really learn the theoretical knowledge and skills of setting up treatment principles and making prescriptions.

Part One   Generalities

1 Principles of Forming a Prescription

A prescription is not just the gathering of drugs of the same properties, and there are strict principles for making prescriptions. "Prescription coming from treatment method" and the combination of "principal, assistant, adjuvant and guiding" drugs are the necessary principles of selecting drugs and making prescriptions.

"Prescription coming from treatment method" explains the relationship between formula and treatment methods. The prescriptions are made according to differentiation and treatment methods. First, establish treatment method and then form a prescription. Treatment methods control prescriptions. The treatment method is the bases for choosing drugs and making prescriptions, and a prescription is a measure for accomplishing the treatment method. A prescription is a method, and no prescriptions will exist without a certain treatment method. Treatment methods and prescriptions rely on each other.

"Principal, assistant, adjuvant and guiding" is the principle for combining drugs, which will lead to the best treatment effect.

Principal drug: A principal drug is one which is aimed at producing the leading effects in treating the cause or the main symptom of a disease. It is the center of a prescription.

Assistant drug: There are two types: (1) helping and strengthening the effect of the principal drug for treating the main symptoms. (2) producing the leading effect for treating accompanying symptoms.

Adjuvant drug: There are three types: (1) strengthening the effects of the principal and assistant drugs. (2) reducing or clearing away the toxicity of the principal and assistant drugs. (3) dealing with possible vomiting in serious cases after taking decoction with too potent effect, possesses the properties opposite to those of the principal drug in compatibility, but produces supplementing effects in the treatment of diseases.

Guiding drug: There are two types: (1) medicinal guide which leads the other drugs in the prescription to the affected site. (2) mediating drug which coordinates or harmonizes the effects of other drugs in the prescription.

To sum up, a principal drug is the leader or dominator in the prescription, indispensable and usually with large dosage. All the other type of drugs do not have to necessarily appear. They are chosen accordingly. When the principal drug does not have toxicity or the effect is not so strong, the adjuvant drug for reducing or weakening the toxicity and controlling the powerful effect will not be necessary. For making a prescription, sometimes the principal drug is combined with the assistant drug, sometimes the principal drug is used together with the adjuvant drug, and sometimes the principal drug is used with the guiding drug. In some prescription, there is only principal drug. Of course, some prescriptions have all type of drugs including the principal, assistant, adjuvant and guiding drugs, such as *Ma Huang Tang*. These different kinds of combination are mainly decided by the treatment method and the situation of the syndrome.

2   Modification of a Prescription

The formation of a prescription is not only based on the strict principles but should also be accommodated in the light of concrete conditions as the state of illness and changing of syndromes. Modification of a prescription includes modification of drugs, modification of dose and modification of dosage forms. Only when the principles and flexibility unite in the clinical application and making prescriptions correspond to the syndromes, can we achieve good therapeutic effect.

2.1   Modification of Drugs

It refers to modifying less important ingredients in accordance with the difference of the secondary symptoms or the accompanying symptoms without any change of the principal drugs and the main indications of the prescription. For instance, *Gui Zhi Tang* (Decoction of Ramulus Cinnamomi) is used for exterior deficiency syndrome due to affection of wind-cold. If the patient also has cough or asthma, *Hou Po* (Cortex Magnoliae Officinalis) and *Xing Ren* (Semen Armeniacae Amarum) can be added to lower the adverse flow of *Qi* and relieve asthma. Now the formula is named *Gui Zhi Jia Hou Po Xing Zi Tang* (Decoction of Ramulus Cinnamomi with Cortex Magnoliae and Semen Armeniacae Amarum). Another example, *Ma Huang Tang* (Decoction of Herba Ephedrae) is used for exterior excess syndrome due to affection of exterior wind-cold. It has a strong effect of inducing perspiration and relieving the exterior. If exterior wind-cold damaged the lung causing nasal obstruction with low speaking voice and cough with a lot of sputum, *Gui Zhi* (Ramulus Cinnamomi) should be removed so that the prescription will mainly has the effect of promoting lung's dispersing and descending function and relieving exterior syndrome. The prescription is changed to *San Ao Tang*. The modification of drugs reflected the flexibility of making prescriptions.

2.2   Modification of Dose

It refers to increasing or decreasing the dose of a drug in a prescription without any change in its ingredients. This method can either change the potency of the original prescription or extend the scope of the treatment, and sometimes the dominant and the subordinate roles of the drugs in a prescription may be changed so as to suit them to new indications. For example, Both *Si Ni Tang* and *Tong Mai Si Ni* Tang are composed of the same drugs. The difference between them is that the former, consisting of a small dose of *Fu Zi* (Radix Aconiti Praeparata) and *Gan Jiang* (Rhizoma Zingiberis), is mainly used to restore *Yang* from collapse, and the latter, having a large dose of *Fu Zi* and *Gan Jiang*, is to be used not only for restoring depleted *Yang* but also for stimulating *Yin* to clear the meridians. Because of different functions, the indications of the prescription are also changed. *Si Ni Tang* is applied for *Yin* excess and *Yang* exhaustion marked by cold limbs, aversion to cold, huddling up in bed, watery diarrhea, and weak or feeble pulse. *Tong Mai Si Ni Tang* is mainly for *Yang* being kept externally by interior excess *Yin*, characterized by cold limbs, watery diarrhea and indistinct pulse.

2.3 Modification of Dosage Forms

It means that some prescriptions should be used differently just because of its dosage form. The modification of dosage form is related to the state of illness. Generally speaking, decoction is of speedy and drastic effect, and pills, bolus and powder forms are of slow-acting and lasting effect. For instance, *Li Zhong Tang* and *Li Zhong Wan* are of the same ingredients, be used to treat middle *Jiao* deficient cold with abdominal pain, smooth defecation or loose and formed stool. Because of different forms of preparation, the two formulas have different functions. *Li Zhong Tang* is used for severe and acute cases, and *Li Zhong Wan* is for mild cases.

The above-mentioned three modifications of prescriptions can either be applied separately or be made simultaneously. Flexibly used the modifications of prescriptions will help you to achieve the expected result.

3 Dosage Forms and Methods of Decocting and Administration

3.1 Dosage Forms

Dosage forms of prescription include: decoction, powder, pill and bolus, extract, ointment and plaster, *Dan*, medicated wine, medicated tea, distilled medicinal water, troche, medicated cake, slender roll of medicated paper, medicated thread, moxa-preparation, syrup, tablet, infusion, and injection etc. Some of them are introduced as follows:

3.1.1 Decoction

Soak the drugs of the prescription in water or yellow wine or the mixture of half water and half wine and then boil them for a certain period of time. After removing the drugs, we will get the fluid which is what we called "Decoction". The characteristics of decoction are quick absorption, powerful effect and easy to make modification according to the state of illness. Decoctions, the most common dosage form in the clinic, are usually used as oral medication, but sometimes they may also be used as enema and external lotion.

3.1.2 Pill and Bolus

Grind the drugs into fine powder and mix it with excipients such as honey, water, rice paste, flour paste, wine, vinegar, herb juices, or bee-wax etc. Then make it into round ball of various sizes. This is "*Wan*" (pill or bolus). Pill or bolus has the characteristics of slow absorption, long-lasting effects, and easy for administration. It is usually used for chronic and deficiency diseases. The common types used in clinic are honeyed bolus (or pill) and water-paste pill.

3.1.2.1 Honeyed Bolus (or Pill)

It refers to pills or boluses prepared by grinding drugs into fine powder, mixing it with the excipient, refined honey.

3.1.2.2 Water-Paste Pill

It refers to medicinal pills prepared manually or mechanically by grinding drugs into fine powder, mixing it with excipients such as cold boiled water, wine, vinegar, or decoction of some drugs.

3.2 Methods of Decocting

Before decocting, put the drugs into earthenware pot and then add water until the drugs are slightly submerged under the water surface and decoct them after the drugs are soaked through. First put the pot on strong fire until the water is boiling, then turn to soft fire. It must not take the pot lid off too frequently so as to reduce the loss of the volatile components. Exterior-relieving, heat-clearing and fragrant drugs should be decocted quickly on strong fire to avoid the volatilization of the effective components. It is preferable to used soft fire for tonic drugs with strong flavour so that the effective components may be completely released. Poisonous drugs should be decocted on soft fire for a longer time to reduce their toxicity.

Some drugs need special way of decocting and they must be noted in the prescription. Here are some of the methods.

3.2.1 To be decocted first:

Some drugs as minerals and shells should be smashed and decocted first. After boiling for 10 to 20 minutes, add other drugs. Some drugs with a lot of sand and mud, such as baked yellow earth and glutinous rice root, should be decocted first to get the fluid. When the fluid is clear, use this fluid instead of water for boiling other drugs.

3.2.2 To be decocted later:

Those drugs with fragrance and active constituents ready to diffuse or evaporate, such as *Bo He* (Herba Menthae) and *Sha Ren* (Fructus Amomi), should be added and decocted for four or five minutes when the decoction is nearly done.

3.2.3 To be decocted in packet:

Some drugs such as *Xin Yi* (Flos Magnoliae) and *Xuan Fu Hua* (Flos Inulae) should be wrapped in a piece of cloth before they are decocted with other drugs in case they may cause the decoction turbid or produce irritation to the throat.

3.2.4 To be decocted alone:

Some rare and expensive drugs should be simmered or decocted alone so as to avoid the destruction of their effective constituents from being absorbed by other drugs when decocted together. For example, ginseng should be sliced into pieces and then decocted in a separate pot with lid for about 2 to 3 hours. Some rare drugs, such as *Ling Yang Jiao* (Cornu Antelopis) with active constituents difficult to decoct out, should also be decocted alone.

3.2.5 To be melted by heating:

Some gluey, viscous and easy-dissolved drugs should be melted alone by heating and then put into the decocted solution of other drugs (after removal of the residue), dissolved by gently boiling or stirring, and then taken orally. Donkey-hide gelatin and antler gelatin is typical drugs of this kind.

3.2.6 To take the drug following its infusion:

Powder, dan, small pill, natural medicinal juice and other fragrant or expensive drugs should be taken after being infused with boiling water, hot decoction or wine, such as Moschus, Notoginseng powder, etc.

3.3 Methods of Taking Drugs

Methods of taking drugs will directly influence the therapeutic effects. It will include both the time and the method of taking medicines.

3.3.1 Time

A. Usually tonic drugs are recommended to be taken before meals while drugs irritant to the gastro-intestinal tract should be taken after meals.

B. Drugs of expelling intestinal parasites and purgatives should be taken with an empty stomach.

C. Sedative drugs should be taken before going to bed.

D. The drugs for acute diseases should be taken at any time while those for chronic cases, such as bolus, powder, extract and wine, should be taken at regular time.

E. Generally, the medicine is taken two times, once in the morning and once in the evening. Sometimes, the drugs can be taken several times a day or be decocted and taken as "tea" in multiple doses.

3.3.2 Methods

Decoction is taken when it is warm. One dose of decoction could be divided into two or three equal portions and taken twice or three times. Decoction for relieving exterior syndromes should be taken when it is hot, and then the patient must be kept warm to induce slight sweat. Cold-natured decoction for heat syndromes should be taken cool while hot-natured decoction for cold syndromes should be taken hot. But for the treatment of heat syndromes with false cold manifestations, the cold-natured decoction should be taken warm while for the treatment of cold syndromes with false heat manifestations, the hot-natured decoction should be taken cool. Patients apt to vomit after taking medicine should take some ginger juice, or chew some tangerine peel, or take the decoction in small doses at intervals. For unconscious patients or patients with lockjaw, nasal feeding should be applied.

Part Two   Particulars

1   Exterior-Relieving Prescriptions

Exterior-relieving prescriptions refer to those principally composed of exterior-relieving herbs which serve to induce diaphoresis, expel pathogenic factors from the muscle and skin, as well as promote eruption for the purpose of relieving exterior syndromes.

In view of the types of exterior syndromes (wind-cold and wind-heat type) and those of patients' physiques (deficiency and excess type), exterior-relieving prescriptions are subdivided into the following three types: acrid and warm, acrid and cool, and strengthening body resistance.

Exterior-relieving herbs should not be boiled for too long time, in case that long decocting time will lead to the volatilization of effective ingredients and the weakening of therapeutic effects. After administration, it is advisable to avoid wind and keep warm so as to induce mild perspiration.

1.1   Exterior-Relieving Prescriptions of Acrid and Warm Type

This type of prescriptions is for the treatment of exterior wind-cold syndrome, characterized by fever and chills, headache and stiff neck, general aching, perspiration or absence of perspiration, floating and tense pulse or floating and slightly slow pulse.

Ma Huang Tang (Decoction of Herba Ephedrae)

- Source: *Shang Han Lun* (Treatise on Cold-Induced Diseases)
- Ingredients: *Ma Huang* (Herba Ephedrae, remove joints) 6g.

    Gui Zhi (Ramulus Cinnamomi) 4g.

    Xing Ren (Semen Armeniacae Amarum, remove skin and tip) 9g.

    Zhi Gan Cao (Radix Glycyrrhizae Praeparata) 3g.

- Administration: Decoct the above herbs in water. After oral administration of the decoction, cover with a quilt for mild perspiration.

- Functions: Induce perspiration to relive exterior syndrome and facilitate the flow of lung *Qi* to relieve asthma.

- Indications: Affection by wind and cold marked by fever and chills, headache, aching pain of the body and joints, absence of perspiration and thirst, or with asthma, thin, white and moist tongue coating, floating and tense pulse.

- Explanation:

Ma Huang: bitter, pungent in taste and warm in nature, serving the principal herb for the functions of inducing perspiration to relieve exterior syndrome and facilitating the flow of the lung-Qi to relieve asthma.

Gui Zhi: pungent and sweet in taste, warm in nature, acting as the assistant drug to have the effects of warming the meridians to ensure the flow of *Yang Qi*, activating Nutrient Qi and Defensive Qi which will resist pathogenic factors at exterior.

Xing Ren: bitter and pungent in taste, warm in nature, functioning as the adjuvant drug for its effects of facilitating the flow of the lung Qi and promoting the circulation of Qi.

Zhi Gan Cao: guiding drug, coordinating the actions of the other drugs and diminish the extremely strong actions of *Ma Huang* and *Gui Zhi*.

○ The above four drugs as a whole have the effects of expelling cold, relieving the exterior, facilitating the flow of the lung Qi and stopping asthma.

● Notes:

(1) Being pungent and warm, this prescription is forceful in inducing perspiration, and clinically it is appropriate for the exterior excess syndromes of affection by wind and cold, represented by such key symptoms of differentiation as fever and chills, absence of perspiration, asthma, floating and tense pulse. In clinical practice, this prescription is used to treat the following diseases accompanied by the above manifestations: common cold, influenza, bronchitis and bronchial asthma.

(2) This prescription is contraindicated for cases with exterior deficiency syndromes of wind and cold, exterior syndromes of wind and heat, as well as cases of Qi and blood deficiency.

Appendix:

(1) *Ma Huang Jia Zhu Tang* (Decoction of Herba Ephedrae Plus Atractylodis Macrocephalae)

● Source: *Jin Gui Yao Lue* (Synopsis of Prescriptions from the Golden Chamber)

● Ingredients: *Ma Huang Tang* Plus

　　　　　　 Bai Zhu (Rhizoma Atractylodis Macrocephalae) 12g.

● Functions and indications: Inducing sweating to relieve exterior condition, dispersing cold and expelling dampness, used to treat cold-dampness affecting the body surface with boring pain of the body.

(2) *Ma Huang Xing Ren Yi Yi Gan Cao Tang* (Decoction of Ephedrae, Apricot Kernel, Job's-tears Seed and Licorice)

● Source: *Jin Gui Yao Lue* (Synopsis of Prescriptions from the Golden Chamber)

● Ingredients: *Ma Huang* (Herba Ephedrae) 6g.

　　　　　　 Xing Ren (Semen Armeniacae Amarum) 6g.

　　　　　　 Yi Yi Ren (Semen Coicis) 15g.

　　　　　　 Zhi Gan Cao (Radix Glycyrrhizae Praeparata) 3g.

● Functions and indications: Relieving the exterior and expelling dampness, used to treat wind-dampness at the body surface, showing general body aching, fever more serious in the afternoon.

(3) *San Ao Tang* (Decoction of Three Crude Drugs)

● Source: *Tai Ping Hui Min He Ji Ju Fang* (Prescriptions of Peaceful Benevolent Dispensary)

● Ingredients: Remove *Gui Zhi* from *Ma Huang Tang*.

● Functions and indications: Promoting lung's functions of dispersing and descending so as to relieve exterior syndrome, used to treat wind evil affecting the surface, manifested as nasal obstruction, heavy voice, aphonia, cough with lots of sputum, fullness in the chest with short breath, headache and general aching.

Gui Zhi Tang (Decoction of Ramulus Cinnamomi)

● Source: *Shang Han Lun* (Treatise on Cold-Induced Diseases)

● Ingredients: *Gui Zhi* (Ramulus Cinnamomi) 9g.

         Shao Yao (Radix Paeoniae) 9g.

         Zhi Gan Cao (Radix Glycyrrhizae Praeparata) 6g.

         Sheng Jiang (Rhizoma Zingiberis Recens) 3 pcs.

         Da Zao (Fructus Ziziphi Jujubae) 4 pcs.

● Administration: Decoct the drugs in water and take the decoction while it is warm. After that, drink some boiled water or hot gruel and is covered with a quilt in winter in order to assist the effects of the drugs. Do not have greasy, raw and cold food.

● Functions: Eliminate the pathogens from the muscle, relieve the exterior and harmonize *Ying* (nutrient) with *Wei* (defence).

● Indications: Affection by external wind, manifested as fever, headache, sweating, aversion to wind, nasal obstruction, nausea, no thirst, white tongue coating, and floating moderate or floating and weak pulse.

● Explanation:

Gui Zhi: acrid and warm in nature, dispersing wind pathogen from the muscle and relieving the surface, used as principal drug.

Gui Zhi: bitter and sour in taste, controlling the dispersing of *Yin* and regulating *Ying* (nutrient), assisting *Gui Zhi* to harmonize *Ying* with *Wei*, used as assistant drug.

Sheng Jiang: acrid and warm in nature, assisting *Gui Zhi* to eliminate wind from the muscle and calming the stomach to stop vomiting.

Da Zao: neutral in nature, combining with *Sheng Jiang* to assist *Gui Zhi* and *Shao Yao* in harmonizing *Ying* with *Wei*.

The above two are used as adjuvant drugs.

Zhi Gan Cao: reinforcing *Qi* and harmonizing the middle *Jiao*, regulating the effects of all the drugs in the prescription, used as guiding drug.

○ The prescription as a whole has the effects of expelling wind pathogen from the superficial muscles and regulating the interior.

● Notes:

(1) This prescription is used for exterior deficient syndrome due to affection of external wind-cold, characterized by fever, sweating and moderate pulse. Clinically, it could be also used to treat cases after delivery, after serious disease, or of endogenous miscellaneous diseases, manifested with fever, sweating, and floating and weak pulse. Good effect can also be obtained for pernicious vomiting due to disharmony between *Ying* and *Wei* and between *Qi* and blood.

(2) The prescription is not suitable for exterior excess syndrome (without sweat) or cases with interior heat.

Appendix:

Gui Zhi Jia Hou Po Xing Zi Tang (Decoction of Ramulus Cinnamomi plus Magnolia Bark and Apricot Kernel)

● Source: *Shang Han Lun* (Treatise on Cold-induced Diseases)

● Ingredients: *Gui Zhi Tang plus*

Hou Po (Cortex Magnoliae Officinalis) 6g.

Xing Ren (Semen Armeniacae Amarum) 6g.

● Functions and indications: Expelling evils from the muscles to relieve the exterior, lowering the rising of *Qi* to stop asthma, used to treat cases of chronic asthma with newly affection by exterior wind-cold, showing a syndrome of *Gui Zhi Tang*, or cases with exterior syndrome accompanied by slight asthma.

Ge Gen Tang (Decoction of Radix Puerariae)

● Source: *Shang Han Lun* (Treatise on Cold-Induced Diseases)

● Ingredients: *Ge Gen* (*Radix Puerariae*) 12g.

Ma Huang (Herba Ephedrae) 9g.

Sheng Jiang (Rhizoma Zingiberis Recens) 9g.

Gui Zhi (Ramulus Cinnamomi) 6g.

Bai Shao (Radix Paeoniae Alba) 6g.

Zhi Gan Cao (Radix Glycyrrhizae Praeparata) 6g.

Da Zao (Fructus Ziziphi Jujubae) 12 pcs.

● Administration: Decoct the drugs in water and take the decoction while it is warm. Cover with a quilt for mild perspiration.

● Functions: Relieve the exterior and expel pathogens from muscles and skin.

● Indications: Affection by external wind-cold, characterized by stiffness of nape and back, no sweat, aversion to wind, or with diarrhea, or with vomiting, floating pulse.

● Explanation:

This prescription is formed from *Gui Zhi Tang* by adding *Ma Huang* and *Ge Gen*.

Ge Gen: sweet and acrid in taste, cool in nature, entering the spleen and stomach meridians, expelling pathogens from muscles and skin of the *Yangming* meridian so as to treat stiffness of nape and back, used as principal drug.

Ma Huang: used together with *Gui Zhi Tang* to induce sweating, as a result to disperse wind-cold from the Taiyang meridian and relieve the exterior syndrome.

○ The combination of all the drugs is suitable for combined syndrome of *Taiyang* and *Yangming*.

● Notes:

(1) This prescription is advisable for stiffness and tension at the nape and back in exterior excess syndrome (no sweating) due to invasion of wind and cold into the body surface, characterized by absence of perspiration and aversion to wind. After variation, it can also be used to treat cervical spondylosis and peripheral arthritis of shoulder with symptoms of mild occipital pain, stiffness of nape and back, pain and numbness of shoulder and arm.

(2) It is contraindicated for aversion to wind with sweating.

Appendix:

Gui Zhi Jia Ge Gen Tang (Decoction of Ramulus Cinnamomi plus Pueraria)

● Source: *Shang Han Lun* (Treatise on Cold-induced Diseases)

● Ingredients: Remove *Ge Gen* from *Ge Gen Tang*.

● Functions and indications: Expelling evils from the muscles, relaxing the tendons, used to treat *Taiyang* syndrome characterized by stiffness and pain of the nape and back, sweating with aversion to wind.

Su Qiang Da Biao Tang (Decoction for Relieving the Exterior with Folium Perillae and Notopterygii)

● Source: *Chong Ding Tong Su Shang Han Lun* (Revised Popular Treatise on Cold-Induced Diseases)

● Ingredients: *Su Ye* (*Folium Perillae*) 6g.

Fang Feng (Radix Ledebouriellae) 3g.

Xing Ren (Semen Armeniacae Amarum) 6g.

Qiang Huo (Rhizoma seu Radix Notoperygii) 3g.

Bai Zhi (Radix Angelicae Dahuricae) 3g.

Ju Hong (Exocarpium Citri Reticulatae) 3g.

Sheng Jiang (Rhizoma Zingiberis Recens) 3g.

Fu Ling Pi (Poria) 6g.

● Administration: Decoct the drugs in water and take the decoction while it is warm.

● Functions: Induce perspiration, relieve the exterior and eliminate dampness.

● Indications: Invasion of external wind-cold complicated with dampness, characterized by headache, stiff neck, nasal obstruction with thin discharge, heaviness and soreness of the body, fever and chills or aversion to wind, absence of perspiration, and floating pulse.

● Explanation:

Su Ye: acrid in taste and warm in nature.

Qiang Huo: bitter and acrid in taste, warm in nature.

The above two are used to disperse exterior wind, cold and dampness, as the principal drugs of the prescription.

Bai Zhi and *Fang Feng*: acrid in taste and warm in nature, helping the principal drugs to expel wind and dampness, relieve the exterior and stop pain, used as assistant drugs.

Xing Ren and *Ju Hong*: slight bitter and acrid, promoting the functions of the lung in dispersing and descending, drying the dampness, as adjuvant drugs.

Sheng Jiang and *Fu Ling Pi*: acrid and tasteless, dispersing so as to expel dampness, used together as guiding drugs.

○ The prescription as a whole plays the functions of inducing sweating, relieving the exterior and expelling dampness.

● Notes:

(1) This prescription is advisable for syndrome caused by external wind, cold and dampness, marked by body aching and no sweat. Influenza and rheumatic arthritis which attribute to exterior wind, cold and dampness could be treated with the modification of this prescription.

(2) Clinically, the dosages of drugs could be increased accordingly. Do not decoct the herbs for too long time.

(3) *Fu Ling Pi* may be omitted or reduce its dosage in treating ordinary common cold.

1.2 Exterior-Relieving Prescriptions of Acrid and Cool Type

This type of prescriptions is used for the treatment of exterior wind-heat syndrome, characterized by fever and slightly aversion to wind and cold, headache, sore throat, thirst and floating rapid pulse.

Sang Ju Yin (Decoction of Folium Mori and Flos Chrysanthemi)

● Source: *Wen Bing Tiao Bian* (Treatise on Differentiation and Treatment of Epidemic Febrile Diseases)

● Ingredients: *Sang Ye* (Folium Mori) 7.5g.

Ju Hua (Flos Chrysanthemi) 3g.

Xing Ren (Semen Armeniacae Amarum) 6g.

Lian Qiao (Fructus Forsythiae) 5g.

Bo He (Herba Menthae) 2.4g.

Jie Geng (Radix Platycodi) 6g.

Gan Cao (Radix Glycyrrhizae) 2.4g.

Wei Gen (Rhizoma Phragmitis) 6g.

● Administration: The drugs are to be decocted in water for oral administration, twice a day.

● Functions: Expel wind, clear heat, promote lung's functions in dispersing and descending so as to stop cough.

● Indications: Beginning of exterior wind-heat syndrome with symptoms of mild fever, cough, slight thirst, and dry throat or sore throat.

● Explanation:

Sang Ye: sweet in taste and cold in nature.

Ju Hua: acrid in taste and cool in nature.

The above two drugs are used as principal drugs for clearing the lung collaterals and dispersing wind-heat from the upper *Jiao*.

Bo He: acrid in taste and cool in nature, having the effect of dispersing, strengthening the action of *Sang Ye* and *Ju Hua* in dispersing wind-heat from the upper *Jiao*.

Xing Ren and *Jie Geng*: combined effect of ascending and descending used to promote lung's functions and stop cough.

The above three are assistant drugs.

Lian Qiao: clearing heat from the surface.

Wei Gen: clearing heat and producing body fluid.

Both are used as adjuvant drugs.

Gan Cao: harmonizing the actions of all the drugs, used as guiding drug, together with *Jie Geng* for clearing the throat.

○ The combination of all the drugs plays the functions of expelling wind, clearing heat and stopping cough.

● Notes:

Influenza and acute bronchitis which attribute to wind-heat could be treated with the modification of this prescription. Besides, by adding *Bai Ji Li* (Fructus Tribuli), *Jue Ming Zi* (Semen Cassiae) and *Xia Ku Cao* (Spica Prunellae), the prescription is used to treat epidemic conjunctivitis, and add *Niu Bang Zi* (Fructus Arctii), *Sheng Di* (Radix Rehmanniae), *Xuan Shen* (Radix Scrophulariae), *Ban Lan Gen* (Radix Isatidis), *Shan Dou Gen* (Radix Sophorae Subprostratae) and *Tu Niu Xi* (Radix Achyranthes Longifolia) etc. to treat acute tonsilitis.

Yin Qiao San (Powder of Lonicera and Forsythis)

● Source: *Wen Bing Tiao Bian* (Treatise on Differentiation and Treatment of Epidemic Febrile Diseases)

● Ingredients: *Yin Hua* (Flos Lonicerae) 9g.

　　　　　　Lian Qiao (Fructus Forsythiae) 9g.

　　　　　　Jie Geng (Radix Platycodi) 6g.

　　　　　　Bo He (Herba Menthae) 6g.

　　　　　　Zhu Ye (Herba Lophatheri) 4g.

　　　　　　Sheng Gan Cao (Radix Glycyrrhizae) 5g.

Jing Jie (Herba Schizonepetae) 5g.

Dan Dou Chi (Semen Sojae Praeparatum) 5g.

Niu Bang Zi (Fructus Arctii) 9g.

Lu Gen (Rhizoma Phragmitis) 9g.

● Administration: The drugs are to be decocted in water for oral administration and take twice a day.

● Functions: Relieve the exterior syndrome with drugs acrid in taste and cool in nature, clear away heat and toxins.

● Indications: Beginning of exterior wind-heat syndrome with symptoms of fever, slightly aversion to wind-cold, no sweat or non-smooth sweating, headache, thirst, cough, sore throat, thin white or thin yellowish tongue coating, redness at the tongue border and tip, floating and rapid pulse.

● Explanation:

Yin Hua and *Lian Qiao*: sweet and acrid taste, cold nature and fragrant smell, clearing away heat and toxins from the surface, used as principal drugs.

Jing Jie and *Dan Dou Chi*: helping the principal drugs to open the pores for expelling pathogens.

Jing Jie and *Dan Dou Chi* are acrid and warm drugs, but when putting into acrid and cool formula, they do not have the disadvantages of warm and dry, but on the other hand they will strengthen the functions of expelling pathogens.

Bo He: acrid in taste and cool in nature, dispersing wind and heat.

The above three ingredients are used as assistant drugs.

Niu Bang Zi, *Jie Geng* and *Gan Cao*: promoting lung's functions of dispersing and descending, eliminating phlegm and clearing the throat.

Zhu Ye and *Lu Gen*: clearing away heat, producing body fluid to stop thirst.

The above five are adjuvant drugs. Since *Gan Cao* has the effect of coordinating all the other drugs, it is also considered as adjuvant drug.

○ The combination of all the drugs has the effects of relieving the exterior syndrome with drugs acrid in taste and cool in nature, and clearing away heat and toxins.

● Notes:

(1) The prescription is used to treat influenza, acute tonsilitis, early stage of measles, and early stage of epidemic cerebral meningitis with exterior wind-heat syndrome. By adding proper dosage of heat-clearing and detoxication drugs, it can also be used to treat early carbuncle and furuncle which have manifestations of exterior wind-heat syndrome.

(2) It is not suitable for cases of headache, aversion to cold, no thirst, and non-rapid pulse.

Qing Jie Tang (Decoction for Clearing Away Heat and Relieving Exterior)

● Source: *Yi Xue Zhong Zhong Can Xi Lu* (Records of Traditional Chinese and Western Medicine in Combination)

● Ingredients: *Bo He* (Herba Menthae) 12g.

Chan Tui (Periostracum Cicadae) 9g.

Sheng Shi Gao (Gypsum Fibrosum) 18g.

Gan Cao (Radix Glycyrrhizae) 5g.

● Administration: The drugs are decocted in water, and *Bo He* should be put in later.

● Functions: Clear away heat from the body surface.

● Indications: Exterior wind-heat syndrome, marked by headache, soreness of joints, high fever, slight cold feeling at the back, no sweat, and floating and slippery pulse.

● Explanation:

Bo He: acrid in taste and cool in nature, dispersing wind-heat at body surface used as principal drug.

Chan Tui: sweet and cold, helping the principal drug to disperse wind and cold.

Shi Gao: acrid in taste and cold in nature, clearing the lung and stomach of heat.

The above two are used as assistant drugs.

Shi Gao, combining with *Bo He* and *Chan Tui* which reach the surface, make the internal heat going out through the surface.

Gan Cao: regulating all the drugs, considered as guiding drug.

○ The combination of the four drugs functions to relieving the exterior and clearing away heat.

● Notes:

(1) Common cold and influenza which attribute to exterior wind-heat syndrome with above mentioned symptoms could be treated with this prescription.

(2) It is not suitable for cases of exterior wind-cold syndrome with symptoms of general aching and pain of joints.

1.3 Exterior-Relieving Prescriptions by Strengthening Body Resistance

This type of prescription is advisable for cases of exterior syndrome with deficiency of body resistance. Since there is *Qi* deficiency, *Yang* deficiency and *Yin* deficiency, the prescriptions are divided into three categories: exterior-relieving prescriptions by reinforcing *Qi*, exterior-relieving prescriptions by building up *Yang* and exterior-relieving prescriptions by nourishing *Yin*.

Ren Shen Bai Du San (Antiphlogistic Powder with Ginseng)

● Source: *Tai Ping Hui Min He Ji Ju Fang* (Prescription of Peaceful Benevolent Dispensary)

● Ingredients: *Ren Shen* (Radix Ginseng) 6g.

　　　　　　or *Dang Shen* (Radix Codonopsis Pilosulae) 9g.

　　　　　　Zhi Qiao (Fructus Aurantii) 6g.

　　　　　　Jie Geng (Radix Platycodi) 6g.

　　　　　　Chai Hu (Radix Bupleuri) 6g.

　　　　　　Qian Hu (Radix Peucedani) 6g.

　　　　　　Qiang Huo (Rhizoma seu Radix Notopterygii) 6g.

　　　　　　Du Huo (Radix Angelicae Pubescentis) 6g.

　　　　　　Chuan Xiong (Rhizoma Ligustici Chuanxiong) 6g.

　　　　　　Fu Ling (Poria) 6g.

　　　　　　Gan Cao (Radix Glycyrrhizae) 6g.

　　　　　　Sheng Jiang (Rhizoma Zingiberis Recens) 2 pcs.

　　　　　　Bo He (Herba Menthae) 3g.

● Administration: Grind the above drugs into powder. Decoct 6g. of the powder together with *Bo He* and *Sheng Jiang*. The above drugs can also be decocted in water for oral administration.

● Functions: Reinforce *Qi*, relieve the exterior, disperse wind and eliminate dampness.

● Indications: Exterior wind, cold and dampness syndrome of *Qi* deficiency patients, marked by headache, stiff neck, chill and high fever, soreness and heaviness of the body and limbs, nasal obstruction with low voice speaking, fullness in the chest, cough with sputum, white greasy tongue coating, and floating and forceless pulse.

● Explanation:

Qiang Huo and *Du Huo*: acrid in taste and warm in nature, dispersing wind, cold and dampness of the whole body in order to treat pain, as the principal drugs.

Chuan Xiong: activating blood circulation and expelling wind.

Chai Hu: acrid in taste, dispersing pathogens from muscles, assisting the principal drugs to stop pain.

The above two are used as assistant drugs.

Qian Hu and *Zhi Qiao*: regulating *Qi* and resolving phlegm.

Jie Geng and *Fu Ling*: promoting lung's dispersing function and removing dampness by diuresis.

The above four drugs are used together to clear the lung, eliminate phlegm-dampness and stop cough.

Ren Shen and *Gan Cao*: reinforcing *Qi*, strengthening the body resistance so as to expel exterior pathogens, used as adjuvant drugs.

Sheng Jiang and *Bo He*: dispersing superficial wind-cold, as adjuvant and guiding drugs.

○ The prescription as a whole plays the functions of reinforcing Qi, relieving the exterior syndrome, dispersing wind and eliminating dampness.

● Notes:

(1) The formula is also suitable for early dysentery with *Qi* deficiency and cold in both exterior and interior.

(2) The dosage of *Ren Shen* in the prescription could be changed accordingly, but it should not be removed. Dysentery which does not have exterior syndrome and pathogenic factor already entered the interior should not be treated by this prescription.

Ma Huang Fu Zi Xi Xin Tang (Decoction of Herba Ephedrae, Radix Aconiti and Herba Asari)

● Source: *Shang Han Lun* (Treatise on Cold-Induced Diseases)
● Ingredients: *Ma Huang* (*Herba Ephedrae*) 6g.

       Fu Zi (Radix Aconiti Praeparata) 9g.

       Xi Xin (Herba Asari) 3g.

● Administration: The drugs are decocted in water and take the decoction when it is warm.

● Functions: strengthen *Yang* and relieve exterior syndrome.

● Indications: *Yang* deficiency patients with attack of exterior wind-cold, characterized by fever and chills, chills more serious than fever, lassitude, desire for lying on bed, wet and smooth tongue coating, and deep thready pulse.

● Explanation:

Ma Huang: acrid in taste and warm in nature, inducing sweating to expel exterior wind-cold.

Fu Zi: acrid in taste and hot in nature, warming the *Yang Qi* of the body.

Xi Xin: connecting the interior with the exterior, helping *Fu Zi* to disperse the interior cold from *Shaoyin* Meridian and assist *Ma Huang* to expel exterior cold.

○ The combination of the three drugs has the effects of inducing perspiration and dispersing cold but not damaging *Yang Qi*, warming the interior and meridians but not hinder the function of relieving the exterior, as a whole, strengthening *Yang Qi* and relieving exterior syndrome.

● Notes:

(1) The prescription is advisable for headache of deficient cold type with affection of external cold, marked by painful throat without redness and swelling.

(2) The prescription is suitable for exterior syndrome complicated with *Yang* deficiency, but *Yang* should not be too deficient. If it is serious *Yang* deficiency with symptoms of

watery diarrhea and feeble and indistinct pulse, the prescription will not be advisable.

Jia Jian Wei Rui Tang (Modified Decoction of
Rhizoma Polygonati Odorati)

- Source: *Tong Su Shang Han Lun* (Popular Treatise on Cold-Induced Diseases)
- Ingredients: *Wei Rui* (or *Yu Zhu*) (Rhizoma Polygonati Odorati) 9g.

  Dan Dou Chi (Semen Sojae Praeparatum) 9g.

  Sheng Cong Bai (Bulbus Allii Fistulosi) 6g.

  Jie Geng (Radix Platycodi) 5g.

  Bai Wei (Radix Cynanchi Atrati) 3g.

  Bo He (Herba Menthae) 5g.

  Zhi Gan Cao (Radix Glycyrrhizae Praeparata) 1.5g.

  Hong Zao (or *Da Zao*) (Fructus Ziziphi Jujubae) 2pcs.

- Administration: The drugs are decocted in water and take the decoction when it is warm.

- Functions: Nourish *Yin*, clear away heat, induce sweating to relieve exterior syndrome.

- Indications: *Yin* deficiency patients with attack of exterior pathogens, characterized by headache, fever, slight aversion to wind-cold, no sweat or little sweat, cough, restlessness, dry throat, thirst, red tongue and rapid pulse.

- Explanation:

Wei Rui: sweet in taste and neutral in nature, nourishing *Yin* and producing body fluid so as to strengthen the source of sweat and moistening the lung, used as principal drug.

Dou Chi, *Bo He*, *Cong Bai* and *Jie Geng*: relieving the exterior, expelling exopathogens, promoting the lung in dispersing and descending, stopping cough and clearing the throat, as assistant drugs.

Bai Wei: helping *Wei Rui* to nourish *Yin* and clear away heat, relieving restlessness and treating thirst.

Gan Cao and *Da Zao*: sweet in taste and moist in property, producing body fluid.

The above three are used as adjuvant drugs.

○ The combination of the drugs has the effects of relieving exterior and inducing perspiration but not damaging *Yin*, nourishing *Yin* but not reserving evil *Qi*, as a whole, nourishing *Yin* and relieving exterior syndrome.

- Notes:

(1) This prescription is used to treat exterior syndrome with *Yin* deficiency, winter-warm cough with dry throat and thick sputum, as well as pulmonary tuberculosis combined with exopathogen affection and manifestations of *Yin* deficiency.

(2) The prescription is contraindicated for common cold without *Yin* deficiency mani-

festations, or common cold complicated with phlegm-dampness.

Summary

10 main exterior-relieving prescriptions are discussed here. According to the functions, they are divided into three types: exterior-relieving prescriptions of acrid and warm type, exterior-relieving prescriptions of acrid and cool type, and exterior-relieving prescriptions by strengthening the body resistance.

(1) Exterior-relieving prescriptions of acrid and warm type

Ma Huang Tang, having a strong effect for inducing perspiration and promoting lung's dispersing and descending functions for relieving asthma, is indicated for exterior excess syndrome caused by external wind-cold, marked by absence of perspiration and slight asthma. *Gui Zhi Tang* has a weaker effect of inducing perspiration, but it is good at expelling pathogens from the muscles and skin and harmonize *Ying*, suitable for exterior deficient syndrome caused by external wind-cold, marked by sweating and aversion to wind. *Ge Gen Tang* is good at inducing perspiration and removing pathogens from muscles, indicated to treat exterior wind-cold syndrome manifested as stiffness of nape and back, no sweat and aversion to wind. *Su Qiang Da Biao Tang* is used to induce sweating, relieve exterior and eliminate dampness, therefore, it is advisable for exterior wind-cold syndrome with dampness.

(2) Exterior-relieving prescriptions of acrid and cool type

Yin Qiao San and *Sang Ju Yin* are the common prescriptions for exterior wind-heat syndrome. *Yin Qiao San* has strong effect of dispersing superficial pathogens and is good at clearing away heat and toxins, thus used to treat cases of more heat and less cold, characterized by cough, sore throat, and thirst etc. *Sang Ju Yin* has a weaker effect of relieving the exterior but is good at stopping cough by helping the lung in dispersing and descending, used to treat wind-heat affecting the lung, marked by cough with slight fever. *Qing Jie Tang*, composed of acrid and cool drugs, plays the functions of relieving the exterior and clearing the interior of heat, suitable for exterior wind-heat syndrome with symptoms of painful joints and high fever.

(3) Exterior-relieving prescriptions by strengthening the body resistance

Ren Shen Bai Du San reinforces *Qi* and relieves the exterior, suitable for cases of exterior wind, cold and dampness syndrome with *Qi* deficiency. *Ma Huang Fu Zi Xi Xin Tang* strengthens *Yang Qi* and relieves the exterior used to treat exterior wind-cold syndrome with *Yang* deficiency. *Jia Jian Wei Rui Tang*, nourishing *Yin* and relieving the exterior, is advisable for exterior wind-heat syndrome with *Yin* deficiency.

Review Questions

(1) Try to compare the ingredients, functions and indications of *Ma Huang Tang* and *Gui Zhi Tang*.

(2) Explain the similarities and differences between *Yin Qiao San* and *Sang Ju Yin*.

(3) What are the types of exterior-relieving prescriptions by strengthening the body resistance? What are their representative prescriptions?

(4) What is the significance of forming *Ren Shen Bai Du San*?

2 Heat-Clearing Prescriptions

Heat-Clearing prescriptions refer to those that are mainly composed of heat-clearing drugs for the treatment of interior heat syndromes, having the functions in heat-clearing, fire-reducing, toxin-removing and blood-cooling.

In view of the difference in interior heat syndrome among Qi system, blood system and the viscera, and the difference in excessive heat and deficient heat, the heat-clearing prescriptions are further classified as the prescriptions for clearing away heat from the Qi system, the prescriptions for removing heat from the $Ying$ system and for cooling the blood, the prescriptions for clearing away heat from both Qi and $Ying$ systems, the prescriptions for clearing away heat and toxins, the prescriptions for removing heat from the $Zang$-fu organs and the prescriptions for clearing away deficient heat.

The heat-clearing prescriptions can be applied to the interior heat syndrome that without exterior superficial pathogenic factor and without hard feces stagnated in the intestines. Pay attention to recognize the deficiency or excess of the heat syndrome, differ to the affected viscera. The suitable and proper dosage of heat-clearing prescriptions can be used according to the degree of heat condition and the constitutional condition so as to conform to pathogenesis and prevent the excessive injury of the spleen and stomach.

2.1 Prescriptions for Clearing Away Heat from the Qi System

This kind of prescriptions can be applied to the syndrome of heat in the Qi system and damage of the body fluid due to excessive heat, characterized by high fever, restlessness, thirst, perspiration, surging and big pulse, or disturbance to the diaphragm due to early invasion of the pathogenic heat in the Qi system, or restlessness caused by remained heat at the later stage of febrile diseases.

Bai Hu Tang (White Tiger Decoction)

- Source: *Shang Han Lun* (Treatise on Cold-Induced Diseases)
- Ingredients: *Shi Gao* (Gypsum Fibrosum) 30g.
    Zhi Mu (Rhizoma Anemarrhenae) 9g.
    Gan Cao (Radix Glycyrrhizae Paeparata) 3g.
    Jing Mi (Semen Oryzae Nonglutionosae) 9g.
- Administration: Decoct the drugs in water until the rice is well-done. Take the decoction warm orally after removal of the residue.
- Functions: Clear away heat, produce body fluid, and treat restlessness and thirst.
- Indications: Excessive heat in the *Yangming* meridian and Qi system, which manifested by high fever, perspiration, flushed face, polydipsia, surging and big pulse with force

or slippery rapid pulse.

● Explanation:

Shi Gao: A principal drug, which is pungent and sweet in flavour and extremely cold in nature, is used to clear away excessive heat in *Yangming* Meridian.

Zhi Mu: An assistant drug, which is bitter in taste and sweet, cold in nature, is to clear away heat, produce body fluid and treat restlessness.

Gan Cao and *Jing Mi*: Adjuvant and guiding drugs that can not only reinforce the stomach and protect the body fluid, but also prevent the stomach from being injured by cold drugs.

○ The four drugs together clear away heat, produce body fluid, treat restlessness and thirst.

● Notes:

(1) This prescription is applied for cases of high fever, perspiration, thirst, surging and big pulse. The recipe can be used to treat those diseases with the above symptoms, such as epidemic cerebrospinal meningitis, epidemic encephalitis B, influenza, pneumonia, summer-heat stroke and infantile measles. The recipe can also be modified to deal with cases with high fever caused by systematic lupus erythematosus, rheumatic fever or bacteria infection which can not be cured by antibiotics.

(2) It is not advisable for cases with aversion to cold, no thirst, no perspiration or perspiration but with pale complexion, big pulse but forceless when pressing heavily.

Appendix:

(1) *Bai Hu Jia Ren Shen Tang* (White Tiger Add Ginseng Decoction)

● Source: *Shang Han Lun* (Treatise on Cold-Induced Diseases)

The prescription is changed from *Bai Hu Tang* by adding *Ren Shen* (Radix Ginseng).

● Functions: Clear away heat, benefit *Qi* and produce body fluid.

● Indications: injury of both *Qi* and body fluid due to interior excessive heat or the cases with injury of both *Qi* and body fluid by summer-heat, marked by fever, thirst, perspiration, slight cold feeling at the back, surging, big and hollow pulse.

(2) *Bai Hu Jia Cang Zhu Tang* (White Tiger Add Atractylodes Rhizome Decoction)

● Source: *Lei Zheng Huo Ren Shu* (A Classified Book on Treating Exogenous Febrile Diseases)

That is to add *Cang Zhu* (Rhizoma Atractylodis) into *Bai Hu Tang* (White Tiger Decoction).

● Functions: Clear away heat and remove dampness.

● Indications: High fever, perspiration, suffocating sensation in the chest, red tongue with greasy coating.

Zhi Zi Chi Tang (Decoction of Capejasmine and Fermented Soybean)

● Source: *Shang Han Lun* (Treatise on Cold-Induced Diseases)

- Ingredients: *Zhi Zi* (Fructus Gardeniae) 10g.

  Dou Chi (Semen Sojae Fermentatum) 10g.
- Administration: All the drugs are to be decocted in water for oral administration.
- Functions: Clear away heat and treat restlessness.
- Indications: Fever, insomnia due to restlessness, slight yellow coating of the tongue, and rapid pulse.
- Explanation:

Zhi Zi: bitter in taste and cold in nature, clearing away heat, reducing fire to treat restlessness.

Dou Chi: pungent, sweet and slight bitter in taste, dispersing accumulated heat at the diaphram.

○ The two drugs are used together to clear away the accumulated heat in order to treat restlessness.

- Notes:

(1) This prescription is advisable for fever, no aversion to cold, no perspiration, restlessness and sleepless due to pathogenic heat in the *Qi* system.

(2) If there is shortness of breath, add *Gan Cao* 6g, vomiting, add *Sheng Jiang* 9g.

(3) *Zhi Zi* is bitter and cold, easy to damage middle-*jiao Yang Qi*. Do not take this formula if there is constitutional *Yang* deficiency, characterized by loose stool.

Liang Ge San (Powder for Removing Heat from the Diaphram)

- Source: *Tai Ping Hui Min He Ji Ju Fang* (Prescriptions of Peaceful Benevolent Dispensary)
- Ingredients: *Lian Qiao* (Fructus Forsythiae) 10g.

  Bo He (Herba Menthae) 10g.

  Zhi Zi (Fructus Gardeniae) 6g.

  Huang Qin (Radix Scutellariae) 10g.

  Jiu Da Huang (Wined Radix et Rhizoma Rhei) 6g.

  Mang Xiao (Natrii Sulphas) 6g.

  Gan Cao (Radix Glycyrrhizae) 3g.

  Zhu Ye (Herba Lophatheri) 3g.
- Administration: Decoct all the drugs in water except *Mang* Xiao which is to be added later. Put into a spoon of honey after removal of the residue. Take the decoction warm orally twice by two separate doses.
- Functions: Clear away heat from the diaphragm.
- Indications: Scorching of pathogenic heat in the chest and diaphragm, fever, irascibility, scorching heat sensation in the chest and diaphragm, dry lips and throat, thirst, or constipation, yellow coating of the tongue, slippery rapid pulse.
- Explanation:

Lian Qiao, *Bo He* and *Zhu Ye*: pungent in taste and cold in nature, clearing and dispersing the heat in the chest and diaphragm.

Zhi Zi and *Huang Qin*: bitter in taste and cold in nature, expelling heat and removing toxins.

Jiu Da Huang and *Mang Xiao*: smoothing bowels and conducting heat to descend.

Gan Cao, *Bai Mi* (honey): relieving acute case and moistening dryness.

○ The combination of all these drugs can clear away heat and conduct it to descend.

● Notes:

(1) The recipe is advisable for fever, irascibility and constipation caused by cholecystitis, cholelithiasis, epidemic encephalitis B and epidemic cerebrospinal meningitis, or toothache, gingival hemorrhage, aphtha, sore throat, tonsilitis and swelling of cervical lymphatic glands.

(2) It is contraindicated in cases without excessive heat.

2.2 Prescriptions for Removing Heat from the *Ying* and Blood Systems

This group of prescriptions has effects of clearing away heat, cooling the blood, and removing blood stasis and toxic materials. They are indicated for syndromes with pathogenic heat in both *Ying* and Blood systems.

Qing Ying Tang (Decoction for Clearing Away Heat in the *Ying* System)

● Source: *Wen Bing Tiao Bian* (Treatise on Differentiation and Treatment of Epidemic Febrile Diseases)

● Ingredients: *Xi Jiao* (Cornu Rhinocerotis; replaced by *Shui Niu Jiao*, Gornu Bubali) 2g.
Sheng Di (Radix Rehmanniae) 15g.
Yuan Shen (Radix Scrophulariae) 9g.
Zhu Ye (Herba Lophatheri) 3g.
Mai Dong (Radix Ophiopogonis) 9g.
Dan Shen (Radix Salviae Miltiorrhizae) 6g.
Huang Lian (Rhizoma Coptidis) 5g.
Yin Hua (Flos Lonicerae) 9g.
Lian Qiao (Fructus Forsythiae) 6g.

● Administration: All the drugs are decocted in water for oral administration. Take orally a day. 20 grams of *Shui Niu Jiao* (Cornu Bubali) can be used to replace *Xi Jiao*. *Shui Niu Jiao* should be decocted prior to other drugs.

● Functions: Clear away heat from the *Ying* system, nourish *Yin* and activate blood.

● Indications: Pathogenic heat invades the *Ying* system, manifested as fever which is severe in the night, irascibility, delirum, dry mouth without desire to drink, or with dull exanthema maculosum, red or deep-red tongue, thready rapid pulse.

● Explanation:

Shui Niu Jiao: salty in flavour and cold in nature.

Sheng Di: sweet in flavour and cold in nature.

They are principal drugs to clear away heat, cool the blood and remove toxin.

Yuan Shen: salty in flavour and cold in nature.

Mai Dong: sweet in flavour and cold in nature.

Both are assistant drugs to nourish *Yin* and clear away heat.

Yin Hua, *Lian Qiao*, *Huang Lian* and *Zhu Ye*: adjuvant drugs, which can clear away heat and remove toxin in order to relieve the pathogenic heat out of the *Qi* system.

Dan Shen: a guiding drug, which can clear away heat, cool blood, activate blood and remove stasis in order to prevent the mingling of blood stasis with heat, and can also guide the other drugs to the heart meridian to clear away heat.

○ The coordination of all the drugs results in clearing away heat from the *Ying* system, removing toxin and nourishing *Yin*.

● Notes:

(1) The recipe can be used for cases with heat in the *Ying* system occurring in epidemic encephalitis B, epidemic cerebrospinal meningitis, summer-heat stroke and septicemia or other febrile diseases.

(2) The recipe takes the red and deep-red tongue as its basis. It is contraindicated for deep-red tongue with white slippery or white greasy coating.

(3) *Xi Jiao* can be replaced by *Shui Niu Jiao* (Cornu Bubali) 30-60g. Decoct *Shui Niu Jiao* first.

Xi Jiao Di Huang Tang (Decoction of Rhinoceros Horn and Rehmannia)

● Source: *Bei Ji Qian Jin Yao Fang* (Prescriptions Worth a Thousand Gold for Emergencies)

● Ingredients: *Xi Jiao* (Cornu Rhinocerotis, replacedby *Shui Niu Jiao*, Corna Bubali) 3g.

                Sheng Di (Radix Rehmanniae) 30g.

                Shao Yao (Radix Paeoniae) 12g.

                Dan Pi (Cortex Moutan Radicis) 9g.

● Administration: All the drugs will be decocted in water for oral administration.

● Functions: Clear away heat, cool the blood, Remove toxins and devolve blood stasis.

● Indications: Syndromes of invasion of the blood system by pathogenic heat.

(1) Bleeding caused by excessive heat, manifested as hematemesis, epistaxis, hemafecia, hematuria and dark purple colour of rashes.

(2) Syndrome of blood retention marked by amnesia, madness, a parched throat with thirst for water, with water in the mouth but no desire to swallow it, restless and pain in the chest and dark smooth stools.

(3) Disturbance of the heart *Ying* by pathogenic heat, which is marked by unconscious-

ness, delirium, or madness, deep-red tongue with prickle-like coating.

● Explanation:

Shui niu Jiao: a principal drug, clearing away heart fire, cooling the blood and removing toxins.

Sheng Di: an assistant drug, clearing away heat and cooling the blood. It not only helps the principal drug to clear away heat and toxin from blood system for the purpose of stopping bleeding, but also tonifies blood and nourishes *Yin*.

Shao Yao and *Dan Pi*: adjuvant and guiding drugs, playing the effect of cooling the blood and removing blood stasis.

○ The combination of these four drugs can cool blood, stop bleeding, activate blood circulation and remove stasis.

● Notes:

(1) The prescription is advisable for hemorrhage syndromes of blood heat type, such as hepatic coma, uremia, various kind of septicemia, carbuncle complicated by septicemia and blood diseases. It can also be used to treat brochiectasis and lobar pneumonia characterized by haemoptysis due to pathogenic heat.

(2) *Xi Jiao* can be replaced by Shui Niu Jiao (Cornu Bubali) 30-60g. Decoct *Shui Niu Jiao* first.

2.3 Prescriptions for Clearing Away Heat from Both *Qi* and Blood Systems

This type of prescriptions is indicated for the syndromes with the pathogenic heat in *Qi*, *Ying* and blood systems.

Jia Jian Yu Nu Jian (Modified Gypsum Decoction)

● Source: *Wen Bing Tiao Bian* (Treatise on Differentiation and Treatment of Epidemic Febrile Diseases)

● Ingredients: *Shi Gao* (Gypsum Fibrosum) 90g.

　　　　　　Zhi Mu (Rhizoma Anemarrhenae) 12g.

　　　　　　Yuan Shen (Radix Scrophulariae) 12g.

　　　　　　Sheng Di (Radix Rehmanniae) 18g.

　　　　　　Mai Dong (Radix Ophiopogonis) 18g.

● Administration: All the drugs are decocted in water for oral administration.

● Functions: Clear away heat from *Qi* system, cool the *Ying* system, nourish *Yin* to produce body fluid.

● Indications: Both *Qi* and *Ying* systems are affected, marked by high fever, thirst, headache, irascibility, macular-eruption on the skin, deep-red tongue with yellow coating, rapid pulse.

● Explanation:

Shi Gao and *Zhi Mu*: Similar to the effect in *Bai Hu Tang* (White tiger Decoction), clearing away heat from *Qi* system, reducing heat and producing body fluid.

Sheng Di, *Mai Dong* and *Yuan Shen*: These drugs form *Zeng Ye Tang* (Fluid-Increasing Decoction), which can nourish *Yin* and clear away heat from *Ying* system.

○ The combination of all the above drugs can clear away heat from *Qi* system, cool *Ying* system, nourish *Yin* and produce body fluid.

● Notes:

(1) The recipe is advisable for febrile diseases of strong evil heat caused by exogenous pathogenic factors, and mild cases of the injury on both *Qi* and *Ying* systems, or it can be modified to treat acute stomatitis and glossitis which have stomatocace.

(2) This recipe is cold and moist, so it is not advisable for cases with loose stool.

Qin Wen Bai Du Yin (Antipyretic and Antitoxic Decoction)

● Source: *Yi Zhen Yi De* (A View of Epidemic Febrile Diseases with Rashes)

● Ingredients: *Sheng Shi Gao* (Gypsum Fibrosum) 60g.

     Sheng Di (Radix Rehmanniae) 30g.

     Xi Jiao (Cornu Rhinocerotis) 10g.

     or *Shui Niu Jiao* (Cornu Bubali) 30g.

     Zhi Zi (Fructus Gardeniae) 10g.

     Huang Qin (Radix Scutellariae) 10g.

     Zhi Mu (Rhizoma Anemarrhenae) 10g.

     Chi Shao (Radix Paeoniae Rubra) 10g.

     Xuan Shen (Radix Scrophulariae) 10g.

     Lian Qiao (Fructus Forsythiae) 10g.

     Dan Pi (Cortex Moutan Radicis) 10g.

     Huang Lian (Rhizoma Coptidis) 6g.

     Jie Geng (Radix Platycodi) 6g.

     Zhu Ye (Herba Lophatheri) 6g.

     Gan Cao (Radix Glycyrrhizae) 3g.

● Administration: *Shui Niu Jiao* and *Shi Gao* should be decocted first before they are mixed and decocted with other drugs.

● Functions: Clear away heat, remove toxins, cool the blood and reduce fire.

● Indications: Epidemic warm toxins filling up the body, affecting both the *Qi* and blood systems. The symptoms are high fever, unconsciousness, splitting-like headache, severe thirst with great desire to drink, dryness of the mouth, sore throat, or hematemesis, epistaxis, or macular-eruption on the skin, or spasm of the four limbs, or syncope, deep rapid pulse, deep-red tongue, and dry lips.

● Explanation:

This prescription is the combination of *Bai Hu Tang* (White Tiger Decoction), *Huang*

Lian Jie Du Tang (Antidotal Decoction of Coptis) and *Xi Jiao Di Huang Tang* (Decoction of Rhinoceros Horn and Rehmannia), which plays corresponding effects.

Shi Gao, *Zhi Mu* and *Gan Cao*: large dosages, clearing away heat and protecting body fluid, taking the effect of *Bai Hu Tang*.

Huang Qin, *Huang Lian* and *Zhi Zi*: reducing the excessive heat from *Sanjiao*, playing the effect of *Huang Lian Jie Du Tang*.

Shui Niu Jiao, *Sheng Di*, *Shao Yao* and *Dan Pi*: forming *Xi Jiao Di Huang Tang*, cooling the blood, stopping bleeding, and removing toxins and blood stasis.

Xuan Shen, *Lian Qiao*, *Jie Geng* and *Gan Cao*: moistening the throat and relieving pain.

Zhu Ye: clearing away heat from the heart, promoting diuresis and conducting heat to descend.

○ The prescription as a whole plays the effect of clearing away heat from both *Qi* and blood systems, reducing fire, cooling blood and removing toxin.

● Notes:

(1) The recipe deals with epidemic encephalitis B, epidemic cerebrospinal meningitis, septicemia and hemorrhagic fever due to invasion of pathogenic heat into both *Qi* and blood systems.

(2) The recipe is extremely cold in nature, therefore it is not advisable for those without excessive heat and toxins.

(3) Dosages here are common dosages used in clinic.

2.4 Prescriptions for Clearing Away Heat and Toxins

This type of prescriptions has the effect of clearing away heat, reducing fire and rmoving toxins, and is indicated for the treatment of domination of toxic fire in the interior and the attack of epidemic pathogens of wind-heat type.

Huang Lian Jie Du Tang (Antidotal Decoction of Coptis)

● Source: *Wai Tai Mi Yao* (The medical Secrets of an Official), but the prescription was made by Dr. *Cui*.

● Ingredients: *Huang Lian* (Rhizoma Coptidis) 9g.

                Zhi Zi (Fructus Gardeniae) 9g.

                Huang Qin (Radix Scutellariae) 6g.

                Huang Bai (Cortex Phellodendri) 6g.

● Administration: All the drugs should be decocted in water for oral administration. Twice a day.

● Functions: Reduce fire and remove toxins.

● Indications: all the syndromes of excessive heat and fire, manifested by high fever, irascibility, dryness of the mouth and throat, or mental disorder, or hematemesis and epistaxis in the course of febrile diseases, skin eruptions, dysentery with fever, jaundice due to damp-heat, sore and carbuncle, red tongue with yellow coating, and rapid pulse.

● Explanation:

All the drugs are bitter in flavour and cold in nature.

Huang Lian: a principal drug, reducing the heart fire in the upper *Jiao* and at the same time reducing the stomach fire in the middle *Jiao*.

Huang Qin: an assistant drug, reducing the lung fire in the upper *Jiao*.

Zhi Zi: a guiding drug, which can reduce the fire in all the *Sanjiao* and conduct the heat to descend.

○ The combination of all the drugs plays the effect of clearing away heat, reducing fire and removing toxins.

● Notes:

(1) This prescription is advisable for septicemia, pyemia, dysentery and pneumonia caused by severe fire and heat-toxin. For treating pustule and furunculosis, it can be decocted in water for oral administration or ground into powder for external use.

(2) The ingredients in the prescription are of bitter and cold properties, therefore it is suitable for cases with overabundance of fire and heat-toxin but no impairment of the body fluid. It may damage the spleen and stomach if it is taken orally for a long time. It is not advisable for those with injury of the body fluid.

Pu Ji Xiao Du Yin (Universal Relief Decoction for Disinfection)

● Source: *Dong Yuan Shi Xiao Fang* (*Dong Yuan's* Effective Prescriptions)
● Ingredients: *Huang Qin* (Radix Scutellariae) 15g.
　　　　　　Huang Lian (Rhizoma Coptidis) 15g.
　　　　　　Niu Bang Zi (Fructus Arctii) 10g.
　　　　　　Lian Qiao (Fructus Forsythiae) 10g.
　　　　　　Bo He (Herba Menthae) 5g.
　　　　　　Xuan Shen (Radix Scrophulariae) 10g.
　　　　　　Ma Bo (Lasiosphaera Seu Calvatia) 6g.
　　　　　　Ban Lan Gen (Radix Isatidis) 10g.
　　　　　　Jie Geng (Radix Platycodi) 6g.
　　　　　　Gan Cao (Radix Glycyrrhizae) 6g.
　　　　　　Chen Pi (Pericarpium Citri Reticulatae) 6g.
　　　　　　Chai Hu (Radix Bupleuri) 6g.
　　　　　　Sheng Ma (Rhizoma Cimicifugae) 3g.
　　　　　　Jiang Can (Bombyx Batryticatus) 6g.
● Administration: All the drugs are to be decocted in water. *Bo He* is put in later. Take the decoction orally twice a day.

● Functions: Clear away heat and remove toxins, dispel wind and other exopathogens.

● Indications: Epidemic febrile diseases marked by aversion to cold, fever, flushed swollen face, heavy eyes, sore throat, restlessness, red tongue with yellow coating, and rapid forceful pulse.

● Explanation:

Huang Qin and *Huang Lian*: principal drugs, bitter in taste and cold in nature, playing the effect of dispelling heat-toxin from the heart and lung in the upper *Jiao*.

Niu Bang Zi, *Bo He*, *Lian Qiao* and *Jiang Can*: assistant drugs, acrid in taste and cold in nature, dispelling wind-heat in the face and head of the upper *Jiao*.

Xuan Shen, *Ma Bo*, *Ban Lan Gen*, *Jie Geng* and *Gan Cao*: adjuvant drugs, clearing away heat-toxin from the throat.

Chen Pi: also adjuvant drug, regulating *Qi* and promoting digestion to dispel accumulation of pathogens.

Sheng Ma and *Chai Hu*: guiding drugs, dispelling accumulated heat and helping the other drugs to come to the face and head.

○ The prescription as a whole performs the effects of clearing away heat and toxic materials, expelling wind and dissipating swelling.

● Notes:

(1) The modified recipe can be used for treatment of diseases with the above symptoms as seen in facial erysipelas, epidemic parotitis, acute tonsilitis, carbuncle and other infectious swelling in the face.

(2) As the drugs are bitter and acrid in taste and cold in nature, the patients should stop taking the recipe when the disease is controlled to prevent the injury of *Yin*.

(3) Plus *Da Huang* if there is constipation.

Sheng Jiang San (Powder of Adjusting the Ascending and Descending)

● Source: *Han Wen Tiao Bian* (Treatise on Differentiation and Treatment of Cold and Febrile Diseases)

● Ingredients: *Jiang Can* (Bombyx Batryticatus) 6g.

     Chan Tui (Periostracum Cicadae) 3g.

     Jiang Huang (Rhizoma Curcumae Longae) 6g.

     Da Huang (Radix et Rhizoma Rhei) 12g.

● Administration: In the original prescription, the drugs are ground into fine powder and mixed with yellow wine and honey to be taken coldly. Two to four times a day. Nowadays it can be decocted in water for oral administration.

● Functions: Disperse stagnation, reduce heat and remove toxins.

● Indications: febrile disease with severe heat in the interior, at the exterior and *Sanjiao*. The symptoms are aversion to cold, high fever, or headache, restlessness, thirst with desire to drink, or sore throat, or general swelling, or distention and fullness in the chest and diaphragm region, or vomiting and diarrhea.

● Explanation:

Da Huang: bitter in taste and cold in nature, entering the *Qi* system and blood, and descending and reducing the interior heat through *Yangming* food passage.

Jiang Can: pungent and bitter in taste, clearing away heat, removing toxins and dispelling masses.

Chan Tui: sweet in taste and cold in nature, expelling wind and cooling the liver; together with *Jiang Can* and owing to its light quality, it ascending to penetrate the pathogens outside.

The above drugs are all principal for eliminating pathogens.

Jiang Huang: as assistant and adjuvant drug, acrid in taste and warm in nature, entering the *Qi* and blood to disperse and remove the stagnation and accumulations.

○ The combination of the four drugs plays the effects of dispersing stagnation, resolving accumulation, reducing heat and removing toxins.

● Notes:

The recipe is characterized by ascending and descending in combination and using cold and cool drugs to clear away heat. It is suitable for the cases of febrile disease with accumulated heat. The modified recipe can be used for the treatment of epidemic encephalitis B, acute tonsillitis, parotitis, pneumonia, pharyngitis, biliary infections, acute epidemic hepatitis and other febrile diseases.

2.5 Prescriptions for Removing Heat from the *Zang-fu* Organs

This kind of prescriptions is indicated for the treatment of fire-heat syndromes caused by overabundance of pathogenic heat in different *Zang-fu* organs.

Dao Chi San (Powder for Treating Dark Urine)

● Source: *Xiao Er Yao Zheng Zhi Jue* (Key to Therapeutics of Children's Diseases)
● Ingredients: *Sheng Di* (Radix Rehmanniae) 15g.

        Mu Tong (Laulis Akebiae) 6g.

        Zhu Ye (Herba Lophatheri) 9g.

        Gan Cao Shao (Tip of Radix Glycyrrhizae) 3g.

● Administration: All the drugs are to be decocted in water for oral administration.
● Functions: Clear away heat from the heart and induce diuresis.
● Indications: Domination of heat in the heart meridian marked by restlessness, thirst with desire to drink cold water, flushed face, and oral ulceration; or transfer of heart heat to the small intestine, manifested as scanty and yellow urine and pain in micturation, red tongue and rapid pulse.
● Explanation:

Sheng Di: a principal drug, sweet in taste and cold in nature, clearing away heat, cooling the blood and nourishing *Yin*.

Mu Tong: bitter in taste and cold in nature.

Zhu Ye: sweet and light in taste and cold in nature.

These two, as assistant drugs in combination, have the effect of clearing away heart fire, stopping restlessness, inducing diuresis for treating stranguria and conducting heat to descend.

Gan Cao: a guiding drug, clearing away heat and toxic materials as well as for coordinating the actions of various ingredients in the recipe.

○ The prescription as a whole functions to clear away heart heat, nourish *Yin* and conduct heat downward through urination.

● Notes:

(1) The recipe can be modified to deal with stomatitis, pyelonephritis, cystitis and infantile mycotic stomatitis which pertain to excessive heat in the heart meridian.

(2) Oral ulceration, scanty and yellow urine, painful micturation, red tongue and rapid pulse are the essential points for diagnosis. The prescription is contraindicated for the cases with difficult urination caused by accumulation of damp-heat in the urinary bladder.

(3) The original prescription uses equal parts of *Sheng Di*, *Mu Tong* and *Sheng Gan Cao Shao*. Grind them into powder. Take 10g each time to be decocted with 1.5g of *Zhu Ye*. Take the decoction warm after meal.

Long Dan Xie Gan Tang (Decoction of Gentian for Reducing Liver Fire)

● Source: *Yi Fang Ji Jie* (Collection of Prescriptions with Notes)
● Ingredients: *Long Dan Cao* (Radix Gentianae) 6g.
　　　　　　Chai Hu (Radix Bupleuri) 6g.
　　　　　　Ze Xie (Rhizoma Alismatis) 12g.
　　　　　　Che Qian Zi (Semen Plantaginis) 9g.
　　　　　　Mu Tong (Caulis Akebiae) 9g.
　　　　　　Huang Qin (Radix Scutellariae) 9g.
　　　　　　Zhi Zi (Fructus Gardeniae) 9g.
　　　　　　Dang Gui (Radix Angelicae Sinensis) 3g.
　　　　　　Sheng Di (Radix Rehmanniae) 9g.
　　　　　　Sheng Gan Cao (Radix Glycyrrhizae) 6g.

● Administration: All the drugs should be decocted in water for oral administration. Twice a day.

● Functions: Reduce excessive fire from the liver and gallbladder and remove damp-heat from the lower *Jiao*.

● Indications: Upward attack of excessive fire in the liver and gallbladder, manifested as hypochondriac pain, bitter taste in the mouth, redness of the eyes, deafness, swelling of the ear, and headache; or downward flow of damp-heat from the liver meridian marked by stranguria with turbid urine, pruritus and swelling of vulva, and damp-heat leukorrhagia.

● Explanation:

Long Dan Cao: a principal drug, bitter in taste and cold in nature, reducing excessive fire in the liver and gallbladder and clearing away damp-heat in the liver meridian.

Huang Qin and *Zhi Zi*: the assistant drugs, strengthening the effect of the principal drug to clear away heat and reduce fire.

Ze Xie, *Mu Tong* and *Che Qian Zi*: helping the principal drug to clear away damp-heat from the liver and gallbladder.

Dang Gui and *Sheng Di*: nourishing the blood and *Yin* so as to benefit the liver.

The above two groups of drugs are used as adjuvant drugs which contains reinforcing within reducing in order not to damage the vital *Qi*.

Chai Hu: regulating liver *Qi* and conducting other drugs into the liver and gallbladder.

Gan Cao: having the effect of coordinating the effect of various ingredients in the recipe.

Both *Chai Hu* and *Gan Cao* are played as guiding drugs.

○ The combination of these drugs can reduce excessive fire and clear away damp-heat without damaging blood because there is reinforcing within reducing.

● Notes:

(1) Nowdays, the prescription is used to treat diseases marked by excessive fire in the liver meridian, such as acute conjunctivitis, acute otitis media, acute hepatitis and acute cholecystitis; or to deal with cases with downward flow of damp-heat in the liver meridian as seen in acute pyelonephritis, cystitis, urethritis, acute pelvic inflamation, vulvitis and orchitis.

(2) The drugs in the recipe are bitter in flavour and cold in nature. Long-term administration of it should be avoided to prevent the injury of the spleen and stomach.

Appendix:

Xie Qing Wan (Pills for Reducing the Liver Fire)

● Source: *Xiao Er Yao Zheng Zhi Jue* (Key to Therapeutics of Children's Diseases).

● Ingredients: *Long Dan Cao* (Radix Gentianae), *Zhi Zi* (Fructus Gardeniae), *Da Huang* (Rhizoma Rhei), *Chuan Xiong* (Rhizoma Ligustici Chuanxiong), *Dang Gui* (Radix Angelicae Sinensis), *Qiang Huo* (Rhizoma seu Radix Notopterygii), *Fang Feng* (Radix Ledebouriellae)

● Administration: All of which are made into honeyed pill.

It has the effect of clearing the liver and reducing fire. It is indicated for cases with wind-heat in the liver and gallbladder, manifested as restlessness during the night, easy to be feared and frightened, redness and swelling pain of the eyes, acute convulsions and spasm.

Ma Xing Shi Gan Tang (Decoction of Ephedrae, Apricot Kernel, Gypsum and Licorice)

● Source: *Shang Han Lun* (Treatise on Cold-Induced Diseases)

- Ingredients: *Ma Huang* (Herba Ephedrae) 6g.

    Xing Ren (Semen Armeniacae Amarum) 9g.

    Sheng Shi Gao (Gypsum Fibrosum) 18g.

    Zhi Gan Cao (Radix Gycyrrhizae Praeparata) 6g.

- Administration: *Sheng Shi Gao* should be decocted first and then add other drugs. Take the decoction orally, twice a day.

- Functions: Clear and disperse the lung heat.

- Indications: Cough and asthma due to lung-heat marked by fever, asthma, cough, rough respiration, or flaring of nares, thirst, sweating or no sweating, thin white or yellow coating of the tongue, slippery rapid pulse.

- Explanation:

Ma Huang: acrid in taste and warm in nature, promoting lung's dispersing and descending functions to relieve asthma.

Shi Gao: pungent in taste and cold in nature, clearing away the lung heat.

Xing Ren: making the *Qi* going downward for relieving asthma.

Sheng Gan Cao: coordinating the effect of various ingredients in the recipe, producing body fluid and treating thirst in combination with *Shi Gao*.

○ The combination of these four drugs plays the effect of dispersing, clearing the lung of heat, and relieving asthma because of its pungent flavor and cold nature.

- Notes:

(1) The formula are used to deal with diseases due to excessive lung-heat, such as upper respiratory infection, pneumonia, acute bronchitis, the acute attack of chronic bronchitis, lobar pneumonia, bronchopneumonia and pneumonia complicated with infantile measles.

(2) It is not advisable for the cases with aversion to cold, fever, thirstless, cough, asthma and profuse sputum.

(3) About the dosage of *Shi Gao*. *Shi Gao* is two times as much as *Ma Huang* in case of asthma without sweating, and *Shi Gao is* five times as much as *Ma Huang* in case of asthma with sweating.

Xie Bai San (Lung-Heat Expelling Powder)

- Source: *Xiao Er Yao Zheng Zhi Jue* (Key to Therapeutics of Children's Diseases)
- Ingredients: *Sang Bai Pi* (Cortex Mori Radicis) 9g.

    Di Gu Pi (Cortex Lycii Radicis) 9g.

    Gan Cao (Radix Glycyrrhizae) 3g.

    Jing Mi (Fructus Oryzae Sativae) 6g.

- Administration: All the ingredients should be decocted in water for oral administration.

- Functions: Reduce the lung-heat to relieve cough and asthma.

- Indications: Cough or asthma due to lung-heat, fever aggravated in the afternoon, red tongue with yellow coating, thready rapid pulse.

● Explanation:

Sang Bai Pi: the principal drug, being sweet in taste and cold in nature, reducing the lung heat so as to relieve cough and asthma.

Di Gu Pi: the assistant drug, mild sweet in taste and cold in nature, reducing latent fire in the lung as well as deficient heat.

Gan Cao and *Jing Mi*: the adjuvant and guiding drugs, nourishing the stomach and harmonizing the middle Jiao to strengthen the lung *Qi*.

○ The combination of these four drugs plays the effects of clearing the lung of heat and relieving cough and asthma.

● Notes:

(1) The recipe is advisable for treating bronchitis, measles, pneumonia, pulmonary tuberculosis and others which manifest as the syndrome of the lung heat.

(2) The recipe is not advisable for the cases with cough caused by exogenous wind cold or cough of deficient cold type.

(3) The original prescription uses *Di Gu Pi*, *Sang Bai Pi* each 30g, *Zhi Gan Cao* 3g. Make into powder and add *Jing Mi*, decoct them in water.

Qing Wei San (Powder for Clearing Stomach Heat)

● Source: *Pi Wei Lun* (Treatise on the Spleen and Stomach)
● Ingredients: *Sheng Di* (Radix Rehmanniae) 12g.

        Dang Gui (Radix Angelicae Sinensis) 6g.

        Huang Lian (Rhizoma Coptidis) 3g.

        Dan Pi (Cortex Moutan Radicis) 9g.

        Sheng Ma (Rhizoma Cimicifugae) 3g.

● Administration: All the ingredients should be decocted in water for oral administration.

● Functions: Clear stomach heat and cool blood.

● Indications: Upward attacking of stomach fire, marked by toothache radiating to the head, feverish cheeks, or bleeding of gum, or ulceration in the gum, or swelling and pain of the lips, tongue and cheeks, or hot and foul breath, dryness of mouth and tongue, red tongue with yellow coating, rapid pulse.

● Explanation:

Huang Lian: the principal drug, being bitter in taste and cold in nature, clearing to reduce stomach fire.

Sheng Di and *Dan Pi*: the assistant drugs, clearing away heat, cooling the blood and nourishing *Yin*.

Dang Gui: the adjuvant drug, can nourishing and activating blood, subduing swelling and relieving pain.

Sheng Ma: the guiding drug, dispelling fire and removing toxins; In combination with *Huang Lian*, balancing the ascending and descending functions so as to treat the upward flaring of fire and dispel the interior accumulated heat.

Both function as a medicinal guide of *Yangming* meridian by guiding other drugs directly to the affected regions.

○ The coordination of all the drugs plays the effect of clearing away the stomach fire and cooling the blood.

● Notes:

(1) The recipe is indicated for trigeminal neuralgia, stomatitis and periodontitis which are caused by upward attacking of stomach fire.

(2) It is not advisable for toothache of wind-cold type or toothache and gingival atrophy with oozing of bloody fluid and pus caused by upward flaring up of fire due to kidney deficiency.

Shao Yao Tang (Peony Decoction)

● Source: *Bao Ming Ji* (Medical Collection for Saving Life)
● Ingredients: *Shao Yao* (Radix Paeoniae) 20g.

    Dang Gui (Radix Angelicae Sinensis) 9g.

    Huang Qin (Radix Scutellariae) 9g.

    Huang Lian (Rhizoma Coptidis) 6g.

    Da Huang (Radix et Rhizoma Rhei) 9g.

    Mu Xiang (Radix Aucklandiae) 6g.

    Bin Lang (Semen Arecae) 6g.

    Guan Gui (Cortex Cinnamomi) 3g.

    Gan Cao (Radix Glycyrrhizae) 6g.

● Administration: All the drugs should be decocted in water for oral administration. Twice a day.

● Functions: Clear stomach heat and cool the blood.

● Indications: Damp-heat in the gastrointestines marked by diarrhea, abdominal pain, pus and blood in the stool, tenesmus, burning sensation in the anus, yellow greasy coating of the tongue.

● Explanation:

Shao Yao: bitter and sour in taste, cold in nature.

Dang Gui: sweet and acrid in taste.

Both are principal drugs to play the effect of regulating nutrient blood and relieving abdominal pain in order to treat diarrhea, pus and blood in the stool.

Da Huang, *Huang Qin* and *Huang Lian*: assistant drugs, being bitter in taste and cold in nature, clearing away heat, drying dampness, removing toxins and stagnation to treat diarrhea.

Mu Xiang and *Bin Lang*: adjuvant drugs, promoting the circulation of *Qi* and removing stagnation.

Gan Cao: regulating middle *Jiao* and relieving pain; together with *Rou Gui* (*Guan Gui*) which is pungent in flavour and hot in nature to play the effect of guiding drugs in order to prevent the injury of *Yin* by *Da Huang*, *Huang Qin* and *Huang Lian*.

○ The combination of these drugs plays the functions of circulating blood and regulating *Qi*. Both cold and hot drugs are used together. In combination of smoothing method, the symptoms can be relieved finally.

● Notes:

(1) This recipe is a special prescription for clearing away damp-heat in the intestines and stomach, regulating *Qi* and blood and treating diarrhea. It is fit for the cases with unsmooth stool and tenesmus due to damp-heat, such as bacillary dysentery, amebic dysentery, allergic colitis and acute enteritis.

(2) It is not advisable for cases with external syndromes at the onset of dysentery.

Bai Tou Weng Tang (Pulsatilla Decoction)

● Source: *Shang Han Lun* (Treatise on Cold-Induced Diseases)
● Ingredients: *Bai Tou Weng* (Radix Pulsatillae) 15g.
　　　　　　　Huang Bai (Cortex Phellodendri) 12g.
　　　　　　　Huang Lian (Rhizoma Coptidis) 5g.
　　　　　　　Qin Pi (Cortex Fraxini) 12g.

● Administration: All the drugs should be decocted in water for oral administration, and take the decoction while it is warm.

● Functions: Clear away heat and toxins, cool the blood to treat dysentery.

● Indications: Dysentery due to heat marked by abdominal pain, tenesmus, burning sensation in the anus, stool with more blood and less mucus, thirst with desire to drink, wiry rapid pulse.

● Explanation:

Bai Tou Weng: the principal drug, being bitter in taste and cold in nature, clearing away heat and toxins and cooling the blood to treat dysentery.

Huang Lian and *Huang Bai*: Bitter in taste and cold in nature, clearing away heat, helping the principal drug to clear away heat and toxins in order to treat dysentery.

Qin Pi: btter and astringent in taste and cold in nature, playing astringenting function to treat dysentery.

Qin Pi, together with *Huang Lian* and *Huang Bai*, plays the effect of assistant and adjuvant drugs.

○ The combination of all the drugs is used to clear away heat and toxins, treat dysentery and relieve tenesmus.

● Notes:

(1) The recipe is a special prescription for treating dysentery due to noxious heat. It is fit for dysentery due to excessive noxious heat, characterized by mucus and blood in stool, such as acute and chronic dysentery, amebic dysentery and bacillary dysentery.

(2) For heat type dysentery with blood deficiency or *Yin* deficiency, this recipe should be added with *E Jiao* (Colla Corii Asini) and *Gan Cao* (Radix Glycyrrhizae) to form *Bai Tou Weng Gan Cao E Jiao Tang* (Pulsatilla, Glycyrrhizae and Colla Corii Asini Decoction).

Zuo Jin Wan (Zuo Jin Bolus)

- Source: *Dan Xi Xin Fa* (Danxi's Experiential Therapy)
- Ingredients: *Huang Lian* (Rhizoma Coptidis) 180g.

  Wu Zhu Yu (Fructus Evodiae) 30g.
- Administration: The boluses are made out of the powdered drug with water. Nowadays the decoction can be done with the decreased dosage according to the scale of the original prescription.
- Functions: Reduce liver fire, lower the rising of the stomach *Qi* to stop vomiting.
- Indications: Invasion to the stomach by liver fire marked by distending pain in the hypochondriac region, gastric discomfort with acid regurgitation, vomiting, bitter taste in the mouth, epigastrium fullness, belching, red tongue with yellow coating, wiry rapid pulse.
- Explanation:

Huang Lian: the principal drug, reducing the fire in the heart and liver.

Wu Zhu Yu: the adjuvant and guiding drug, having the effect of dispersing due to its pungent flavour, warming and dredging in order to promote the movement of *Qi*, and lowering the upward peversion of *Qi* to nausea.

○ About these two drugs, one is cold in nature and the other is hot, one is pungent in flavour which can disperse and the other is bitter which can descend in order to disperse the accumulated fire. The combination of them plays the functions of clearing and reducing the liver fire, lowering the upward peversion of *Qi* to stop nausea.

- Notes:

(1) This prescription is commonly used for acute and chronic gastritis, marked by invasion to the stomach by liver fire. For cases with stomach heat associated with stagnation of the liver Qi, the recipe can be used together with modified *Si Ni San* (Powder for Treating Cold Limbs) to strengthen the effect of relieving liver *Qi* stagnation and regulating the stomach.

(2) Pay attention that the ratio of dosage for *Huang Lian* and *Wu Zhu Yu* is 6:1.

2.6 Prescriptions for Clearing Away Heat of Deficient Type

This group of prescriptions is suitable for syndromes at later stage of febrile diseases that there is remaining heat in the *Yin* system and consumption of *Yin* fluid, or hectic fever with feeling of heat steaming out from the bone due to liver and kidney *Yin* deficiency and persistent fever resulting from *Yin* deficiency.

Qin Hao Bie Jia Tang (Sweet Wormwood and Turtle Shell Decoction)

● Source: *Wen Bing Tiao Bian* (Treatise on Differentiation and Treatment of Epidemic Febrile Diseases)

● Ingredients: Qing Hao (Herba Artemisiae) 6g.

Bie Jia (Carapax Trionycis) 15g.

Sheng Di (Radix Rehmanniae) 12g.

Zhi Mu (Rhizoma Anemarrhenae) 6g.

Dan Pi (Cortex Moutan Radicis) 9g.

● Administration: All the drugs should be decocted with five cups of water and finally two cups of decoction left. Drink it twice a day.

● Functions: Nourish *Yin* and expel pathogenic heat from the interior.

● Indications: Consumption of *Yin* fluid and remaining of latent heat in the *Yin* system in the late stage of febrile disease manifested by fever at night, absence of perspiration after fever subsides, polyphagia with emaciation, red tongue with less coating, deep thready and rapid pulse.

● Explanation:

Bie Jia : salty in taste and cold in nature, nourishing *Yin* and clearing away heat.

Qing Hao : bitter in taste and cold and fragrant in nature, clearing heat out of the body.

The combination of these two drugs plays the effect of principle drugs which nourish *Yin*, clear away heat and expel pathogenic heat out of *Yin* system.

Sheng Di : sweet in taste and cool in nature.

Zhi Mu : bitter in flavour and cold in nature.

Both of them help *Bie Jia* to nourish *Yin* and clear away heat.

Dan Pi : subducing latent heat in the blood and supporting *Qing Hao* to expel heat out of collaterals.

In the recipe, *Sheng Di*, *Zhi Mu* and *Dan Pi* are used as assistant and adjuvant drugs.

○ The combination of all the drugs shows the effect of nourishing *Yin* and clearing away heat, treating both the root cause and symptoms.

● Notes:

The recipe is modified to deal with infantile summer fever, unreasonable persistent fever, and chronic prelonephritis, renal tuberculosis marked by perisitent low fever due to *Yin* deficiency.

Qing Gu San (Powder for Clearing Bone Heat)

● Source: *Zheng Zhi Zhun Sheng* (Standards of Diagnosis and Treatment)

- Ingredients: *Yin Chai Hu* (Radix Stellariae) 5g.

  Bie Jia (Carapax Trionycis) 3g.

  Di Gu Pi (cortex Lycii Radicis) 3g.

  Zhi Mu (Rhizoma Anemarrhenae) 3g.

  Qin Jiao (Radix Gentianae Macrophyllae) 3g.

  Qing Hao (Herba Artemisiae) 3g.

  Hu Huang Lian (Rhizoma Picrorhizae) 3g.

  Zhi Gan Cao (Radix Glycyrrhizae Praeparata) 2g.

- Administration: All the drugs should be decocted in water for oral administration. Twice a day.

- Functions: Clear away deficient heat and remove hectic fever due to *Yin* deficiency.

- Indications: Steaming sensation in the bones and interior heat due to *Yin* deficiency, marked by hectic fever in the afternoon or during the night, hot sensation in the palms and soles, restlessness, dryness of the mouth, red tongue with little coating, thready rapid pulse or forceless and rapid pulse.

- Explanation:

Yin Chai Hu: a principal drug, being sweet in flavour and cold in nature, clearing "bone-heat" and deficient heat.

Hu Huang Lian, *Zhi Mu* and *Di Gu Pi*: assistant drugs, being bitter and sweet in taste and cold in nature, playing the effect of reducing deficient fire by entering the *Yin* system.

Qing Hao and *Qin Jiu*: expelling latent heat.

Bie Jia: nourishing *Yin* and clearing heat.

Gan Cao: coordinating various effects of the drugs.

These three drugs play the effect of adjuvant and guiding drugs.

○ The combination of all the drugs can play the function of clearing away deficient heat and bone-steaming heat.

- Notes:

(1) This prescription is mainly to clear bone-steaming heat, associated with nourishing *Yin* and expelling heat. The recipe can be modified to deal with low fever, hectic fever, hot sensation in the palms and soles in the process of tuberculosis and some chronic diseases which manifest milder *Yin* deficiency and severe heat condition.

(2) It is not advisable for cases with severe *Yin* deficiency and milder hectic fever.

(3) Clinically, *Bie Jia* is decocted first with dosage from 9-18g.

Summary

Twenty main heat-clearing prescriptions are selected. According to their functions, they are classified as the prescriptions for clearing away heat from *Qi* system, the prescriptions for removing heat from the *Ying* and blood systems, the prescriptions for clearing away heat from both *Qi* and *Ying* (blood) systems, the prescriptions for clearing heat and toxins, the prescriptions for removing heat from the *Zang-fu* organs and the prescriptions for clearing away deficient heat.

(1) The prescription for clearing away heat from the *Qi* System

Bai Hu Tang plays the effect of clearing away heat and producing body fluid. It is indicated for excessive heat in *Yangming* meridians marked by high fever, perspiration, thirst, surging and big pulse. It is a typical prescription for treating excessive heat in *Qi* system. *Zhi Zi Chi Tang* has the effect of clearing away heat and treating restlessness, indicating for early invasion of pathogenic heat to *Qi* system which manifests as restlessness and insomnia. *Liang Ge San* plays the effect of clearing away heat from diaphragm, associating with purgation. It is advisable for scorching heat sensation in the chest and diaphragm, irascibility, aphthous stomatitis and constipation, etc.

(2) The prescriptions for removing heat from the *Ying* and blood systems

Qing Ying Tang has the effect of clearing heat from the *Ying* system, nourishing *Yin* and activating blood. It is indicated for invasion of pathogenic heat to *Ying* system manifested as fever which is severe in the night, delirium and with dull exanthema maculosum. *Xi Jiao Di Huang Tang* has the effect of clearing heat, removing toxin, cooling blood and removing blood stasis. It is indicated for the syndrome of invasion of pathogenic heat to the blood system which causes quick circulation of the blood.

(3) The prescriptions for clearing away heat from both *Qi* and *Ying* (blood) systems

Both *Jia Jian Yu Nu Jian* and *Qing Wen Bai Du Yin* play the effect of clearing heat from both *Qi* and *Ying* (blood) systems, indicating that *Qi* system syndrome is not fully cured, but together with the syndromes of *Ying* and blood systems. The former has mild strength, which is suitable for slight case of the injury of *Qi* and *Ying* systems, and the latter can clear away heat from *Qi* system, cool the blood, reduce fire and remove toxin, indicating for severe cases with toxins in both interior and exterior and heat disturbing at both *Qi* and blood systems.

(4) The prescriptions for clearing away heat and toxins

Huang Lian Jie Du Tang, *Pu Ji Xiao Du Yin* and *Sheng Jiang San* have the effect of clearing away heat and toxins. The first one is mainly to reduce fire and remove toxin by its bitter flavour and cold nature. It is indicated for excessive heat of fire toxin in *San Jiao*. The second one is associated with the effect of expelling wind and removing pathogens, indicating for syndomes with epidemic wind-heat toxins manifested on the head and face. The third one plays the effect of both ascending and descending, associated with the effect of dispersing stagnation and reducing heat. It is suitable for toxic heat syndromes resulting from accumulation of heat.

(5) The prescriptions for removing heat from *Zang-fu* organs

This group of prescriptions is applied according to the organ that pathogenic heat affects. *Dao Chi San* has the effect of clearing heat from the heart and inducing diuresis, indicating for syndromes with transmission of heart fire into the small intestine. *Long Dan Xie Gan Tang* plays the effect of reducing excessive fire of liver and gallbladder and clearing damp-heat of lower *Jiao*. It is indicated for syndromes with upward attack of excessive fire in the liver and gallbladder and downward flow of damp-heat from the liver meridian. *Zuo Jin Wan* has the effect of clearing liver fire, descending upward perversion and stopping vomiting, indicating invasion to the stomach by liver fire. *Ma Xing Shi Gan Tang* plays the effect of clearing and dispersing lung heat, indicating for cough due to heat accumulated in the lung. The functions of *Xie Bai San* is clearing lung heat, indicating for cough and asthma caused by latent fire and accumulated heat in the lung. Both *Zuo Jin Wan* and *Ma Xing Shi Gan Tang* play the effect of clearing away lung heat, but the former is mainly to clear and disperse, and the latter is mainly to clear and reduce. *Qing Wei San* has the effect of clearing away stomach heat and cooling blood, indicating for toothache or gingival atrophy with oozing of bloody fluid and pus due to accumulated heat in the stomach which disturbs upward along the meridians. Both *Bai Tou Weng Tang* and *Shao Yao Tang* have the functions of clearing away heat and removing toxin and can treat dysentery. The former is also associated with the effect of cooling blood to treat dysentery, indicating for dysentery of heat-toxin type with more blood and less pus in the stool. While the latter mainly plays the effect of regulating *Qi* and blood in order to treat dysentery of damp-heat type with both blood and pus in the stool.

(6) The prescriptions for clearing away deficient heat

Qing Hao Bie Jia Tang and *Qing Gu San* have the effect of nourishing *Yin* and reducing heat. Both are used to treat deficient heat. The former has the effect of both nourishing *Yin* and expelling heat, indicating for syndromes with latent pathogens in *Yin* system in the later period of febrile diseases. The latter mainly plays the effect of clearing away deficient heat, associating with the effect of nourishing *Yin* and expelling heat. It is indicated for consumptive bone-steaming heat.

Review Questions

(1) How many types can heat-clearing prescriptions be divided into? What are their indications?

(2) Please recount the ingredients, functions and indications of *Bai Hu Tang* and analyse the effects of individual drugs.

(3) Please recount the ingredients, functions and indications of *Qing Ying Tang* and explain the functions of some drugs for *Qi* System such as *Yin Hua*, *Lian Qiao*, *Zhu Ye* and *Huang Lian*.

(4) Please recount the ingredients, functions and indications of *Huang Lian Jie Du Tang* and analyse the effect of individual drugs in the prescription.

(5) What are the ingredients, functions and indications of *Long Dan Xie Gan Tang*?

Why *Sheng Di* and *Dang Gui* which are for nourishing blood are used in this prescription?

(6) Both *Bai Tou Weng Tang* and *Shao Yao Tang* are representative prescriptions for treat dysentery. What are the differences between them in function and indications?

(7) Which drugs compose *Qing Hao Bie Jia Tang* ? Please explain the effects of the drugs in the prescription.

3 Prescriptions for Clearing Away Summer-Heat

The prescriptions which consist of herbs having the functions of clearing away summer-heat, being used to treat the diseases due to summer-heat, are called the prescriptions for clearing away summer-heat.

Based on the characteristics that when summer-heat invades the body, it tends to consume Qi and damage body fluid and it is easy to be accompanied by dampness and exterior cold syndrome, the prescriptions for clearing away summer-heat are divided into three categories: clearing away summer-heat and relieving the exterior syndrome, clearing away summer-heat and eliminating dampness, and clearing away summer-heat and reinforcing Qi.

While the prescriptions for clearing away summer-heat are used, we should pay attention that do not use too cold drugs in case they may encourage dampness and do not use too dry drugs for eliminating dampness in case they may damage body fluid.

3.1 Clearing Away Summer-Heat and Relieving Exterior Syndrome

The prescriptions for clearing away summer-heat and relieving exterior syndrome are advisable for cases with summer-heat and dampness who are again affected by wind-cold.

Xiang Ru Yin (Decoction of Elsholtziae seu Moslae)

● Source: *Tai Ping Hui Min He Ji Ju Fang* (Prescriptions of Peaceful Benevolent Dispensary)

● Ingredients: *Xiang Ru* (Herba Elsholtziae Seu Moslae) 9g.

Bai Bian Dou (Semen Dolichoris Album) 6g.

Hou Po (Cortex Magnoliae Officinalis) 6g.

● Administration: The drugs are decocted in water or with some wine for oral administration.

● Functions: Clear away summer-heat, expel exopathogenic evils, eliminate dampness and regulate the middle *Jiao*.

● Indications: For cases caused by affection of exogenous cold and endogenous dampness during the hot summer time, manifested as headache, chills and fever, anhidrosis, abdominal fullness, vomiting, diarrhea, white greasy tongue coating, floating pulse.

● Explanation:

Xiang Ru: the principal drug, acrid in taste and warm in nature, fragrant in smell, expelling the evil in the superficies, eliminating summer-heat and dampness.

Hou Po: the assistant drug, acrid in taste and warm in nature, promoting the circulation of Qi to relieve fullness, and eliminating dampness.

Bai Bian Dou: the adjuvant and guiding drug, sweet and mild in taste, strengthening the spleen and the stomach, eliminating summer-heat and dampness from the middle *Jiao*, descending turbidity and ascending clearity.

○ These three drugs as a whole perform the functions of clearing away summer-heat, expelling the evil from the body surface, eliminating the dampness and regulating the functions of the middle *Jiao*.

● Notes:

(1) The nature of drugs in this prescription is warm. It is indicated for the cases caused by cold and dampness in summer. Chills and anhidrosis are the main symptoms. Clinically, this prescription is suitable for cases of influenza in summer and gastroenteritis attributive to the symptoms mentioned above.

(2) This prescription is not applicable to the case with fever, chills and hidrosis.

Appendix:

Xin Jia Xiang Ru Yin (Newly Added Decoction of Elsholtziae seu Moslae)

● Source: *Wen Bing Tiao Bian* (Treatise on Differentiation and Treatment of Epidemic Febrile Diseases)

● Ingredients: *Xiang Ru Yin* (Decoction of Elsholtziae seu Moslae) plus:

        Jin Yin Hua (Flos Lonicerae) 9g.

        Lian Qiao (Fructus Forsythiae) 9g.

● Functions and indications: It has the effects of expelling summer-heat and eliminating dampness, and is indicated for the syndrome of summer-heat and dampness with external cold, manifested as fever and chills, hidrosis, headache, general pain, thirst, red face, white and greasy tongue coating, floating and rapid pulse.

3.2 Clearing Away Summer-Heat and Eliminating Dampness

The prescriptions for clearing away summer-heat and eliminating dampness are indicated for cases with summer-heat and dampness.

Liu Yi San (Six to One Powder)

● Source: *Shang Han Zhi Ge* (The Principles of Cold-induced Diseases)

● Ingredients: *Hua Shi* (Talcum) 30g.

        Gan Cao (Radix Glycyrrhizae) 5g.

● Administration: Ground into powder, 10g. each time. It is wrapped in cloth and decocted in water, or take the powder with warm water. 2-3 times a day. This recipe is often put in other prescriptions for making decoction.

● Functions: Clear away summer-heat and eliminate dampness.

● Indications: syndrome of summer-heat and dampness, manifested as fever, thirst, dysuria, and diarrhea.

● Explanation:

Hua Shi: the principal drug, mild sweet in taste and cold in nature, clearing away summer-heat, eliminating dampness, and promoting diuresis.

Sheng Gan Cao: clearing away heat and regulating the middle *Jiao*, used with *Hua Shi* to strengthen the effect of clearing away summer-heat and inhibiting the cold nature of *Hua Shi*.

○ The combination of the two drugs eliminates summer-heat and dampness from the lower part, and as a result, fever will be reduced and thirst be stopped.

● Notes:

(1) The prescription is used for the syndrome of summer-heat and dampness, manifested as fever, thirst, irritability, scanty and redish urine. Clinically, this prescription can also be used with other drugs for cases of stranguria with difficult and painful urination due to damp-heat or stone in the urinary bladder.

(2) Since the dose of *Hua Shi* is 6 times as much as *Gan Cao*, the recipe is named *Liu Yi San* (6:1 powder). The proportion of the drugs in the prescription is important.

Appendix:

(1) *Yi Yuan San* (Powder Beneficial to *Yuan*-Primary *Qi*)

● Source: *Shang Han Zhi Ge* (The Principles of Cold-Induced Diseases)

● Administration: Add *Chen Sha* (Cinnabaris) into the prescription and take with decoction of Medulla Junci.

● Functions and indications: It has the effects of clearing away summer-heat and tranquilizing the mind, and is indicated for the syndrome of summer-heat and dampness with symptoms of palpitation, irritability, insomnia, and dream-disturbed sleep.

(2) *Bi Yu San* (Green Jade Powder)

● Source: *Shang Han Zhi Ge* (The Principles of Cold-Induced Diseases)

● Ingredients: *Liu Yi San* plus *Qing Dai* (Indigo Naturalis).

● Functions and indications: It has the effects of clearing away summer-heat, and is indicated for the syndrome of summer-heat and dampness combined with accumulation of the liver and gallbladder heat marked by sore throat, red eyes, and oral ulcer etc.

(3) *Ji Su San* (Cock-waking Powder)

● Source: *Shang Han Zhi Ge* (The Principles of Cold-Induced Diseases)

● Ingredients: *Liu Yi San* plus *Bo He* (Herba Menthae).

● Functions and indications: It has the effects of expelling wind and clearing away summer-heat, and is indicated for the syndrome of summer-heat and dampness with slight aversion to wind and cold, headache, feeling of distention in the head, and difficult cough.

3.3   Clearing Away Summer-Heat and Strengthening *Qi*

The prescriptions for clearing away summer-heat and strengthening *Qi* is suitable for cases with the consumption of body fluid and *Qi* by summer-heat.

Wang Shi Qing Shu Yi Qi Tang (Wang's Decoction for Clearing Away Summer-Heat and Reinforcing *Qi*)

- Source: *Wen Re Jing Wei* (Compendium of Seasonal Febrile Diseases)
- Ingredients: *Xi Yang Shen* (Radix Panacis Guinquefolli) 5g.

  Shi Hu (Herba Dendrobii) 15g.

  Mai Dong (Radix Ophiopogonis) 9g.

  Huang Lian (Rhizoma Coptidis) 3g.

  Zhu Ye (Herba Lophatheri) 6g.

  He Geng (Petiolus Nelumbinis) 15g.

  Zhi Mu (Rhizoma Anemarrhenae) 6g.

  Gan Cao (Radix Glycyrrhizae) 3g.

  Jing Mi (Fructus Oryzae Sativae) 15g.

  Xi Gua Cui Yi (Exocarpium Citrulli) 30g.

- Administration: The drugs are decocted in water for oral administration.
- Functions: Clear away summer-heat, reinforce *Qi*, promote the production of body fluid.
- Indications: syndrome of consumption of body-fluid and *Qi* by summer-heat, marked by fever, irritability, thirst, hidrosis, yellow urine, fatigue, shortness of breath, and forceless pulse.
- Explanation:

Xi Gua Pi: sweet in taste and cool in nature, clearing away summer-heat, stopping thirst and promoting urination.

Xi Yang Shen: bitter in taste and cool in nature, reinforcing *Qi*, promoting the production of the body fluid to stop thirst.

These two drugs perform the main function as the principal drugs in the prescription.

He Geng: helping *Xi Gua Cui Yi* to clear away summer-heat.

Shi Hu: sweet and mild in taste.

Mai Dong: sweet in taste and cold in nature.

Both *Shi Hu* and *Mai Dong* help *Xi Yang Shen* to reinforce *Yin* and clear away heat. The above three are used as assistant drugs.

Zhi Mu: bitter in taste and cold-moist in nature, nourishing *Yin* and clearing away heat.

Zhu Ye: sweet and mild in taste and cold in nature, clearing away heat and stopping irritability.

Huang Lian: bitter in taste and cold in nature, clearing away heat.

The above three are adjuvant drugs.

Gan Cao and *Jing Mi*: the guiding drugs, reinforcing *Qi* and regulating middle *Jiao*.

○ The prescription is an excellent decoction for clearing away summer-heat and reinforcing both.

Qi and *Yin*.

● Notes:

(1) The decoction is for cases caused by summer-heat with consumption of both *Qi* and body fluid, mainly manifested as fatigue, shortness of breath, thirst, hidrosis, forceless and rapid pulse. Clinically, it can also be used as a basic prescription for treating prolonged summer fever in children with symptoms of *Qi* and body fluid deficiency.

(2) Some drugs in the prescription are used for nourishing *Yin*, therefore the recipe is not advisable for cases of summer-heat with dampness.

Appendix:

Qing Shu Yi Qi Tang (Decoction for Clearing Away Summer-Heat and Reinforcing Qi)

● Source: *Pi Wei Lun* (Treatise on the Spleen and Stomach)

● Ingredients: *Huang Qi* (Radix Astragali seu Hedysari) 6g.

Cang Zhu (Rhizoma Atractylodis) 3g.

Sheng Ma (Rhizoma Cimicifugae) 3g.

Chao Shen Qu (Baked Massa Fermentata Medicinalis) 3g.

Bai Zhu (Rhizoma Atractylodis Macrocephalae) 3g.

Mai Men Dong (Radix Ophiopogonis) 3g.

Huang Bai (Certex Phellodendri) 3g.

Ge Gen (Radix Puerariae) 3g.

Ze Xie (Rhizoma Alismatis) 3g.

Wu Wei Zi (Fructus Schisandrae) 3g.

Ren Shen (Radix Ginseng) 1.5g.

Ju Pi (Pericarpium Citri Reticulatae) 1.5g.

Dang Gui (Radix Angelicae Sinensis) 1g.

Zhi Gan Cao (Radix Glycyrrhizae Praeparata) 1g.

● Administration: The drugs are decocted in water for oral administration.

● Functions and indications: used to clear away summer-heat, reinforce *Qi*, promote the production of body fluid, strengthen the spleen and eliminate dampness, manifested as headache, fever, thirst, spontaneous sweating, tiredness, anorexia, fullness in the chest, heavy sensation of the body, deep-coloured urine, watery stool, greasy tongue coating and forceless pulse.

Summary

There are three main prescriptions discussed here. According to the effects, the three prescriptions for clearing summer-heat are divided into three categories: clearing away summer-heat and relieving exterior syndrome, clearing away summer-heat and eliminating dampness, and clearing away summer-heat and reinforcing *Qi*.

(1) Clearing away summer-heat and relieving exterior syndrome

Xiang Ru Yin has the effects of clearing summer-heat and expelling exogenous evils, eliminating dampness and regulating the middle *Jiao*. It is advisable for the cases due to cold and dampness in summer.

(2) Clearing away summer-heat and eliminating dampness

Liu Yi San is the basic prescription for clearing summer-heat and eliminating dampness, which is advisable for the cases with summer-heat and dampness.

(3) Clearing away summer-heat and reinforcing *Qi*

Wang's Qing Shu Yi Qi Tang has the effects of clearing away summer-heat, reinforcing *Qi* and promoting the production of body fluid. It is advisable for the cases with consumption of body fluid and *Qi* by summer-heat.

Review Questions

(1) What are the indications, pathogenesis, ingredients of *Xiang Ru Yin*? What is the commonly used prescription which is formed on the basis of *Xiang Ru Yin*?

(2) What are the commonly used prescriptions which are formed on the basis of *Liu Yi San*? Write out the ingredients, functions and indications of these prescriptions.

(3) Briefly explain the effects of the individual drugs in *Wang's Qing Shu Yi Qi Tang*.

4　Prescriptions for Expelling Cold

The prescriptions which consist of drugs with warm-hot nature, having the effects of warming *Yang*, expelling cold, clearing meridians, being used for treating internal cold syndromes, are named the prescriptions for expelling cold, also known as the prescriptions for warming the interior.

The interior cold syndromes are caused by exterior cold which invades the *Zang-fu* organs and meridians directly, or interior cold due to *Yang* deficiency. For either exterior cold or interior cold, warming *Yang* to expel cold is the main principle. According to the effect of the prescription, the seriousness of the syndrome and the affected position, the prescriptions are divided into three categories: Warming the Middle *Jiao* to Expel cold, Expelling Cold from Meridians, and Recuperating Depleted *Yang* and Rescuing the Patient from Collapse.

Most drugs in the prescription for expelling cold have acrid taste, warm or hot and dry nature, and they are prohibited for heat syndromes with pseudo-cold manifestations at the exterior. Therefore, distinguishing the false manifestations of cold or heat from true is necessary. On the other hand, the drugs with acrid taste and dry nature may impair the *Yin* of the body, thus over-using of this type of prescriptions is undesirable.

4.1　Warming the Middle Jiao to Expel Cold

The prescriptions of warming the middle *Jiao* to expel cold are used for cases with deficient type cold syndrome in the middle *Jiao*.

Li Zhong Wan (*Tang*) (Pill or Decoction for Regulating the Function of the Middle *Jiao*)

- Source: *Shang Han Lun* (Treatise on Cold-Induced Diseases)
- Ingredients: *Ren Shen* (Radix Ginseng) 6g.
  Gan Jiang (Rhizoma Zingiberis) 5g.
  Bai Zhu (Rhizoma Atractylodis Macrocephalae) 9g.
  Zhi Gan Cao (Radix Glycyrrhizae Praeparata) 6g.
- Administration: The drugs are decocted in water. The original form of the prescription is pill and now it is usually prepared as decoction.
- Functions: Warm the middle *Jiao* to expel cold, reinforce *Qi* and the spleen.
- Indications: Deficient type cold of the spleen and stomach with manifestations of abdominal pain, diarrhea, vomiting, anorexia, no thirst, pale tongue, deep thready or slow pulse.
- Explanation:

Gan Jiang: the principal drug, acrid in taste and hot in nature, warming the middle *Jiao* to expel cold.

Ren Shen: the assistant drug, sweet in taste and warm in nature, reinforcing *Qi* and invigorating the spleen.

Bai Zhu: the adjuvant drug, reinforcing the spleen for eliminating dampness, promoting the functions of the spleen and stomach in ascending clarity and descending turbidity and receiving and transformation of food.

Zhi Gan Cao: the guiding drug, reinforcing *Qi* and regulating the middle *Jiao*.

○ The prescription as a whole has the effects of warming the middle *Jiao* to expel cold, reinforcing *Qi* and invigorating the spleen.

● Notes:

(1) It is the representative prescription for warming the middle *Jiao* to expel cold. Clinically, it can be used for the cases as chronic dysentery, chronic gastroenteritis, indigestion, insufficient gastrointestinal function, gastric duodenal ulcer resulting from deficiency of the spleen and stomach *Yang*. It can also be used as a basic prescription for treating the cases of obstruction of *Qi* in the chest, chronic infantile convulsions, dysfunctional uterine bleeding due to deficiency of the spleen and stomach Yang.

(2) The function of honeyed pill of the prescription is not as strong as the decoction, so it is suitable for the mild cases. For acute cases, decoction is advisable.

Appendix:

Fu Zi Li Zhong Wan (*Tang*) (Bolus or Decoction of Aconiti Praeparata for Regulating the Middle *Jiao*)

● Source: *Yan Shi Xiao Er Fang Lun* (Yan's Treatise on Prescriptions for Children)

● Ingredients: The prescription is formed by adding *Fu Zi* (Radix Aconiti Praeparata).

● Functions and indications: Warming *Yang* to expel cold, reinforcing *Qi* and the spleen. It is used for the cases due to deficient cold of the spleen and the stomach, manifested as diarrhea, feeble pulse, cold extremities, etc..

Xiao Jiang Zhong Tang (Minor Decoction for Strengthening the Middle *Jiao*)

● Source: *Shang Han Lun* (Treatise on Cold-Induced Diseases)
● Ingredients: *Shao Yao* (Radix Paeoniae) 18g.
  Gui Zhi (Ramulus Cinnamomi) 9g.
  Zhi Gan Cao (Radix Glycyrrhizae Praeparata) 6g.
  Sheng Jiang (Rhizoma Zingiberis Recens) 9g.
  Da Zao (Fructus Ziziphi Jujubae) 4pcs.
  Yi Tang (Saccharum Granorum) 30g.

● Administration: The first five drugs are decocted in water twice. After getting the decoction, add *Yi Tang* into the decoction which will be divided into two doses and take the two doses for two times in a day when the decoction is warm.

● Functions: Warm the middle *Jiao*, reinforce the deficiency, regulate the interior to stop spasm.

● Indications: Deficient cold of the spleen and stomach with manifestations of abdominal pain at times, lessened by pressure and warmth, pale tongue with white coating; or deficiency of both *Qi* and blood marked by palpitation, restlessness, insomnia, lack of luster on the face, lassitude, etc.

● Explanation:

Yi Tang: sweet in taste and warm and moist in nature, invigorating the spleen *Qi* and nourishing the spleen *Yin*, warming the middle *Jiao* to relieve spasm, used as the principal drugs in the prescription.

Gui Zhi: warming *Yang Qi*.

Shao Yao: reinforcing *Yin* and blood.

The above two are used as assistant drugs.

Zhi Gan Cao: sweet in taste and warm in nature, helping *Yi Tang* to reinforce *Qi*, combined with *Shao Yao*, "sour and sweet for transforming *Yin*", benefiting the liver and nourishing the spleen, relieving the spasm to stop pain, used as adjuvant drug.

Sheng Jiang and *Da Zao*: reinforcing the spleen and regulating *Ying*, also used as adjuvant drugs.

○ This prescription has drugs of acrid, sweet and sour taste. "Acrid and sweet transforms to *Yang*, while sour and sweet transforms to *Yin*". The prescription as a whole performs the functions of warming the middle *Jiao*, regulating the interior and stopping spasm.

● Notes:

(1) Abdominal pain of deficient cold type seen in duodenal ulcer and intestinal spasm, or chronic hepatitis, chronic peritonitis and neurasthenia with the above-mentioned symptoms could be treated with this formula.

(2) The dosage of *Yi Tang* should be large and the dosage of *Shao Yao* should be larger than that of *Gui Zhi*.

Appendix:

(1) *Huang Qi Jian Zhong Tang* (Decoction of Astragalus for Tonifying Middle *Jiao*)

● Source: *Jin Gui Yao Lue* (Synopsis of Prescriptions of the Golden Chamber)

● Ingredients: Add *Huang Qi* (Radix Astragali seu Hedysari) into *Xiao Jian Zhong Tang*.

● Functions and indications: warming the middle *Jiao* and reinforcing *Qi*, used to treat intestinal spasm due to deficiency.

(2) *Dang Gui Jian Zhong Tang* (Decoction of Radix Angelicae Sinensis for Tonifying Middle *Jiao*)

● Source: *Qian Jin Yi Fang* (A Supplement to the Essential Prescriptions Worth a Thousand Gold)

● Ingredients: Add *Dang Gui* (Radix Angelicae Sinensis) into *Xiao Jian Zhong Tang*.

● Functions and indications: warming and reinforcing *Qi* and blood, relieving spasm to stop pain, advisable for continuous colicky pain in the lower abdomen, lassitude and lack of energy due to *Qi* and blood deficiency after delivery, or lower abdominal pain at times and referring to the whole abdomen and the back due to deficient cold of the internal organs.

Da Jian Zhong Tang (Major Decoction for Tonifying the Middle *Jiao*)

● Source: *Jin Gui Yao Lue* (Synopsis of Prescriptions of the Golden Chamber)
● Ingredients: *Chuan Jiao* (Pericarpium Zanthoxyli) 3g.

                Gan Jiang (Rhizoma Zingiberis) 4.5g.

                Ren Shen (Radix Ginseng) 6g.

                Yi Tang (Saccharum Granorum) 30g.

● Administration: The first three drugs are decocted in water. After getting the decoction, add *Yi Tang* into the decoction which will be divided into two doses and take one dose when it is warm.

● Functions: Warm the middle *Jiao* to reinforce middle *Yang*, lower the rising of *Qi* and relieve pain.

● Indications: Weakness of the middle Yang, excess of cold in the interior, marked by severe coldpain over the heart and chest, vomiting, distention and tenderness sensation in chest and abdomen, borborygmus, white and glassy tongue coating, wiry slow or thready and tense pulse.

● Explanation:

Yi Tang: the principal drug, sweet in taste and warm in nature, warming *Yang*, reinforcing the middle *Jiao* and relieving pain.

Ren Shen: the assistant drug, tonifying *Yuan*-primary *Qi*, strengthening *Yi Tang*'s function of reinforcing the middle *Jiao*.

Chuan Jiao and *Gan Jiang*: *Chuan Jiao* is related to the liver and *Gan Jiang* is related to the spleen and stomach. Both of them are assistant and guiding drugs, having the effects of smoothing the *Qi* movement of Jueyin and warming the middle *Jiao* to expel cold.

○ The prescription as a whole has the effects of warming the middle *Jiao*, tonifying deficiency, descending adverse-rising *Qi*, and expelling cold to relieve pain.

● Notes:

(1) It is a representative prescription for treating *Yang* deficiency in the middle *Jiao*. It is indicated for the cases of abdominal pain caused by intestinal spasm, hernia which belongs to the type of *Yang* deficiency in the middle Jiao.

(2) After taking the decoction, it is necessary to have a good rest and keeping warm. The hard digested food is prohibited.

(3) *Dang Shen* (Radix Angelicae Sinensis) can be used to replace *Ren Shen*.

Wu Zhu Yu Tang (Decoction of Evodia Fruit)

- Source: *Shang Han Lun* (Treatise on Cold-Induced Diseases)
- Ingredients: *Wu Zhu Yu* (Fructus Evodiae) 6g.

  Ren Shen (Radix Ginseng) 6g.

  Da Zao (Fructus Ziziphi Jujubae) 4pcs.

  Sheng Jiang (Rhizoma Zingiberis Recens) 20g.
- Administration: The drugs are decocted in water for oral dose.
- Functions: Warm the liver and stomach, lower the adverse rise of *Qi* to stop vomiting.
- Indications: deficient-cold of the liver and stomach deficiency, adverse rising of turbid *Yin*, manifested as stomachache, vertical headache, vomiting of fluid, or vomiting with diarrhea, or nausea, etc.
- Explanation:

Wu Zhu Yu: the principal drug, acrid, bitter in taste and dry and hot in nature, warming the liver and stomach, expelling cold, descending turbidity.

Sheng Jiang: used as assistant drug, acrid in taste, expelling cold, warming the stomach to stop vomiting.

Ren Shen and *Da Zao*: sweet in taste and warm in nature, reinforcing middle *Jiao Qi*, used as adjuvant and guiding drugs.

○ The prescription as a whole has the effects of warming the middle *Jiao* and tonifying deficiency, eliminating *Yin* evil to strengthen *Yang Qi*, and descending adverse-rising *Qi* to stop vomiting.

- Notes:

(1) It is indicated for chronic gastritis, nervous headache, otogenic vertigo, vomiting of pregnancy which belongs to the type of deficient cold of the liver and stomach.

(2) Vomiting can be caused by either heat or cold. This prescription is prohibited for cases due to heat. Pale tongue, white glassy tongue coating, thready and slow or wiry-thready pulse are the main clinical manifestations of this prescription.

4.2 Warming the Meridians to Expel Cold

The prescriptions for warming the meridians to expel cold are indicated for cases with deficiency of *Yang* and blood and invasion of cold into the meridians.

Dang Gui Si Ni Tang (Chinese Angelica Decoction for Restoring *Yang*)

- Source: *Shang Han Lun* (Treatise on Cold-Induced diseases)
- Ingredients: *Dang Gui* (Radix Angelicae Sinensis) 9g.

  Shao Yao (Radix Paeoniae Alba) 9g.

  Gui Zhi (Ramulus Cinnamomi) 9g.

Xi Xin (Herba Asari) 3g.

Zhi Gan Cao (Radix Glycyrrhizae Praeparata) 6g.

Tong Cao (Medulla Tetrapanacis) 6g.

Da Zao (Fructus Ziziphi Jujubae) 8 pcs.

- Administration: The drugs are decocted in water for oral administration.
- Functions: Warm the meridians to expel cold, nourish blood and clear the meridians.
- Indications:

(1)Blood deficiency and *Yang* deficiency with attack of external cold, manifested as cold extremities, pale tongue and white tongue coating, deep thready or faint pulse.

(2) Invasion of cold into the meridians showing pain at lower back, thigh, lower limbs and foot.

- Explanation:

Dang Gui: the principal drug, sweet and acrid in taste and warm in nature, related to the liver, promoting blood circulation and nourishing blood.

Bai Shao: regulating Ying and blood.

Gui Zhi: warming *Yang* to promote blood circulation.

Xi Xin: acrid in taste and warm in nature, expelling cold.

All above are assistant drugs, helping *Dang Gui* to clear the Jueyin meridian interiorly and regulating *Ying* and *Wei* exteriorly.

Tong Cao: the adjuvant drug, clearing away heat to prevent from injury of *Yin* by the acrid-heat drugs.

Mu Xiang and *Gan Cao*: reinforcing the middle Jiao.

○ The prescription as a whole has the effects of warming the meridians to expel cold, nourishing blood and dredging the meridians.

- Notes:

(1) The prescription is indicated for cold limbs, extremities pain, irregular menstruation, cold pain in abdomen and lumbar region, cold colic, which are attributive to deficiency of *Yang* and blood with attack of cold.

(2) It is also applicable to thromboangiitis obliterans, Raynaud's phenomenon, arthritis, pulseless disease, which are attributive to blood deficiency and affection of cold.

(3) In the primary prescription, the dosage of *Xi Xin* is the same to *Gui Zhi*. Clinically, the dosage of *Xi Xin* should be decided according to the syndrome.

Mu Tong (Caulis Akebiae) can be used to replace *Tong Cao*.

4.3 Recuperating Depleted *Yang* and Rescuing the Patient from Collapse

The prescriptions for recuperating depleted *Yang* and rescuing the patient from collapse are indicated for cases with excess of *Yin* and exhaustion of *Yang*.

Si Ni Tang (Decoction for Resuscitation)

● Source: *Shang Han Lun* (Treatise on Cold-Induced Diseases)

● Ingredients: *Sheng Fu Zi* (Crude Radix Aconiti) 10g.

Gan Jiang (Rhizoma Zingiberis) 6g.

Zhi Gan Cao (Radix Glycyrrhizae Praeparata) 12g.

● Administration: The drugs are decocted in water. Take the decoction till it is cold if vomiting appear.

● Functions: Recuperate depleted *Yang* and rescue the patient from collapse.

● Indications: Exhaustion of *Yang* and excess of *Yin*, marked by cold limbs, tiredness, sleepiness, cold pain in abdomen, watery diarrhea with indigested food, white glassy tongue coating, deep or faint pulse.

● Explanation:

Fu Zi: the principal drug, acrid in taste and hot in nature, strengthening general *Yang Qi*.

Gan Jiang: the assistant drug, acrid in taste and hot in nature, warming the middle *Jiao* to expel cold, strengthening the effect of recuperating the depleted *Yang* of the principal drug.

Gan Cao: the adjuvant drug, sweet in taste and warm in nature, reinforcing *Qi* and relieving the acrid and drastic nature of *Fu Zi* and *Gan Jiang*.

○ The prescription as a whole has the effects of recuperating the depleted *Yang* and rescuing the patient from collapse.

● Notes:

(1) It is an important prescription for recuperating the depleted *Yang* and rescuing the patient from collapse, also one of the prescriptions of TCM for emergency treatment. It is applicable for cases with exhaustion of *Yang*, seen in cardiac infarction with shock, cerebral accident with coma, severe bleeding with cold limbs, hidrosis and shock, cardiac failure attributive to *Yang* collapse. It is also indicated to treat chronic diarrhea, disfunction of gastrointestine.

(2) It is indicated for the cases with cold limbs due to *Yang* deficiency and excess of *Yin*. If cold limbs due to accumulation of *Yang Qi* in the interior and *Yang* can not reach the surface, this prescription will not be used.

Appendix:

Tong Mai Si Ni Tang (Decoction of Clearing the Meridians and Treating Cold Limbs)

● Source: *Shang Han Lun* (Treatise on Cold-Induced Diseases)

● Ingredients: Increase the dosages of *Sheng Fu Zi* (15g) and *Gan Jiang* (9-12g) in *Si Ni Tang*.

● Functions and indications: Rescue *Yang* and clear the meridians, used to treat *Shaoyin* syndrome characterized by diarrhea of undigested food, interior cold and exterior heat, cold hands and feet, feeble and indistinct pulse, not aversion to cold, red face, or diarrhea stopped but pulse remaining the same.

Shen Fu Tang (Decoction of Ginseng and Prepared Aconite)

- Source: *Fu Ren Liang Fang* (The Effective Prescriptions for Women)
- Ingredients: *Ren Shen* (Radix Ginseng) 12g.

    Pao Fu Zi (Radix Aconiti Praeparata) 9g.
- Administration: Decoct *Ren Shen* and *Shou Fu Zi* in water separately, take the mixed decoction.
- Functions: Recuperate *Yang*, reinforce *Qi*, and stop collapse.
- Indications: Sudden exhausting of *Yang Qi* with cold limbs, hidrosis, short breath, dyspnea, faint pulse at *Guan* and *Chi* positions.
- Explanation:

Ren Shen: the principal drug, sweet in taste and warm in nature, reinforcing the *Yuan*-primary *Qi*.

Fu Zi: the assistant drug, acrid in taste and hot in nature, warming and reinforcing the *Yuan*-primary *Yang*.

○ Two drugs together have the effects of recuperating *Yang* and reinforcing *Qi*.

- Notes:

(1) It is used for cases with shock due to heart failure or the syndromes of *Yang* depletion due to bleeding after delivery, metrorrhagia and metrostaxis, or bleeding resulting from diabrosis of carbuncle and furuncle.

(2) It is one of the prescriptions for emergency treatment, therefore, stop using the prescription when the emergency situation is over.

Summary

According to the effect, the seven main prescriptions for expelling cold mentioned above are divided into three categories: warming the middle *Jiao* to expel cold, expelling cold from the meridians, recuperating depleted *Yang* and rescuing the patient from collapse.

(1) Warming the middle *Jiao* to expel cold :

This kind of prescription is indicated for the cases of *Yang* deficiency in middle *Jiao*. *Li Zhong Wan* has the effects of warming the middle *Jiao* to expel cold, reinforcing *Qi* and spleen. It is a main prescription for treating the cases of *Yang* deficiency in middle *Jiao* manifested as abdominal pain, vomiting and diarrhea. *Da Jian Zhong Tang* has the effects of warming the middle *Jiao* to expel cold, reinforcing deficiency to stop pain, used for severe cold and pain in the heart and chest due to *Yang* deficiency in middle *Jiao* and interior excess of cold. Both *Xiao Jian Zhong Tang* and *Da Jian Zhong Tang* have the effects of warming the middle *Jiao*, reinforcing the deficiency, expelling cold and stopping pain. *Xiao Jian Zhong Tang* tends to reinforcement such as warming *Yang*, nourishing *Yin*, relieving spasm to stop pain, used to treat abdominal pain due to *Yang* deficiency with *Yin* deficiency, while *Da Jian Zhong Tang* tends to reduce pathogens such as warming *Yang* to expel cold, lower the rise of *Qi* to stop pain. *Wu Zhu Yu Tang* has the effects of warming the middle *Jiao*, reinforcing deficiency, descending adverse rising *Qi* to stop vomiting. It is used for cases with vomiting and headache due to adverse rising of cold.

(2) Expelling cold from the meridians

Dang Gui Si Ni Tang is a representative prescription for expelling cold from the meridians, indicated for cases of cold limbs due to deficiency of *Yang* and blood with invasion of cold into the meridians.

(3) Recuperating depleted *Yang* and rescuing the patient from collapse

Si Ni Tang and *Shen Fu Tang* are the prescriptions for emergency treatment, having the effects of recuperating depleted *Yang* and rescuing the patient from collapse. They can be used to treat the cases with chills, huddling up in bed, vomiting, diarrhea, and abdominal pain due to deficiency of *Yang Qi*, excessive cold in the interior. *Si Ni Tang* has the functions of restoring *Yang*, particularly for the cases of excessive cold in the interior with exhaustion of *Yang*. Besides the effect of restoring *Yang*, *Shen Fu Tang* also has the effect of reinforcing *Qi*, and its effect of emergency treatment is stronger and quicker, used for the cases of exhaustion of vital *Qi* and *Yang Qi*.

Review Questions

(1) Write out the ingredients, functions and indications of *Li Zhong Wan*.

(2) Briefly explain the effects of the drugs in *Wu Zhu Yu Tang*.

(3) Write out the ingredients, functions and indications of *Dang Gui Si Ni Tang*.

(4) Explain the differences of ingredients, functions and indications between *Si Ni Tang* and *Shen Fu Tang*.

5 Prescriptions for Eliminating Dampness

The prescriptions which consist of drugs for eliminating dampness, having the effects of resolving dampness and promoting diuresis, treating stranguria, removing turbidity, are named the prescriptions for eliminating dampness.

According to the position of dampness and its cold or heat nature, the prescriptions for eliminating dampness are divided into five categories: drying dampness and regulating the stomach, clearing away heat and dampness, warming *Yang* to resolve dampness, dispelling wind and dampness, and removing dampness by promoting diuresis.

When choosing the prescriptions for eliminating dampness, distinguishing the position of pathogens (upper, lower, interior or exterior) and making sure of deficiency or excess, cold or heat, are necessary. Meanwhile, we should pay attention to the regulation of the functions of the *Zang-fu* organs and using of the drugs for promoting *Qi* movement, because "*Qi* has the function of promoting water circulation, stagnation of *Qi* will cause retention of water". On the other hand, the prescriptions for eliminating dampness should be used carefully for weak patients and pregnant women.

5.1 Drying the Dampness and Regulating the Stomach

The prescriptions for drying dampness and regulating the stomach are indicated for the cases caused by stagnation of dampness in the middle *Jiao* (the spleen and stomach).

Huo Xiang Zheng Qi San (Powder of Agastachis for Restoring Health)

● Source: *Tai Ping Hui Min He Ji Ju Fang* (Prescriptions of Peaceful Benevolent Dispensary)

● Ingredients: *Huo Xiang* (Herba Agastachis) 12g.
    Fu Ling (Poria) 12g.
    Zi Su (Folium Perillae) 10g.
    Da Fu Pi (Pericarpium Arecae) 10g.
    Chao Bai Zhu (Rhizoma Atractylodis Macrocephalae) 10g.
    Ban Xia Qu (Massa Pinelliae Fermentatae) 10g.
    Bai Zhi (Radix Angelicae Dahuricae) 6g.
    Chen Pi (Pericarpium Citri Reticulatae) 6g.
    Hou Po (Cortex Magnoliae Officinalis) 5g.
    Jie Geng (Radix Platycodi) 5g.
    Zhi Gan Cao (Radix Glycyrrhizae Preaparata) 5g.

● Administration: The original prescription is used as powder which is taken with fluid for decocting *Sheng Jiang* (Rhizoma Zingiberis Recens) and *Da Zao* (Fructus Ziziphi Jujubae). Now, the drugs, together with 3 pcs. of *Sheng Jiang* and 2 pcs of *Da Zao*, are decocted in water for two times. The decoction of the two times are mixed and again be divided into two doses, one dose for the morning and the other for the evening.

● Functions: Expel exterior pathogens and eliminate dampness, regulating Qi and the middle *Jiao*.

● Indications: For cases due to the affection of wind-cold and stagnation of dampness in the interior, manifested as vomiting, diarrhea, fever and chills, headache, stuffiness in the chest, borborygmus, abdominal pain, and white sticky tongue coating.

● Explanation:

Huo Xiang: the principal drug, acrid in taste, warm in nature and fragrant in smell, expelling exterior pathogens, regulating the middle *Jiao*, removing dampness.

Zi Su and *Bai Zhi*: the assistant drugs, acrid in taste, warm in nature and fragrant in smell, strengthening the effects of *Huo Xiang*.

Ban Xia Qu, *Chen Pi*, *Hou Po* and *Da Fu Pi*: acrid and bitter in taste, expelling external pathogens and descending turbidity, promoting Qi and eliminating dampness, lowering the adverse rising of Qi to stopping vomiting, and relieving distension in the stomach.

Bai Zhu and *Fu Ling*: reinforcing Qi and spleen, dispelling dampness, stopping diarrhea.

Jie Geng: promoting lung's dispersing function so as to promote the circulation of water, used as adjuvant drug.

Sheng Jiang, *Da Zao* and *Gan Cao*: the guiding drugs, regulating the functions of the spleen and stomach and harmonizing the effects of the drugs in the prescription.

○ The prescription as a whole performs the effects of expelling exterior wind cold and eliminating the interior dampness, regulating Qi and the middle *Jiao*.

● Notes:

(1) This prescription is indicated for cases of common cold (digestive type), acute gastroenteritis due to the affection of exogenous wind-cold and stagnation of dampness in the interior. It is especially effective for the cases with disfunction of gastrointestine due to external pathogens in summer. The prescription is also applicable for cases of sunstroke due to summer-heat and dampness, manifested as sudden irritability, or even coma and deafness and for vomiting and diarrhea appearing when a person is not acclimatized.

(2) In the prescription, there are a lot of drugs which are of acrid taste, fragrant smell and warm and dry nature, and they are good at treating dampness in the spleen and stomach accompanied by cold. Cases of severe internal heat or *Yin* deficiency without dampness should not be treated with this recipe.

(3) There are fluid and capsule forms of this formula. They are very convenient for common use.

Ping Wei San (Peptic Powder)

● Source: *Tai Ping Hui Min He Ji Ju Fang* (Prescriptions of Peaceful Benevolent Dispensary)

● Ingredients: *Cang Zhu* (Rhizoma Atractylodis) 15g.

Hou Po (Cortex Magnoliae Officinalis, fried with ginger juice) 9g.

Chen Pi (Pericarpium Citri Reticulatae) 9g.

Zhi Gan Cao (Radix Glycyrrhizae Praeparata) 5g.

Sheng Jiang (Rhizoma Zingiberis Recens) 2 pcs.

Da Zao (Fructus Ziziphi Jujubae) 2 pcs.

● Administration: Ground the drugs into powder, 6g. each time, taking with fluid for decocting *Sheng Jiang* and *Da Zao*. Now, it is often used as decoction.

● Functions: Eliminate dampness and promote the circulation of *Qi*, strengthen the spleen and regulate the stomach.

● Indications: For disorders of the spleen and stomach due to stagnation of dampness in the middle *Jiao*, manifested as abdominal distension, anorexia, vomiting, nausea, loose stools, tiredness, thick and sticky tongue coating, and moderate pulse.

● Explanation:

Cang Zhu: the principal drug, bitter in taste and warm in nature, drying dampness and promoting the functions of the spleen.

Hou Po: the assistant drug, bitter and acrid in taste and warm in nature, promoting the circulation of *Qi*, drying dampness, and relieving distension.

Chen Pi: the adjuvant drug, fragrant in smell and warm in nature, promoting *Qi* circulation, eliminating dampness, and regulating the functions of the stomach.

Zhi Gan Cao: reinforcing the middle *Jiao*, regulating the nature of the drugs in the prescription.

Sheng Jiang and *Da Zao*: the guiding drugs, regulating the functions of the spleen and stomach.

○ The prescription as a whole performs the functions of eliminating dampness, regulating the circulation of *Qi*, strengthening the functions of the spleen and stomach.

● Notes:

(1) This is a representative prescription for treating the cases with stagnation of dampness in the middle *Jiao*. It is indicated for abdominal distension appearing in chronic gastritis, gastroptosis, gastrointestinal neurosis, acute gastroenteritis.

Cases of un-acclimatization just arrived to a damp place with affection of mountainous evil air can also be treated by this prescription.

(2) This prescription is suitable for the treatment of excessive syndromes, and it should not be used often as tonics for reinforcing the spleen. Spleen deficiency without dampness, *Yin* deficiency and pregnant women should not be treated with this prescription.

5.2 Clearing Away Heat and Eliminating Dampness

The prescriptions for clearing away heat and eliminating dampness are indicated for syndromes of internal or external damp-heat, or damp-heat flowing downward.

Yin Chen Hao Tang (Oriental Wormwood Decoction)

● Source: *Shang Han Lun* (Treatise on Cold-Induced Diseases)
● Ingredients: *Yin Chen* (Herba Artemisiae Capillaris) 30g.
　　　　　　　Zhi Zi (Fructus Gardeniae) 15g.
　　　　　　　Da Huang (Radix et Rhizoma Rhei) 9g.
● Administration: The drugs are decocted in water, and *Yin Chen* should be decocted first for some time and then put in *Zhi Zi* and *Da Huang*.
● Functions: Clear away heat, eliminate dampness and relieve jaundice.
● Indications: Damp-heat type jaundice, characterized by fever, bright yellowish colour of the sclera and skin, constipation, yellow urine, distension in the chest and abdomen, dry mouth, yellow sticky tongue coating, slippery rapid or deep and forceful pulse.
● Explanation:
Yin Chen: the principal drug, bitter in taste and cold in nature, clearing away heat, eliminating dampness and relieving jaundice.
Zhi Zi: the assistant drug, bitter in taste and cold in nature, dredging *Sanjiao*, eliminating damp-heat through urination.
Da Huang: the adjuvant drug, bitter in taste and cold in nature, promoting bowel movement so as to remove heat and stagnation and to make damp-heat going out from the stool.
○ The prescription as a whole enters the *Qi* and blood systems to clear away heat, eliminate dampness and treat jaundice.
● Notes:
(1) The prescription is applicable to cases of acute icteric hepatitis, cholecystitis, cholelithiasis, acute pancreatitis, etc., which are attributive to stagnation of damp-heat and also for cases of early cirrhosis of liver, and cancer of the liver.
(2) It is not applicable to cases of *Yin* type jaundice.

Er Miao Wan (Two Wonderful Drugs Pill)

● Source: *Dan Xi Xin Fa* (Danxi's Experiential Therapy)
● Ingredients: *Cang Zu* (Rhizoma Atractylodis) 15g.
　　　　　　　Huang Bai (Cortex Phellodendri) 15g.
● Administration: Grind the drugs into powder or be prepared into water pills. Taking 5g. each time with water. Now the drugs can also be decocted in water for oral administration.

- Functions: Clear away heat and dry dampness.
- Indications: syndromes of downward-attacking of damp-heat, manifested as flaccidity of the lower limbs, redness, swelling and hot sensation over the knees and legs, and yellow greasy tongue coating. Eczema at leg, morbid leukorrhea due to damp-heat, stranguria with turbid urine can also be treated with this prescription.
- Explanation:

Huang Bai: bitter in taste and cold in nature, clearing away heat and drying dampness.

Cang Zhu: bitter in taste and warm in nature, drying dampness.

○ Two drugs together perform the effects of clearing the heat and drying the dampness.
- Notes:

(1) It is a common prescription for clearing away damp-heat from the lower *Jiao*, used as a basic prescription for the cases of rheumatic arthritis, beriberi, vulvitis, eczema at scrotum region which are due to damp-heat.

(2) It is not applicable for cases due to stagnation of cold-dampness in the lower *Jiao*.
Appendix:

San Miao Wan (Three Wonderful Drugs Pill)
- Source: *Yi Xue Zheng Zhuan* (Orthodox Medical Problems)
- Ingredients: *Huang Bai* (Certex Phllodendri) 120g.

        Cang Zhu (Rhizoma Atractylodis) 180g.

        Chuan Niu Xi (Radix Cyathulae) 60g.
- Administration: Ground into powder and prepared in pills as the size of Chinese parasol seed, 50-70 pills per dose. Take the pills with ginger soup or salty water while the stomach is empty.
- Functions: It has the effects of clearing away heat and drying dampness, for the cases of numbness of foot or with burning heat due to damp-heat flowing downward.

San Ren Tang (Decoction of Three Kinds of Kernels)

- Source: *Wen Bing Tiao Bian* (Treatise on Differentiation and Treatment of Epidemic Febrile Diseases)
- Ingredients: *Xing Ren* (Semen Armeniacae Amarum) 15g.

        Hua Shi (Talcum) 18g.

        Bai Tong Cao (Medulla Tetrapanacis) 6g.

        Bai Kou Ren (Semen Amomi Rotundus) 6g.

        Zhu Ye (Herba Lophatheri) 6g.

        Hou Po (Cortex Magnoliae Officinalis) 6g.

        Sheng Yi Ren (Semen Coicis) 18g.

        Ban Xia (Rhizoma Pinelliae) 10g.
- Administration: The drugs are decocted in water for oral dose.

- Functions: Promote functional activities of Qi, clear away damp-heat.

- Indications: For the initial stage of damp-heat syndrome, marked by chills, less sweating, heavy sensation over the head and body, oppression feeling in the chest and epigastric region, afternoon fever, white sticky tongue coating, wiry, thready and soft pulse.

- Explanation:

Xing Ren: acrid and bitter in taste, warm in nature, promoting the dispersing function of the lung.

Bai Kou Ren: resolving dampness with its fragrant smell, activating Qi to ease the middle *Jiao*.

Yi Yi Ren: Sweet, mild in taste, eliminate dampness through urination. The above three are the principal drugs.

Hua Shi, *Tong Cao* and *Zhu Ye*: sweet in taste and cold in nature, helping *Yi Yi Ren* to clear away damp-heat, used as assistant drugs.

Ban Xia and *Hou Po*: the adjuvant and guiding drugs, regulating Qi to remove dampness and relieving stuffy sensation in the abdomen.

○ The prescription as a whole has the functions of promoting lung's dispersing function at the upper *Jiao*, regulating the middle *Jiao*, and removing the dampness from the lower *Jiao* through urination, and clearing away heat.

- Notes:

(1) It is applicable for cases of ileotyphus typhoid, gastroenteritis, pyelonephritis, which are attributive to the type of more dampness and less heat with stagnation of Qi, and the prescription may also be for cases after infusion with heavy sensation of the body, oppression in the chest, and white and greasy tongue coating, etc.

(2) It is not advisable for the cases of damp-heat disease that heat is more than dampness.

Ba Zheng San (Eight Health Restoring Powder)

- Source: *Tai Ping Hui Min He Ji Ju Fang* (Prescriptions of Peaceful Benevolent Dispensary)

- Ingredients: *Qu Mai* (Herba Dianthi) 10g.

  Mu Tong (Caulis Akebiae) 5g.

  Bian Xu (Herba Polygoni Avicularis) 10g.

  Che Qian Zi (Semen Plantaginis) 10g.

  Hua Shi (Talcum) 10g.

  Sheng Shan Zhi (Fructus Gardeniae) 6g.

  Shou Da Huang (Radix et Rhizoma Rhei, roasted) 6g.

  Gan Cao (Radix Glycyrrhizae) 3g.

  Deng Xin Cao (Medulla Junci) 1.5g.

- Administration: The drugs will be decocted in water for oral administration.

● Functions: Clear away heat, reduce fire, promote urination to relieve stranguria.

● Indications: For cases of stranguria caused by heat, urinary stone, or stranguria with blood due to heat-dampness, manifested as dysuria, dripping of urine, or even retention of urine, fullness of lower abdomen, thirst, irritability, yellow greasy tongue coating, slippery rapid pulse.

● Explanation:

Qu Mai and *Bian Xu*: the principal drugs, bitter in taste and cold in nature, promoting urination to relieve stranguria, clearing away damp-heat from the lower *Jiao*.

Che Qian Zi, *Hua Shi* and *Deng Xin Cao*: the assistant drugs, clearing away heat and eliminating dampness, promoting urination to relieve stranguria.

Zhi Zi and *Da Huang*: the adjuvant drugs, bitter in taste and cold in nature, clearing away heat and reducing fire.

Gan Cao: coordinating the actions of various ingredients in the prescription, and relieving pain.

○ The prescription as a whole has the effects of clearing away heat, reducing fire, promoting urination and relieving stranguria.

● Notes:

(1) It can be used for treating cystitis, urethritis, urinary stone, acute nephritis, pyelonephritis, which are attributive to attack of damp-heat in the lower *Jiao*, also for the cases of bladder cancer with stranguria due to heat.

(2) Most ingredients in the prescription are bitter and cold, having the effects of promoting urination, therefore the prescription is indicated for cases of stranguria due to damp-heat, but not for cases of persistent stranguria with deficiency of antipathogenic *Qi*.

5.3 Warming *Yang* to Eliminate Dampness

The prescriptions for warming *Yang* to eliminate dampness are indicated for the cases of edema due to cold-dampness or *Yang* deficiency.

Zhen Wu Tang (Decoction for Strengthening the Spleen and Kidney *Yang*)

● Source: *Shang Han Lun* (Treatise on Cold-Induced Diseases)
● Ingredients: *Fu Zi* (Radix Aconiti Praeparata) 9g.

             Fu Ling (Poria) 9g.

             Bai Shao (Radix Paeoniae Alba) 9g.

             Bai Zhu (Rhizoma Atractylodis Macrocephalae) 6g.

             Sheng Jiang (Rhizoma Zingiberis Recens) 9g.

● Administration: Decoct the drugs in water for oral administration.
● Functions: Warm *Yang*, promot urination.
● Indications: For cases due to deficiency of the spleen and kidney *Yang* and retention

of dampness in the interior, marked by dysuria, pain and heavy sensation of limbs, general edema, abdominal pain, diarrhea, unthirst, white tongue coating, and deep pulse.

● Explanation:

Fu Zi: the principal drug, acrid in taste and hot in nature, warming the spleen and kidney *Yang*.

Fu Ling and *Bai Zhu*: the assistant drugs, reinforcing the spleen and promoting water metabolism.

Bai Shao: the adjuvant drug, relieving pain and promoting urination.

Sheng Jiang: the guiding drug, acrid in taste and warm in nature, dispersing water.

○ The prescription as a whole has the effects of warming the kidney *Yang* to eliminate cold, strengthening the function of the spleen to promote water metabolism.

● Notes:

(1) It is indicated for the cases of chronic enteritis, cardiogenic edema, nephritic edema, auditory vertigo, chronic hepatic edema, which are due to deficiency of the spleen and kidney.

(2) *Fu Zi* used in the prescription should be specially prepared.

5.4 Dispelling Wind and Dampness

The prescriptions for dispelling wind and dampness are indicated for cases with *Bi* syndrome due to wind-dampness.

Gui Zhi Shao Yao Zhi Mu Tang (Decoction of Cinnamomi, Paeoniae and Anemarrhenae)

● Source: *Jin Gui Yao Lue* (Synopsis of Prescriptions of the Golden Chamber)
● Ingredients: *Gui Zhi* (Ramulus Cinnamomi) 12g.

    Bai Shao (Radix Paeoniae Alba) 9g.

    Zhi Mu (Anemarrhena) 12g.

    Sheng Jiang (Rhizoma Zingiberis Recens) 15g.

    Bai Zhu (Rhizoma Atractylodis Macrocephalae) 15g.

    Fang Feng (Radix Ledebouriellae) 12g.

    Ma Huang (Herba Ephedrae) 6g.

    Zhi Fu Pian (Radix Aconiti Praeparata) 6g.

    Zhi Gan Cao (Radix Glycyrrhizae Praeparata) 6g.

● Administration: The drugs are decocted in water. One decoction per day, taking in 3 times.

● Functions: Dispel wind and dampness, clear away heat and relieve pain.

● Indications: *Bi* syndrome due to wind, cold and dampness, changing to heat and mixture of cold and heat, manifested as pain, swelling and burning sensation of the joints, emaciation and weakness of the body, dizziness, and short breath, etc.

● Explanation:

Gui Zhi, *Ma Huang* and *Fang Feng*: the principal drugs, acrid in taste and warm in nature, warming *Yang* and dispelling wind-cold.

Fu Zi: acrid in taste and hot in nature.

Bai Zhu: bitter in taste and warm in nature.

Both of them are the assistant drugs, warming the meridians and dispelling cold and dampness.

Bai Shao and *Zhi Mu*: the adjuvant drugs, regulating *Yin* to prevent the transformation of wind, cold and dampness into heat.

Sheng Jiang and *Gan Cao*: the guiding drugs, regulating the function of the middle *Jiao*.

○ The prescription as a whole performs the functions of dispelling wind and cold, clearing heat and relieving pain.

● Notes:

(1) It is indicated for the cases of *Bi* syndrome due to wind, cold and dampness, and the pathogens just start to transform to heat, seen in rheumatoid arthritis and ankylosing spondylitis.

(2) Both cold and hot nature drugs are used in the prescription, therefore clinically it is necessary to make a variation to the prescription according to patients' conditions. If the main symptom is pain and stiffness of joints which may be relieved with warmth, use more drugs with acrid in taste and hot in nature, such as *Ma Huang*, *Fu Zi*, *Gui Zhi*. If the pain with obvious burning sensation, use more *Bai Shao*, *Zhi Mu*, *Gan Cao* and plus *Sheng Di* (Radix Rehmanniae) and *Ren Dong Teng* (Caulis Lonicerae).

Du Huo Ji Sheng Tang (Pubescent Anbgelica and Loranthus Decoction)

● Source: *Qian Jin Fang* (Prescriptions Worth a Thousand Gold for Emergencies)
● Ingredients: *Du Huo* (Radix Angelicae Pubescentis) 10g.

                Sang Ji Sheng (Ramulus Loranthi) 15g.

                Qin Jiao (Radix Gentianae Macrophyllae) 10g.

                Fang Feng (Radix Ledebouriellae) 10g.

                Xi Xin (Herba Asari) 3-6g.

                Dang Gui (Rhizoma Angelicae Sinensis) 10g.

                Chuan Xiong (Rhizoma Ligustici Chuanxiong) 10g.

                Gan Di Huang (Radix Rehmanniae) 12g.

                Niu Xi (Radix Achyranthis Bidentatae) 10g.

                Du Zhong (Cortex Eucommiae) 10g.

                Fu Ling (Poria) 10g.

                Gui Xin (Lignum Cinnamomi) 3g.

                Ren Sheng (Radix Ginseng) 5g.

Shao Yao (Radix Paeoniae Alba) 6g.

Gan Cao (Radix Glycyrrhizae) 5g.

● Administration: The drugs are decocted in water. One decoction per day, taking in twice.

● Functions: Dispel wind and dampness, relieve pain, reinforce the liver and kidney, nourish *Qi* and blood.

● Indications: For the wind-cold *Bi* syndrome due to deficiency of the liver and kidney and deficiency of *Qi* and blood, marked by cold pain in lumbar region and knee, limited mobility, flaccidity, numbness of joints, aversion to cold and desire for warmth, palpitation, short breath, pale tongue with white coating, thready weak pulse.

● Explanation:

Du Huo: the principal drug, acrid and bitter in taste, warm in nature, entering the kidney meridian, dispelling wind, cold and dampness in the lower *Jiao* and between tendons and bones.

Xi Xin and *Fang Feng*: acrid in taste and warm in nature.

Qin Jiao: bitter and acrid in taste and little cold in nature.

Both are used to dispel wind-cold and relieve pain.

Sang Ji Sheng, *Du Zhong* and *Niu Xi*: dispelling wind and dampness, reinforcing the kidney and liver, strengthening lumbum and knee, as the assistant drugs.

Dang Gui, *Ren Shen*, *Fu Ling*, *Sheng Di*, *Chuan Xiong* and *Bai Shao*: nourishing *Qi* and blood.

Gui Xin: warming the meridians to promote the circulation of blood.

The above seven are used as the adjuvant drugs.

Gan Cao: the guiding drug, coordinating the actions of all ingredients in the prescription.

○ The prescription has the functions of dispelling wind and dampness, relieving pain, reinforcing the liver and kidney, and nourishing *Qi* and blood.

● Notes:

(1) The prescription has both functions of strengthening the body resistance and eliminating pathogens, indicated for the cases with prolonged *Bi* syndrome with combination of excess and deficiency, marked by cold pain in lumbar and knee, pale tongue with white coating, thready weak pulse. It can be used for the cases of rheumatic arthritis, over strain of lumbar muscles, sciatica, hyperosteogeny, etc. which are due to deficiency of the liver and kidney and deficiency of *Qi* and blood. It is also used for pregnant women whoes lumbar and leg pain aggravated during the pregnancy.

(2) The dosage of *Xi Xin* is usually 2-3g.

5.5　Removing Dampness by Promoting Diuresis

The prescriptions for removing dampness and promoting diuresis are indicated for the cases of dysuria, stranguria with turbid urine, edema, diarrhea, etc. which are due to reten-tion of water and dampness in the body.

Wu Ling San (Powder of Five Drugs with Poria)

- Source: *Shang Han Lun* (Treatise on Cold-Induced Diseases)
- Ingredients: *Fu Ling* (Poria) 9g.

  Zhu Ling (Polyporus Umbellatus) 9g.

  Ze Xie (Rhizoma Alismatis) 15g.

  Bai Zhu (Rhizoma Atractylodis Macrocephalae) 9g.

  Gui Zhi (Ramulus Cinnamomi) 6g.

- Administration: Make the above into powder and take 3-6g. each time or the drugs will be decocted in water for oral administration.
- Functions: Strengthe the spleen to eliminate dampness, activate Qi-transforming function to induce diuresis.
- Indications: For cases due to retention of water and dampness in the interior and affection of wind-cold at the exterior, manifested as headache, fever, dysuria, or restlessness with desire for drinks, vomiting after drinking, white and greasy tongue coating, and floating pulse; also for cases of edema, heavyness sensation over the body, dysuria, diarrhea caused by retention of water and dampness in the interior or vomiting, diarrhea attributive to summer-heat and dampness.
- Explanation:

Ze Xie: the principal drug, sweet and mild in taste and cold in nature, removing dampness and promoting diuresis.

Fu Ling and *Zhu Ling*: the assistant drugs, sweet and mild in taste and neutral in nature, strengthening the effect of the principal drugs.

Bai Zhu: reinfrocing the functions of the spleen and drying dampness.

Gui Zhi: warming *Yang*, activating *Qi* and promoting diuresis.

The above two are the adjuvant and guiding drugs.

○ The prescription as a whole performs the functions of reinforcing the functions of the spleen to eliminate dampness, activating Qi-transforming function to induce diuresis.

- Notes:

(1) It is commonly used for cases of nephritic edema, vomiting and diarrhea in gastroenteritis, cardiopathy, cirrhosis with dysuria etc. Dysuria and retention of urine due to spasm of sphincter vesicae after abdominal operation can also be treated with this prescription.

(2) It is forbidden for the cases of dysuria which belong to the type of *Yin* deficiency.

Wu Pi Yin (Decoction Containing Five Kinds of Peel)

- Source: *Hua Shi Zhong Zang Jing* (Hua's Precious Classics)

- Ingredients: *Fu Ling Pi* (Poria) 9g.

    Chen Pi (Pericarpium Citri Reticulatae) 9g.

    Sheng Jiang Pi (Cortex Zingiberis) 9g.

    Da Fu Pi (Pericarpium Arecae) 9g.

    Sang Bai Pi (Cortex Mori Radicis) 9g.

- Administration: The drugs are to be decocted in water for oral administration.

- Functions: Strengthen the function of the spleen, regulate *Qi*, promote diuresis to relieve edema.

- Indications: Retention of dampness due to deficiency of the spleen, general edema, distention in chest and abdomen, asthma, short breath, dysuria, edema during pregnancy, white and greasy tongue coating, and deep moderate pulse.

- Explanation:

Fu Ling Pi: the principal drug, mild sweet in taste and neutral in nature, dispelling dampness, strengthening the spleen and regulating the middle *Jiao*.

Chen Pi: the assistant drug, fragrant smell which is good to eliminate dampness and regulate *Qi* and the middle *Jiao*.

Sang Bai Pi: descending the adverse rising of the lung *Qi*, regulating water metabolism.

Da Fu Pi: activating *Qi* to relieve distention and eliminating dampness.

Sheng Jiang Pi: dispeling the water retention in the body by acrid taste.

○ The prescription as a whole performs the functions of strengthening the spleen and promoting diuresis, activating *Qi* and relieving edema.

- Notes:

The prescription is used to treat subcutaneous edema and applicable to cases of mild edema which affects only the shallow portion, such as edema due to nephritis, heart diseases which belongs to the type of water retention due to spleen deficiency, and ascites of early cirrhosis.

Zhu Ling Tang (Umbellate Pore Decoction)

- Source: *Shang Han Lun* (Treatise on Cold-Induced Diseases)
- Ingredients: *Zhu Ling* (Polyporus Umbellatus) 9g.

    Fu Ling (Poria) 9g.

    Ze Xie (Rhizoma Alismatis) 9g.

    E Jiao (Colla Corii Asini) 9g.

    Hua Shi (Talcum) 9g.

- Administration: The drugs are decocted in water, but *E Jiao* should be melted with the hot decoction.

- Functions: Promote diuresis, clear away heat and nourish *Yin*.

- Indications: For cases due to retention of water and heat in the interior, manifested as dysuria, fever, irritability, insomnia, or hematuria, stranguria, and lower abdominal distension, etc.

● Explanation:

Zhu Ling: the principal drug, sweet and mild in taste, eliminating dampness and promoting diuresis.

Fu Ling: strengthening the spleen to eliminate dampness.

Ze Xie and *Hua Shi*: sweet and mild in taste, cold in nature, promoting diuresis and clearing heat.

The above three are assistant drugs.

E Jiao: the adjuvant and guiding drug, nourishing the kidney *Yin* to prevent impairment of *Yin* by drugs for eliminating dampness and promoting diuresis.

○ The prescription as a whole performs the functions of promoting diuresis without impairing *Yin*, nourishing *Yin* without retaining evil factors, and clearing away heat.

● Notes:

It can be used for cases of urinary infection, urinary stone, nephritis, cystitis manifested as frequent urination, stranguria and hematuria, which belong to the type of retention of water and heat with impairment of *Yin*.

Summary

The 12 main prescriptions for eliminating dampness are subdivided into 5 categories: drying dampness and regulating the stomach, clearing away heat and dampness, warming *Yang* to resolve dampness, dispelling wind and dampness, and removing dampness by promoting diuresis.

(1) Drying dampness and regulating the stomach

Both *Ping Wei San* and *Huo Xiang Zheng Qi San* are the prescriptions for drying dampness and regulating the stomach. *Ping Wei San* is particularly for drying dampness and activating *Qi*, and it is the basic prescription for cases due to stagnation of dampness in the spleen and stomach. *Huo Xiang Zheng Qi San* also has the effect of dispelling wind-cold and is a commonly used prescription for cases of stagnation of dampness in the body with affection of external wind-cold.

(2) Clearing away heat and dampness

Yin Chen Hao Tang has the effects of clearing the heat and dampness, relieving jaundice. It is a special prescription for damp-heat type jaundice. *Er Miao San* is used to clear the heat and dry the dampness, a basic prescription for cases with flaccidity of lower limbs, sores due to dampness, morbid leukorrhea due to retention of damp-heat in lower *Jiao*. *Ba Zheng San* is to clear heat and reduce fire, promote diuresis and relieve stranguria. It is a representative prescription for *Lin* Stranguria) syndrome, the cases with stranguria due to retention of damp-heat in the lower *Jiao*. *San Ren Tang* is good to activate *Qi* circulation, clear the dampness and heat. It is commonly used for cases in the initial stage of damp-heat syndrome with more dampness and less heat.

(3) Warming *Yang* to resolve dampness

Zhen Wu Tang has the effect of warming *Yang* to eliminate dampness. It is a common prescription for cases with general edema, dysuria, pain and heavy sensation in limbs due to retention of water in the body caused by *Yang* deficiency.

(4) Dispelling wind and dampness

Gui Zhi Shao Yao Zhi Mu Tang has the effects of dispelling wind and dampness, clearing away heat and relieving pain. It is indicated for *Bi* syndromes with pain, swelling and hot sensation of joints due to accumulation of wind, cold and dampness, or in the early stage of formation of heat. *Du Huo Ji Sheng Tang* is used to dispel wind-dampness, relieve pain, reinforce the liver and kidney, strengthen *Qi* and blood, indicated for cases with cold pain in lumbar region and knee, soreness and weakness of legs due to deficiency of the liver and kidney and insufficiency of *Qi* and blood.

(5) Removing dampness by promoting diuresis

Wu Ling San and *Zhu Ling* Tang are all the prescriptions for promoting diuresis, and they can be used for cases with dysuria (scanty urine). *Wu Ling San* also has the effects of warming *Yang*, activating *Qi* and expelling evils from the body surface. It is indicated for syndrome due to accumulation of water in the body, both *Taiyang* meridian and its organ are affected. *Zhu Ling Tang* is used to clear away heat and nourish *Yin* so that to treat cases due to retention of water and heat, injury of *Yin* by heat. *Wu Pi Yin* has the effect of reinforcing the spleen and regulating *Qi*, promoting diuresis to relieve edema, indicated for cases of general edema due to deficiency of the spleen and excess of dampness.

Review Questions

(1) What are the indications of the prescriptions for drying dampness and regulating the stomach? Write out the explanation and indications of *Ping Wei San*.

(2) Analyze the functions, indications and ingredients of *Yin Chen Hao Tang*.

(3) What are the indications of *San Ren Tang*? Analyze the effects and ingredients.

(4) What are the differences and similarities between *Wu Ling San* and *Zhu Ling Tang* in ingredients and indications?

(5) What are the ingredients of *Du Huo Ji Sheng Tang*? What kind of *Bi* syndrome is it indicated for?

(6) Try to write out the indications, functions and explanation of *Zhen Wu Tang*.

6　Phlegm-Eliminating Prescriptions

Those composed of phlegm-eliminating drugs, with the effect of removing the retention of phlegm and fluids and for the treatment of various phlegm diseases, are generally known as phlegm-eliminating prescriptions.

According to the nature, phlegm can be divided into damp phlegm, heat phlegm and wind phlegm, etc. Phlegm-eliminating prescriptions can be divided into four kinds: the prescriptions for warming and resolving phlegm-fluid, the prescriptions for clearing away heat and removing phlegm, the prescriptions for treating wind and resolving phlegm and the prescriptions for eliminating phlegm-fluid.

Phlegm-eliminating prescriptions should be associated with drugs for regulating Qi because smooth movement of Qi will help to resolve phlegm. In addition, phlegm-eliminating drugs are those with effects for circulating and reducing, which can not be taken for a long time. Stop taking it as soon as the disease is cured.

6.1　Prescriptions for Warming and Resolving Phlegm-fluid

This group of recipes is indicated for syndromes caused by damp-phlegm and cold-phlegm.

Er Chen Tang (Two Old Drugs Decoction)

● Source: *Tai Ping Hui Min He Ji Ju Fang* (Prescriptions of Peaceful Benevolent Dispensary)

● Ingredients: *Ban Xia* (Rhizoma Pinelliae) 15g.

　　　　　　　Ju Hong (Pericarpium Citri Reticulatae) 15g.

　　　　　　　Fu Ling (Poria) 9g.

　　　　　　　Zhi Gan Cao (Radix Glycyrrhizae Praeparata) 5g.

　　　　　　　Sheng Jiang (Rhizoma Zingiberis Recens) 3g.

　　　　　　　Wu Mei (Fructus Mume) 1pcs.

● Administration: All the drugs should be decocted in water for oral use. Generally, *Wu Mei* may not be used.

● Functions: Dry dampness and remove phlegm, regulate Qi and harmonize the middle *Jiao*.

● Indications: Damp-phlegm syndrome manifested by cough with profuse sputum, nausea, vomiting, fullness and suffocation sensation in the chest and diaphragm, dizziness, palpitation, white and moist or thin greasy coating of the tongue and slippery pulse.

● Explanation:

Ban Xia: the principal drug, acrid in taste and warm in nature, having the effect of drying dampness to remove phlegm and reducing upward perversion of Qi to stop vomiting.

Ju Hong: the assistant drug, acrid and bitter in taste and warm in nature, playing the effect of regulating Qi, drying dampness and removing phlegm.

Fu Ling: an adjuvant drug which can invigorate the spleen and resolve dampness to prevent the gathering of dampness and production of phlegm.

Zhi Gan Cao: harmonizing the middle *Jiao* and invigorating the spleen.

Sheng Jiang: lowering the upward perversion to remove phlegm and also reducing the toxic effect of *Ban Xia*.

Wu Mei: small dosage, used to prevent the dispersing of the lung Qi.

The above three dugs are used as guiding drugs.

○ The combination of all these drugs plays the effect of drying dampness to remove phlegm, regulating Qi and harmonizing the middle *Jiao*.

● Notes:

This is a basic recipe to treat phlegm-damp syndrome, or to treat all kinds of phlegm syndrome by adding or omitting some drugs. Clinically it is often used to treat damp-phlegm syndrome, such as chronic bronchitis, pulmonary emphysema, chronic gastritis, otogenic dizziness, cerebral-vascular accident, pregnant morning sickness, sleepiness and infantile salivation. By adding some other drugs, this recipe can also treat heavyness, pain and numbness of the arm after drinking alcohol.

Appendix:

(1) *Jin Shui Liu Jun Jian* (Decoction of Metal-Water Six Ingredients)

● Source: *Jing Yue Quan Shu* (Complete Works of *Zhang Jing Yue*)

● Ingredients: *Er Chen Tang* plus

        Dang Gui (Radix Angelicae Sinensis) 10g.

        Shu Di (Rehmanniae Praeparata) 10g.

● Functions and indications: nourishing *Yin* and removing phlegm, indicated for phlegm due to upward attacking of water-dampness caused by deficient cold of the lung and kidney, or cough with a lot of sputum due to interior excess of damp-phlegm, or cough with nausea and profuse sputum, dyspnea, thick white and greasy tongue coating and slippery pulse, seen in aged people with *Yin* and blood deficiency and affection of external wind-cold.

(2) *Ling Zhu Er Chen Jian* (Polyporus Umbellatus and Rhizoma Atractylodis Macrocephalae Two Old Drugs Decoction)

● Source: *Jing Yue Quan Shu* (Complete Works of *Zhang Jing Yue*)

● Ingredients: *Er Chen Tang* plus:

        Zhu Ling (Polyporus Umbellatus) 5g.

        Bai Zhu (Rhizoma Atractylodis Macrocephalae) 3g.

        Ze Xie (Rhizoma Alismatis) 5g.

        Gan Jiang (Rhizoma Zingiberis) 1.5g.

● Functions and indications: invigorating the spleen, removing phlegm, warming the middle *Jiao*, removing stagnation, circulating *Qi* and inducing diuresis, indicated for retention of phlegm-fluid due to deficient cold of the spleen and stomach, manifested as diarrhea, semi-liquid stool, anorexia, lassitude, cough with white and thin sputum.

(3) *Wen Dan Tang* (Decoction for Clearing Gallbladder Heat)

● Source: *Qian Jin Fang* (Prescriptions Worth a Thousand Gold For Emergencies)

● Ingredients: *Er Chen Tang* minus *Wu Mei* and plus:

Zhu Ru (Caulis Bambusae in Taeniam) 10g.

Zhi Shi (Fructus Aurantii Immaturus) 10g.

Da Zao (Fructus Ziziphi Jujubae) 4pcs.

● Functions and indications: regulating *Qi*, removing phlegm, clearing gallbladder heat and harmonizing stomach, indicated for interior disturbance of phlegm heat caused by disharmony between gallbladder and stomach, manifested as restlessness of deficient type, insomnia, bitter taste in the mouth, suffocation in the chest, nausea, vomiting, or palpitation and epilepsy.

Xiao Qing Long Tang (Small Blue Dragon Decoction)

● Source: *Shang Han Lun* (Treatise on Cold-Induced Diseases)

● Ingredients: *Ma Huang* (Herba Ephedrae) 9g.

Shao Yao (Radix Paeoniae) 9g.

Xi Xin (Herba Asari) 3g.

Gan Jiang (Rhizoma Zingiberis) 6g.

Zhi Gan Cao (Radix Glycyrrhizae Praeparata) 6g.

Gui Zhi (Ramulus Cinnamomi) 9g.

Ban Xia (Rhizoma Pinelliae) 9g.

Wu Wei Zi (Fructus Schisandrae) 3g.

● Administration: All the drugs should be decocted in water for oral use.

● Functions: Relieve exterior syndrome, eliminate fluid, stop cough and relieve asthma.

● Indications: Suffering from exogenous wind-cold, together with interior phlegm fluid, manifestd as aversion to cold, fever, no perspiration, cough, asthma, spitting of thin and profuse sputum, or heavy sensation of the body, edema on the head, face and four limbs, white and moist coating of the tongue and floating pulse.

● Explanation:

Ma Huang and *Gui Zhi*: the principal drugs, acrid in taste and warm in nature, relieving exterior syndrome and inducing diaphoresis, expelling exogenous cold and promoting the functions of the lung in dispersing.

Gang Jiang and *Xi Xin*: the assistant drugs, acrid in taste and hot in nature, warming the lung to remove fluid and helping the principal drugs to relieve exterior syndrome.

Wu Wei Zi: astringenting *Qi*.

Shao Yao: nourishing blood.

Ban Xia: eliminating phlegm, harmonizing stomach and dispelling masses.

These three drugs are adjuvant drugs.

Zhi Gan Cao: the guiding drug which can benefit Qi, harmonize the middle *Jiao* and coordinate the effects of the other drugs.

○ The prescription as a whole plays the effect of dispelling exogenous wind-cold, eliminating interior water-fluid, stopping cough and relieving asthma.

● Notes:

(1) This is a recipe for inducing diaphoresis and eliminating phlegm. The modified recipe can treat common cold, influenza, chronic bronchitis, bronchial asthma and pulmonary emphysema which complicated with exogenous pathogens showing exterior cold and interior fluid.

(2) It is contraindicated in cases with dry cough or with little thick sputum, or cough with yellow sticky sputum.

Appendix:

She Gan Ma Huang Tang (Decoction Rhizoma Belamcandae and Herba Ephedrae)

● Source: *Jin Gui Yao Lue* (Synopsis of Prescriptions of the Golden Chamber)

● Ingredients: *She Gan* (Rhizoma Belamcandae) 6g.

        Ma Huang (Herba Ephedrae) 9g.

        Sheng Jiang (Rhizoma Zingiberis Recens) 9g.

        Xi Xin (Herba Asari) 3g.

        Zi Yuan (Radix Asteris) 6g.

        Kuan Dong Hua (Flos Farfarae) 6g.

        Ban Xia (Rhizoma Pinelliae) 9g.

        Wu Wei Zi (Fructus Schisandrae) 3g.

        Da Zao (Fructus Ziziphi Jujubae) 3pcs.

● Functions and indications: promoting lung's dispersing function, eliminating phlegm, descending Qi and stopping cough, indicated for cough with inspiratory dyspnea and a sound in the throat resembling the croaking of a frog.

Ling Gui Zhu Gan Tang (Decoction Poria, Ramulus Cinnamomi, Rhizoma Atractylodis Macrocephalae and Radix Glycyrrhizae)

● Source: *Jin Gui Yao Lue* (Synopsis of Prescriptions of the Golden Chamber)

● Ingredients: *Fu Ling* (Poria) 12g.

        Gui Zhi (Ramulus Cinnamomi) 9g.

        Bai Zhu (Rhizoma Atractylodis Macrocephalae) 6g.

        Zhi Gan Cao (Radix Glycyrrhizae) 6g.

● Administration: All the drugs should be decocted in water for oral administration.

● Functions: Invigorate the spleen, resolve dampness, warm and remove phlegm-fluid.

● Indications: Phlegm fluid disease caused by insufficiency of middle *Yang* manifested as distentional fullness in the chest and costal region, cough, shortness of breath, palpitation, vertigo, white greasy tongue coating, and wiry slippery pulse.

● Explanation:

Fu Ling: the principal drug, mild sweet in taste, invigorating the spleen, inducing diuresis and resolving dampness.

Gui Zhi: the assistant drug, pungent in taste and warm in nature, warming *Yang*, resolving fluid and promoting *Qi*-transforming function of the urinary bladder to induce diuresis.

Bai Zhu: the adjuvant drug, bitter and sweet in taste and warm in nature, benefiting *Qi*, invigorating the spleen and drying dampness in order to remove the source of producing phlegm.

Zhi Gan Cao: the guiding drug, benefiting *Qi* and harmonizing the middle *Jiao*.

○ The prescription as a whole plays the effect of invigorating the spleen, resolving dampness, warming and removing phlegm fluid.

● Notes:

(1) As a mild recipe to treat phlegm fluid, it is characterized by warming but not hot, gently inducing diuresis but the drugs are not of drastic effects. The modified recipe can treat phlegm syndrome due to spleen deficiency such as chronic bronchitis, bronchial asthma, pleurisy and hydrothorax or treat diarrhea due to deficiency of spleen and excess of dampness.

(2) This recipe is a little bit warm in nature. It is not advisable for phlegm fluid syndrome with hot nature.

6.2 Heat-clearing and Phlegm-eliminating Prescriptions

This group of prescriptions is indicated for heat-phlegm syndrome.

Qing Qi Hua Tan Wan (Bolus for Clearing *Qi* and Phlegm)

● Source: *Yi Fang Kao* (Textual Research on Prescriptions)
● Ingredients: *Dan Nan Xing* (Arisaema cum Bile) 45g.

          Jiang Ban Xia (Rhizoma Pinelliae, prepared with ginger) 45g.

          Gua Lou Ren (Semen Trichosanthis) 30g.

          Chen Pi (Pericarpium Citri Reticulatae) 30g.

          Huang Qin (Radix Scutellariae) 30g.

          Xing Ren (Semen Pruni Armentiacae) 30g.

          Zhi Shi (Fructus Aurantii Immaturus) 30g.

          Fu Ling (Poria) 30g.

● Administration: The above drugs are ground into powder and mixed with ginger juice to make bolus. Take 6g. each time. These drugs can also be decocted in water for oral administration with the dosage decreased.

- ● Functions: Clear away heat, eliminate phlegm, regulate *Qi* and relieve cough.
- ● Indications: Interior accumulation of phlegm-heat manifested as cough with sticky yellow sputum which is difficult to spit out, rapid breath, nausea, fullness and stuffiness sensation in the chest and hypochondrium, scanty yellow urine, red tongue with yellow greasy coating and slippery rapid pulse.
- ● Explanation:

Dan Nan Xing: the principal drug, bitter in taste and cold in nature, clearing away heat and eliminating phlegm.

Huang Qin: bitter in taste and cold in nature.

Gua Lou: sweet in taste and cold in nature.

Both are assistant drugs which reduces the lung-fire and removes phlegm-heat.

Chen Pi and *Zhi Shi*: regulating *Qi* movement, resolving phlegm and dispelling accumulation.

Fu Ling and *Ban Xia*: invigorating the spleen to harmonize the middle *Jiao*, eliminating dampness and removing phlegm.

Xing Ren: promoting lung's dispersing function and relieving cough.

The above drugs are adjuvant and guiding drugs.

- ○ The prescription as a whole has the effects of clearing away heat, eliminating phlegm, regulating *Qi* and relieving cough.
- ● Notes:

(1) This is a commonly-used recipe for heat phlegm, which emphasizes on clearing *Qi* of heat and smoothing the movement of *Qi* in order to eliminate phlegm. The recipe can treat pneumonia and chronic bronchitis which belong to interior obstruction of phlegm-heat.

(2) It is contraindicated for cold phlegm syndrome and dry phlegm syndrome.

Xiao Xian Xiong Tang (Minor Decoction for Relieving Stuffiness in the Chest)

- ● Source: *Shang Han Lun* (Treatise on Cold-Induced Diseases)
- ● Ingredients: *Huang Lian* (Rhizoma Coptidis) 6g.

  Ban Xia (Rhizoma Pinelliae) 12g.

  Gua Lou Shi (Fructus Trichosanthis) 30g.
- ● Administration: All the drugs are decocted in water for oral administration.
- ● Functions: Clear away heat, resolve phlegm, ease the chest and disperse lumps.
- ● Indications: Phlegm and heat accumulated below the heart, marked by fullness and stuffiness in the chest and epigastrium and with pain by pressing, or cough with thick yellow sputum, yellow greasy tongue coating, floating slippery or slippery rapid pulse.
- ● Explanation:

Gua Lou Shi: the principal drug, sweet in taste and cold in nature, clearing away heat, resolving phlegm, easing the chest and benefiting *Qi*.

Huang Lian: the assistant drug, bitter in taste and cold in nature, clearing stuffiness below the heart.

Ban Xia: descending upward perversion, eliminating stuffiness, removing lumps below the heart, and together with *Huang Lian* to eliminate stuffiness and dispel accumulation because acrid taste has the effect of dispersing and bitter taste has the effect of descending.

○ The combination of all the drugs plays the effect of clearing heat, eliminating phlegm, dispelling accumulation, dispersing stuffiness and easing the chest.

● Notes:

(1) As a common recipe for treating accumulation of phlegm-heat in the chest, this prescription is characterized by the combination of dispersing with the acrid drugs and descending with the bitter drugs. The clinical diagnostic points are uncomfortable sensation below the heart and painful sensation by pressing. The modified prescription can treat syndromes of phlegm-heat accumulation seen in exudative pleurisy, bronchial pneumonia, cholecystitis and acute gastritis.

(2) This prescription is suitable for phlegm-heat syndrome in the chest and epigastrium, which takes yellow greasy tongue coating with root as its basis. If the yellow greasy tongue coating is easy to be scraped out (without root), this is deficiency of the middle *Qi* associated with damp-heat, and the prescription will not be applicable.

6.3 Prescriptions for Treating Wind and Resolving Phlegm

This group of prescriptions is indicated for wind-phlegm syndrome, which can be divided into endogenous type and exopathic type. Calming wind and resolving phlegm are good to treat phlegm produced by endogenous wind. Expelling wind and resolving phlegm are good to treat phlegm produced by exogenous wind.

Ban Xia Bai Zhu Tian Ma Tang (Decoction of Pinellia, Bighead Atractylodes and Gastrodia)

● Source: *Yi Xue Xin Wu* (Medicine Comprehended)
● Ingredients: *Ban Xia* (Rhizoma Pinelliae) 9g.
             Fu Ling (Poria) 6g.
             Bai Zhu (Rhizoma Atractylodis Macrocephalae) 15g.
             Ju Hong (Exocarpium Citri Reticulatae) 6g.
             Tian Ma (Rhizoma Gastrodiae) 6g.
             Gan Cao (Radix Glycyrrhizae) 4g.
             Sheng Jiang (Rhizoma Zingiberis Recens) 1pc.
             Da Zao (Fructus Ziziphi Jujubae) 2pc.
● Administration: All the drugs should be decocted in water for oral administration.
● Functions: Resolve phlegm, calm wind, invigorate the spleen and dry dampness.

● Indications: Upward disturbance of wind-phlegm, marked by dizziness and vertigo, headache, suffocation in the chest, nausea, white greasy tongue coating, and wiry slippery pulse.

● Explanation:

Ban Xia: acrid in taste and warm in nature, drying dampness, resolving phlegm, reducing upward peversion of *Qi* to stop vomiting.

Tian Ma: calming the liver and stopping wind.

Both are principal drugs to treat wind-phlegm.

Bai Zhu and *Fu Ling*: invigorating spleen and drying dampness.

Ju Hong: regulating *Qi* and resolving phlegm.

These three drugs are assistant drugs.

Sheng Jiang, *Da Zao* and *Gan Cao*: the adjuvant and guiding drugs, regulating the spleen and stomach and coordinate the effects of the other drugs.

○ The combination of all the drugs plays the effects of resolving phlegm, stopping wind and relieving dizziness.

● Notes:

(1) The modified prescription are used to treat auditory dizziness and vertigo, dizziness and headache due to neurasthenia associated with gastrointestinal symptoms, cerebral arteriosclerosis and cerebrovascular accident which belong to the pathology of upward disturbance of windphlegm.

(2) It is contraindicated for dizziness and headache caused by preponderance of liver *Yang*.

Zhi Sou San (Stopping Cough Powder)

● Source: *Yi Xue Xin Wu* (Medicine Comprehended)
● Ingredients: *Bai Bu* (Radix Stemonae) 9g.

　　　　　　Bai Qian (Rhizoma Cynanchi Stauntonii) 9g.

　　　　　　Zi Yuan (Radix Asteris) 9g.

　　　　　　Chen Pi (Pericarpium Citri Reticulatae) 6g.

　　　　　　Jing Jie (Herba Schizonepetae) 6g.

　　　　　　Gan Cao (Radix Glycyrrhizae) 4.5g.

　　　　　　Jie Geng (Radix Platycodi) 9g.

● Administration: All the drugs are decocted in water for oral administration.

● Functions: Relieve cough, resolve phlegm, expel exterior syndrome and promote lung's dispersing function.

● Indications: Cough due to exogenous factors, itching sensation in the throat, difficult to spit out sputum, or with slight aversion to cold, fever, thin white tongue coating.

● Explanation:

Bai Zhu, *Bai Qian* and *Zi Yuan*: the principal drugs, pungent, bitter and sweet in taste and neutral in nature, relieving cough and resolving phlegm.

Jie Geng: bitter and pungent in taste and neutral in nature, promoting the functions of the lung in dispersing so as to eliminate phlegm.

Ju Hong: regulating Qi and resolving phlegm.

Both are assistant drugs.

Jing Jie: the adjuvant drug, expelling wind to relieve exterior syndrome.

Gan Cao: a guiding drug, coordinating the effect of other drugs, with *Jie Geng* to clear the throat.

○ The prescription as a whole performs the functions of relieving cough, resolving phlegm, expelling exterior syndrome and promoting the functions of the *lung* in dispersing.

● Notes:

(1) This prescription is neutral in nature and good at relieving cough and resolving phlegm. Clinically, it treats many kinds of cough, and with modification of the prescription, we can treat cough of cold type and cough of heat type. The recipes are suitable for common cold, influenza and acute bronchitis which belong to invasion of pathogenic wind into the lung.

(2) It is not advisable for cough due to *Yin* deficiency.

6.4 Prescriptions for Eliminating Phlegm-fluid

This group of prescriptions is indicated for excess syndrome with excessive phlegm-saliva in the interior.

Kong Xian Dan (Controlling Phlegm-fluid Pill)

● Source: *San Yin Ji Yi Bing Zheng Fang Lun* (Prescriptions Assigned to the Three Categories of Pathogenic Factors of Diseases)

● Ingredients: *Gan Sui* (Radix Euphorbiae Kansui) 60g.

          Da Ji (Radix Knoxiae) 60g.

          Bai Jie Zi (Semen Sinapos Albae) 60g.

● Administration: All the drugs are ground into powder and made into pills which sizes are as big as seed of Chinese parasol. Take 5 to 7 pills each time with ginger decoction before going to bed.

● Functions: Eliminate phlegm and remove fluid.

● Indications: Phlegm-fluid retains in the chest and diaphragm region, manifested as sudden pain in the chest, back, hands, feet, waist, rib, neck and nape which is unbearable, and there is drawing and moving pain at the tendons and bones, or heavy sensation and cold pain of hands and feet, or mental lassitude and sleepiness, or poor appetite, or profuse sputum and running saliva.

● Explanation:

Da Ji: bitter and pungent in taste and cold in nature, removing water-dampness of the

Zang-fu organs.

Gan Sui: bitter and sweet in taste and cold in nature, eliminating water-dampness of meridians.

Bai Jie Zi: acrid in taste and warm in nature, expelling the phlegm inside the skin and outside membrane.

○ The combination of all the drugs plays the effect of eliminating phlegm-saliva and water fluid.

● Notes:

(1) The prescription can treat excessive phlegm-fluid caused by tracheitis and pneumonia, ascites due to cirrhosis, as well as scrofula, subcutaneous nodule, *Yang* type phlegmon, and pyogenic infection of bone, which have the above-mentioned manifestations.

(2) It is not advisable for patients with loose stool and with weak constitution.

Summary

Phlegm-eliminating prescriptions here include eight prescriptions which are divided into four types according to their functions. They are: the prescriptions for warming and resolving phlegm-fluid, the prescriptions for clearing heat and removing phlegm, the prescriptions for treating wind and resolving phlegm and the prescriptions for eliminating phlegm-fluid.

(1) Prescriptions for warming and resolving phlegm-fluid

This group of prescriptions is indicated for damp-phlegm and cold phlegm. *Er Cheng Tang* has the effects of drying dampness, removing phlegm, regulating *Qi* and harmonizing the middle *Jiao* and is a basic recipe for treating damp-phlegm. It is mainly indicated for interior obstruction of damp-phlegm, marked by cough, nausea, vomiting, dizziness and vertigo. *Ling Gui Zhu Gan Tang* has the effects of invigorating the spleen, resolving dampness, warming and removing phlegm fluid and is a typical recipe to treat gathering of dampness into phlegm caused by insufficiency of the middle *Yang*. *Xiao Qing Long Tang* has the effects of warming the lung, dispelling cold and stopping asthma and is indicated for cough and asthma in cases which have a constitution of phlegm-fluid and are affected again by exogenous cold.

(2) Prescriptions for clearing away heat and removing phlegm

Qing Qi Hua Tan Wan has the effects of clearing away heat, removing phlegm, regulating *Qi* and relieving cough and is indicated for interior accumulation of phlegm-heat, marked by cough with yellow sticky sputum. *Xiao Xian Xiong Tang* has the effects of clearing away heat, resolving phlegm, relaxing the chest and dispelling lumps, indicating for syndrome of minor stuffiness in the chest caused by accumulation of phlegm-heat below the heart.

(3) Prescriptions for treating wind and resolving phlegm

Ban Xia Bai Zhu Tian Ma Tang has the effects of drying dampness, resolving phlegm, calming the liver to stop the wind, and is good at treating dizziness and headache due to upward perversion of wind-phlegm. *Zhi Sou San* has the effects of relieving cough, resolving phlegm, expelling exterior syndrome and promoting the function of the lung in dispersing, and is a common recipe for exogenous cough.

(4) Prescriptions for eliminating phlegm-fluid

Kong Xian Dan has the effects of eliminating phlegm and removing fluid and is indicated for retention of phlegm fluid in the chest and diaphragm, marked by a dull pain in the chest and hypochondrium, sticky and greasy tongue coating, wiry, slippery pulse. The force will become mild when pill form is used.

Review Questions

(1) How many types are phlegm-eliminating prescriptions divided into? And what phlegm syndrome are they indicated for?

(2) Please state the ingredients, indications and explanation of *Er Chen Tang*.

(3) What are the functions and indications of *Ling Gui Zhu Gan Tang*?

(4) Please state the ingredients, functions and indications of *Qing Qi Hua Tan Wan* and explain the meaning of associating with drugs for regulating *Qi*.

(5) What kind of dizziness and headache does *Ban Xia Bai Zhu Tian Ma Tang* treat? And state its ingredients and explanation.

(6) Both *Zhi Sou San* and *Sang Ju Yin* are used to treat exogenous cough. What are their differences in indications?

7 Mediating Prescriptions

Mediating prescriptions refer to the prescriptions which have the effects of mediation and regulation and are indicated for treating *Shaoyang* syndromes or disharmony between the liver and spleen, and disharmony between the intestine and stomach.

According to their functions, this group of prescriptions are divided into three types: the prescriptions for treating *Shaoyang* syndromes by mediation, the prescriptions for regulating the liver and spleen, and the prescriptions for regulating the intestine and stomach.

Mediating prescriptions have strict indications. They are forbidden to be used for pathogenic factors only in the exterior without invading *Shaoyang* meridians or pathogenic factors already in the interior with excessive heat in *Yangming* meridians.

7.1 Prescriptions for Treating *Shaoyang* Syndrome by Mediation

The prescriptions for treating *Shaoyang* syndrome by mediation are indicated for *Shaoyang* syndrome that the pathogenic factors are neither located in the exterior nor in the interior but in between.

Xiao Chai Hu Tang (Minor Decoction of Bupleurum)

- Source: *Shang Han Lun* (Treatise on Cold-Induced Diseases)
- Ingredients: *Chai Hu* (Radix Bupleuri) 12g.

  Huang Qin (Radix Scutellariae) 6g.

  Ren Shen (Radix Ginseng) 6g.

  Ban Xia (Rhizoma Pinelliae) 9g.

  Gan Cao (Radix Glycyrrhizae Praeparata) 5g.

  Sheng Jiang (Rhizoma Zingiberis Recens) 9g.

  Da Zao (Fructus Ziziphi Jujubae) 4pcs.
- Administration: All the drugs should be decocted in water for oral administration.
- Functions: Treat *Shaoyang* syndrome by mediation.
- Indications: *Shaoyang* syndrome, manifested as alternate attacks of chills and fever, fullness in the chest and hypochondriac region, poor appetite, restlessness, vomiting, bitter taste in the mouth, dry throat, dizziness, white tongue coating and wiry pulse.
- Explanation:

Chai Hu: a principal drug, bitter and acrid in taste and slight cold in nature, having mild effects of clearing, ascending and dispersing to expel pathogenic factor out of exterior.

Huang Qin: an assistant drug, dispersing and discharging by its bitter taste and cold nature.

The combination of the two drugs, one for dispelling pathogen, and the other for clearing away heat, removes pathogenic factors from *Shaoyang* meridians.

Ban Xia: harmonizing stomach, descending upward perversion of *Qi* to stop vomiting.

Ren Shen and *Gan Cao*: harmonizing the middle *Jiao* by sweet taste, benefiting *Qi* and supporting antipathogenic energy to expel evil factors out from the body.

The above three drugs are adjuvant drugs.

Sheng Jiang and *Da Zao*: guiding drugs, acrid and sweet in taste, regulating *Ying* and *Wei*.

○ The combination of these drugs mainly expels pathogenic factors associated with the effect of supporting anti-pathogenic *Qi* in order to cure the patients by harmonizing *Shaoyang*.

● Notes:

This is a representative prescription for treating *Shaoyang* syndrome. It is clinically advisable for various miscellaneous diseases, such as malaria, jaundice, chronic hepatitis as well as "heat entering the blood Chamber" due to affection of exogenous pathogens after delivery or during menstruation.

Hao Qin Qing Dan Tang (Decoction of Artemisiae Aunuae and Scutellaria for Clearing away Damp-heat from Gallbladder)

● Source: *Chong Ding Tong Su Shang Han Lun* (Revised Popular Treatise on Cold-Induced Diseases)

● Ingredients: *Qing Hao* (Herba Artemisiae Aunuae) 6g.

Huang Qin (Radix Scutellariae) 9g.

Zhu Ru (Caulis Bambusae in Taeniam) 9g.

Zhi Ban Xia (Rhizoma Pinelliae Praeparata) 5g.

Chi Fu Ling (Red Poria) 9g.

Zhi Qiao (Fructus Aurantii) 5g.

Chen Pi (Pericarpium Citri Reticulatae) 5g.

Bi Yu San (Green Jade Powder*) 9g. (Packed)

* Green Jade Powder is composed of Six to One Powder plus *Qing Dai* (Natural Indigo).

● Administration: All the drugs should be decocted in water for oral administration.

● Functions: Clear away damp-heat from the gallbladder, harmonize stomach and remove phlegm.

● Indications: Damp-heat in *Shaoyang* meridian and disharmony between gallbladder and stomach, marked by alternate fever and chills like malaria, severe fever and slight chills, stuffy chest, nausea and vomiting, bitter taste in the mouth, acid regurgitation or vomiting yellow saliva, red tongue with white greasy coating, rapid pulse with slippery on the right side and wiry on the left.

● Explanation:

Qing Hao: the principal drug, bitter in taste, cold in nature and fragrant in smell, clearing away pathogenic heat from *Shaoyang meridian*.

Huang Qin: an assistant drug, bitter in taste and cold in nature, clearing away heat from gallbladder meridian.

Zhu Ru: clearing away heat, removing phlegm, treating restlessness and stopping vomiting.

Chen Pi, *Ban Xia* and *Zhi Qiao*: regulating Qi, removing dampness, harmonizing the stomach and lowering the upward-rising of *Qi*.

These four drugs are adjuvant drugs.

Chi Fu Ling and *Bi Yu San*: the guiding drugs, clearing away damp-heat and conducting pathogenic heat to descend.

○ The combination of all the drugs plays the effect of clearing away damp-heat from gallbladder, harmonizing stomach, removing phlegm, and clearing away exogenous heat from *Shaoyang* meridian.

● Notes:

The modified prescription can treat acute cholecystitis, acute and chronic hepatitis, chronic pancreatitis and gastritis due to damp-heat of gallbladder meridian. In addition, it is also advisable for vomiting due to disharmony between the liver and stomach, dizziness and vertigo caused by obstruction of phlegm-dampness in the middle *Jiao*, night sweating due to disturbance of *Yin* by damp-heat of the liver and gallbladder, and palpitation and insomnia caused by phlegm-heat.

7.2 Prescriptions for Regulating the Liver and Spleen

This group of prescriptions is indicated for disharmony between the liver and spleen.

Si Ni San (Powder for Treating Cold Limbs)

● Source: *Shang Han Lun* (Treatise on Cold-Induced Diseases)
● Ingredients: *Chai Hu* (Radix Bupleuri) 6g.

          Zhi Shi (Fructus Aurantii Immaturus) 6g.

          Shao Yao (Radix Paeoniae Alba) 9g.

          Zhi Gan Cao (Radix Glycyrrhizae Praeparata) 6g.

● Administration: All the drugs are decocted in water for oral administration.

● Functions: Disperse pathogens and relieve depression, soothing the liver and regulate the spleen.

● Indications: Interior accumulation of pathogenic heat, marked by cold limbs, gastric and abdominal pain, or diarrhea with tenesmus.

● Explanation:

Chai Hu: the principle drug, bitter and acrid in taste and slight cold in nature, soothing the liver to relieve depression, regulating *Qi* movement to disperse accumulated heat out of the body.

Zhi Shi: the assistant drug, reducing with its bitter taste and normalizing *Qi* movement of the liver and spleen; *Zhi Shi* combining with *Chai Hu* to regulate the ascending and descending of *Qi*.

Bai Shao: the adjuvant drug, nourishing *Yin*, harmonizing the interior, relieving spasm to stop pain.

Zhi Gan Cao: the guiding drug, in combination with *Bai Shao*, tonifying the liver and spleen, and coordinating the effects of all the drugs in the prescription.

○ The combination of all the drugs plays the effect of dispersing heat, relieving depression and harmonizing the liver and spleen.

● Notes:

(1) The prescription can treat stagnation of liver *Qi*, seen in such diseases as chronic hepatitis, intercostal neuralgia, gastritis, diseases of biliary tract, pleurisy and acute pancreatitis.

(2) It is contraindicated for cold limbs caused by *Yang* deficiency and *Yin* excess.

Xiao Yao San (Ease Powder)

● Source: *Tai Ping Hui Min He Ji Ju Fang* (Prescription of Peaceful Benevolent Dispensary)

● Ingredients: *Chai Hu* (Radix Bupleuri) 9g.

　　　　　　Dang Gui (Radix Angelicae Sinensis) 9g.

　　　　　　Bai Shao (Radix Paeoniae Alba) 9g.

　　　　　　Bai Zhu (Rhizoma Atractylodis Macrocephalae) 9g.

　　　　　　Fu Ling (Poria) 12g.

　　　　　　Zhi Gan Cao (Radix Glycyrrhizae Praeparata) 5g.

　　　　　　Bo He (Herba Menthae) 2g.

　　　　　　Wei Jiang (Rhizoma Zingiberis Recens Praeparata) 2g.

● Administration: All the drugs should be decocted in water for oral administration.

● Functions: Soothe the liver to relieve depression, invigorate the spleen and nourish blood.

● Indications: Liver *Qi* stagnation with blood deficiency, and dysfunction of the spleen to transport, marked by hypochondriac pain, dizziness, headache, dryness of the mouth and throat, mental lassitude, poor appetite, or alternate attacks of chills and fever or irregular menstruation, distention in the breast, light red tongue, wiry and forceless pulse.

● Explanation:

Chai Hu: the principal drug, bitter and acrid in taste and slight cold in nature, regulating the liver *Qi* to relieve depression.

Dang Gui: sweet and acrid in taste and slight warm in nature.

Bai Shao: bitter and sour in taste and slight cold in nature.

Both of them nourish and harmonize the blood and tonifying the liver.

Fu Ling, *Bai Zhu*, *Zhi Gan Cao* and *Wei Jiang*: invigorating the spleen, harmonizing the middle *Jiao* and benefiting *Qi*.

These six drugs are assistant drugs.

Bo He: the adjuvant drug, helping *Chai Hu* to regulate liver *Qi* to treat depression.

○ The combination of all the drugs plays the effect of regulating the liver, relieving depression, invigorating the spleen and harmonizing *Ying*.

● Notes:

This is a common prescription for coordinating the liver and spleen, which treats both the liver and spleen and takes care of both *Qi* and blood. It is advisable for cases with liver *Qi* stagnation and blood deficiency, seen in such diseases as chronic hepatitis, chronic gastritis, pleurisy, neurasthenia, menstrual catatony of women and infertility. By adding some drugs, the prescription can also treat hectic fever and night sweating in the infiltration stage of pulmonary tuberculosis, central chorioretinopathy, infantile blindness of retrobulbar neuritis caused by high fever.

● Appendix:

(1) *Jia Wei Xiao Yao Wan* (Ease Pills Added with Other Drugs)

● Source: *Nei Ke Zhai Yao* (Abstracts of Internal Disease)

● Ingredients: *Xiao Yao San* plus 3 grams of *Dan Pi* (Cortex Montan Radicis) and 3 grams of *Zhi Zi* (Fructus Gardeniae).

● Functions and indications: soothing the liver, invigorating the spleen, harmonizing blood and regulating menstruation; indicated for blood deficiency of the liver and spleen with transformation of fire-heat, marked by irascibility, or spontaneous sweating and night sweating, or headache and dryness of the eyes, or red cheeks and dryness of the mouth, or irregular menstruation with lower abdominal pain, or abdominal distention and heaviness, difficult and painful in micturition.

(2) *Hei Xiao Yao San* (Black Ease Powder)

● Source: *Yi Lue Liu Shu-Nu Ke Zhi Yao* (Six Essential Medical Books, Essentials of Gynecology)

● Ingredients: *Xiao Yao San* plus *Sheng Di* (Radix Rehmanniae) or *Shu Di* (Radix Rehmanniae Praeparata).

● Functions and indications: soothing the liver, invigorating the spleen, nourishing blood and regulating menstruation, indicated for blood deficiency of the liver and spleen, marked by abdominal pain during menstruation, wiry and forceless pulse.

Tong Xie Yao Fang (Prescription of Importance for Diarrhea with Pain)

● Source: *Jing Yue Quan Shu* (Complete Works of Zhang Jing Yue)

● Ingredients: *Chao Bai Zhu* (Stir-baked Rhizoma Atractylodis Macrocephalae) 9g.

                Chao Bai Shao (Stir-backed Radix Paeoniae Alba) 6g.

Chen Pi (Pericarpium Citri Reticulatae) 4.5g.

Fang Feng (Radix Ledebouriellae) 6g.

- Administration: All the drugs should be decocted in water for oral administration.
- Functions: Reinforce the spleen, reduce the liver, relieve pain and stop diarrhea.
- Indications: Excess of the liver and deficiency of the spleen, marked by borborygmus, abdominal pain not be relieved by diarrhea, but be induced or become severe by emotions, thin white tongue coating and wiry pulse.
- Explanation:

Bai Zhi: the principal drug, bitter and sweet in taste and warm in nature, invigorating the spleen, drying dampness and stopping diarrhea.

Bai Shao: the assistant drug, sour in taste and slight cold in nature, nourishing blood reducing the liver to relieve pain.

Chen Pi: regulating *Qi* and wakening the spleen to support transportation and transformation.

Fang Feng: dispersing stagnant liver *Qi*, strengthening the spleen and resolving dampness.

They are adjuvant and guiding drugs.

- The combination of all the drugs plays the effect of reinforcing the spleen, reducing the liver, regulating *Qi* movement and relieving pain and diarrhea.
- Notes:

(1) This prescription is suitable for diarrhea caused by excess of the liver and deficiency of the spleen. The modified prescription can treat chronic enteritis, allergic enteritis, intestinal functional disorder, tuberculous enteritis and chronic dysentery which give rise to abdominal pain and diarrhea due to disharmony between the liver and spleen.

(2) It is contraindicated for diarrhea caused by damp-heat of intestines and stomach.

7.3 Prescriptions for Regulating the Intestine and Stomach

This group of prescriptions is fit for the treatment of suffocation, fullness, vomiting and diarrhea caused by disharmony between the intestine and stomach with manifestations of alternate chills and fever and dysfunction of ascending and descending.

Ban Xia Xie Xin Tang (Pinellia Decoction for Reducing Stomach-fire)

- Source: *Shang Han Lun* (Treatise of Cold-Induced Diseases)
- Ingredients: *Ban Xia* (Rhizoma Pinelliae) 9g.

    Huang Qin (Radix Scutellariae) 6g.

    Huang Lian (Rhizoma Coptidis) 3g.

    Gan Jiang (Rhizoma Zingiberis) 6g.

    Ren Shen (Radix Ginseng) 6g.

    Zhi Gan Cao (Radix Glycyrrhizae Praeparata) 6g.

Da Zao (Fructus Ziziphi Jujubae) 4pcs.

● Administration: All the drugs should be decocted in water for oral administration.

● Functions: harmonize the stomach, lower the upward perversion of *Qi* to relieve accumulation and remove flatulence.

● Indications: Disharmony between the intestine and stomach and accumulation of cold and heat, marked by suffocation and hard sensation below the heart without pain, nausea or vomiting, diarrhea, thin yellow and greasy coating of the tongue.

● Explanation:

Ban Xia and *Gan Jiang*: acrid in taste and warm in nature, dispelling cold.

Huang Qin and *Huang Lian*: bitter in taste and cold in nature, clearing away heat and drying dampness.

Ren Shen, *Da Zao* and *Gan Cao*: sweet in taste and warm in nature, benefiting Qi and tonifying the body.

○ In this prescription, cold and hot drugs are used together. The drugs of acrid nature are used for dispersing and those of bitter taste are used for descending. The combination of all the drugs plays the effects of reinforcing *Qi*, harmonizing the stomach, lowering the rising of *Qi*, and dispersing the lumps to relieve fullness.

● Notes:

This is a representative prescription for the treatment of suffocation and fullness in the epigastrium, vomiting and diarrhea caused by deficiency in the middle *Jiao*, coldness in the lower part and heat in the upper part of the body. The modified prescription can treat acute gastroenteritis and chronic enteritis, which show the above symptoms.

● Appendix:

(1) *Sheng Jiang Xie Xin Tang* (Ginger Decoction for Reducing Stomach)

● Source: *Shang Han Lun* (Treatise on Cold-Induced Diseases)

● Ingredients: Remove 6 grams of *Gan Jiang* (Rhizoma Zingiberis) from *Ban Xia Xie Xin Tang* and add 12 grams of *sheng Jiang* (Rhizoma Zingiberis Recens).

● Functions and indications: harmonizing the stomach, removing flatulence, dispersing accumulation and eliminating water, indicated for accumulation of water-heat, marked by suffocation and hard sensation in the epigastrium, borborygmus, diarrhea, belching with foul smell and a thunder-like sound in the abdomen.

(2) *Gan Cao Xie Xin Tang* (Liquorice Root Decoction for Reducing Stomach-fire)

● Source: *Shang Han Lun* (Treatise on Cold-induced Diseases)

● Ingredients: *Ban Xia Xie Xin Tang* plus 3g. of *Gan Cao* (Radix Glycyrrhizae) (altogether 9 grams).

● Functions and indications: benefiting qi, harmonizing stomach, removing flatulence and stopping vomiting, indicated for weakness of the stomach *Qi*, marked by a thunder-like sound in the abdomen, diarrhea with undigested food, suffocation, hard and fullness in the epigastrium, nausea and restlessness.

(3) *Huang Lian Tang* (Chinese Goldthread Decoction)

● Source: *Shang Han Lun* (Treatise on Cold-Induced Diseases)

● Ingredients: *Huang Lian* (Rhizoma Coptidis) 5g

      Gan Cao (Radix Glycyrrhizae) 6g

      Gan Jiang (Rhizoma Zingiberis) 5g

      Gui Zhi (Ramulus Cinnamomi) 5g

      Ren Shen (Radix Ginseng) 3g

      Ban Xia (Rhizoma Pinelliae) 9g

      Da Zao (Fructus Ziziphi Jujubae) 4pcs.

● Functions and indications: regulating to balance cold and heat, harmonizing the stomach and lowering the rising of Qi, indicated for heat in the chest and cold in the stomach, manifested as restlessness and hot sensation in the chest with suffocation, upward attacking of Qi with tendency of vomiting, abdominal pain, or borborygmus and diarrhea, white greasy coating of the tongue and wiry pulse.

Summary

Six main mediating prescriptions are selected. According to their functions, the prescriptions can be divided into three types: the prescriptions for treating *Shaoyang* syndrome by mediation, the prescriptions for regulating the liver and spleen, and the prescriptions for regulating the intestine and stomach.

(1) The prescriptions for treating *Shaoyang* syndrome by mediation

Xiao Chai Hu Tang is a principal prescription for *Shaoyang* syndrome. It is good at mediating *Shaoyang* and eliminating pathogenic factors and supporting anti-pathogenic Qi, indicated for alternate chills and fever, fullness in the chest and hypochondriac region, and restlessness and vomiting. *Hao Qin Qing Dan Tang* is mainly to clear away damp-heat from gallbladder, but also harmonize the stomach and remove phlegm. It is indicated for invasion to *Shaoyang* meridian by pathogenic factors and deficiency of middle Qi, associated with interior obstruction of phlegmdampness, marked by severe heat and slight chills, distention and fullness in the chest and diaphragm, vomiting, acid regurgitation or spitting of yellow and sticky sputum, etc.

(2) The prescriptions for regulating the liver and spleen.

Si Ni San, *Xiao Yao San* and *Tong Xie Yao Fang* have the effects of regulating the liver and spleen, indicating for disharmony between the liver and spleen. *Si Ni San* is associated with the effects of relieving depression and dispersing pathogens, used for cold limbs, abdominal pain and diarrhea which are caused by interior stagnation of *Yang Qi*. *Xiao Yao San* nourishes blood, regulates liver Qi, invigorates the spleen and harmonizes *Ying*, indicating for hypochondriac pain, poor appetite, lassitude, irregular menstruation which are caused by liver Qi stagnation and blood deficiency. *Tong Xie Yao Fang* strengthens the spleen and calms the liver is indicated for abdominal pain and diarrhea caused by excess of the liver and deficiency of the spleen.

(3) The prescriptions for regulating the intestine and stomach

Ban Xia Xie Xin Tang is a representative prescription for regulating the intestine and stomach. It has the effects of dispersing with acrid taste, descending with bitter taste, combining cold and hot drugs to regulate the stomach and intestines. It is fit for fullness, vomiting, abdominal pain and diarrhea due to mingling of cold and heat and abnormal ascending and descending.

Review Questions

(1) What do mediating prescriptions mean? How many types can they be divided into? And what are their indications?

(2) Please state the ingredients, functions, indications and explanation of *Xiao Chai Hu Tang*.

(3) Please state the ingredients, functions and indications of *Si Ni San* and *Xiao Yao San* and their differences.

(4) What are the characteristics of *Tong Xie Yao Fang* in pathology and symptoms? And why is *Fang Feng* used in the prescription?

(5) Please state the ingredients, functions and indications of *Ban Xia Xie Xin Tang* and list out its modified prescriptions.

8　Purgative Prescriptions

Purgative prescriptions are mainly composed of purgative drugs with the effects of relieving constipation, removing intestinal and gastric stagnation, purging away water and fluid and accumulation of cold, being used for the treatment of interior excess syndrome.

Since the interior excess syndromes varies with the accumulation of heat, cold, dryness and fluid, purgative prescriptions can be divided into four types: purgative prescriptions of cold nature, purgative prescriptions of warm nature, emollient prescriptions for causing laxation and prescriptions for eliminating retained fluid.

Purgative prescriptions are harmful to the stomach-*Qi*, therefore, immediate withdrawal is indicated once the effect attained for the treatment of interior excess syndrome. Over-administration is prohibited. For aged people, weak constitution and insufficiency of body fluid and blood, or pregnant women, or women after delivery, purgatives should not be used alone even though they have pathogenic evils in the interior.

8.1　Purgative Prescriptions of Cold Nature

This group of prescriptions is indicated for excess syndrome of interior heat and accumulation.

Da Cheng Qi Tang (Major Decoction for Purging down Digestive *Qi*)

- Source: *Shang Han Lun* (Treatise on Cold-Induced Diseases)
- Ingredients: *Da Huang* (Radix et Rhizoma Rhei) 12g.
  　　　　　Hou Po (Cortex Magnoliae Officinalis) 15g.
  　　　　　Zhi Shi (Fructus Aurantii Immaturus) 12g.
  　　　　　Mang Xiao (Natrii Sulphas) 9g.
- Administration: All the drugs should be decocted in water for oral administration.

Hou Po and *Zhi Shi* are to be decocted prior to *Da Huang*. *Mang Xiao* is infused in the decoction before administration.

- Functions: Evacuate accumulation of heat with drastic purgatives.
- Indications:

(1) Excess syndrome of *Yangming-fu* organ, marked by constipation, fullness in the epigastrium and abdomen, abdominal pain which can't be pressed, and even hectic fever, delirium, polyhidrosis of hands and feet, prickled tongue with yellow dry coating or dry black tongue with fissures, deep and forceful pulse.

(2) Watery discharge of terribly foul odor, pain in the abdomen with mass felt when pressing.

(3) Cold limbs, convulsions or mania due to excess of interior heat.

● Explanation:

Da Huang: the principal drug, bitter in taste and cold in nature, reducing heat, loosening the bowels and cleaning accumulation of wastes and heat in the gastric and intestinal tract.

Mang Xiao: the assistant drug, salt in taste and cold in nature, softening hard mass and moistening the dryness.

Hou Po and *Zhi Shi*: the adjuvant and guiding drugs, promoting the circulation of *Qi* to relieve fullness, dispersing the stagnation to help the principal drug releasing the obstruction of wastes in the stomach and intestines, and promoting the downward-moving of the *Qi* in *Yangming Fu* organs.

○ The combination of all the drugs plays the effect of evacuating the *Fu* organs of heat stagnation with drastic purgatives.

● Notes:

(1) The diagnostic points of this prescriptions are distention, fullness, dryness, excess and hard mass. The modified prescriptions can treat excess syndrome of *Yangming Fu* organs, seen in such diseases as acute simple ileus, adhesive ileus, acute cholecystitis and acute appendicitis. For high fever of some febrile diseases with unconsciousness, convulsion and mania belonging to dry excess syndrome in the stomach and intestine, the modified prescriptions will be applied.

(2) It is not advisable for the cases without gastrointestinal accumulation of heat.

● Appendix:

(1) *Xiao Cheng Qi Tang* (Minor Decoction for Purging Down Digestive *Qi*)

● Source: *Shang Han Lun* (Treatise on Cold-Induced Diseases)

● Ingredients: *Da Huang* (Radix et Rhizoma Rhei) 12g.

　　　　　　Hou Po (Cortex Magnoliae Officinalis) 6g.

　　　　　　Zhi Shi (Fructus Aurantii Immaturus) 9g.

● Functions and indications: relieving heat accumulation by its mild effect, indicating for mild cases of excess syndrome of *Yangming Fu* organ, marked by constipation, hectic fever, abdominal pain, deep and slippery pulse; or the onset of dysentery with distention pain in the abdomen, or epigastric distention and fullness, tenesmus and so on.

(2) *Tiao Wei Cheng Qi Tang* (Purgative Decoction for Coordinating the Function of the Stomach)

● Source: *Shang Han Lun* (Treatise on Cold-induced Diseases)

● Ingredients: *Da Huang* (Radix et Rhizoma Rhei) 12g.

　　　　　　Zhi Gan Cao (Radix Glycyrrhizae Praeparata) 6g.

　　　　　　Mang Xiao (Natrii Sulphas) 12g.

● Functions and indications: purging the stagnation of heat by laxative action, indicating for gastrointestinal dryness and heat, characterized by constipation, thirst, restlessness, and steaming fever as well as subcutaneous bleeding, hematemesis, epistaxis, and swelling and pain of gum and throat resulting from gastrointestinal dry heat.

8.2　Purgative Prescriptions of Warm Nature

This group of prescriptions is indicated for the treatment of interior excess syndrome due to accumulation of cold in the stomach and intestine.

Da Huang Fu Zi Tang (Decoction of Rhubarb and Aconite)

- Source: *Jin Gui Yao Lue* (Synopsis of Prescriptions of the Golden Chamber)
- Ingredients: *Da Huang* (Radix et Rhizoma Rhei) 6g.
  　　　　　Pao Fu Zi (Radix Aconiti Praeparata) 9g.
  　　　　　Xi Xin (Herba Asari) 3g.
- Administration: All the drugs are to be decocted in water for oral administration.
- Functions: Warm *Yang*, dispel cold, purge accumulation and remove stagnation.
- Indications: Interior excess syndrome of cold accumulation, manifested as abdominal pain, constipation, hypochondriac pain, fever, cold limbs, white greasy coating of the tongue and tense wiry pulse.
- Explanation:

Fu Zi: the principal drug, acrid in taste and hot in nature, warming *Yang* and dispelling cold.

Xi Xin: acrid in taste and warm in nature, removing cold and dispelling accumulation.

Da Huang: bitter in taste and cold in nature, eliminating accumulation of food.

Both of them are assistant and adjuvant drugs.

When *Da Huang* is used together with *Fu Zi* and *Xi Xin*, its nature of bitter and cold will be controlled but the purgative effect remains.

○ The prescription as a whole plays the effect of purgation with warm nature.

- Notes:

(1) The prescription is used to treat constipation due to stagnation of "cold-excess". Diseases such as acute appendicitis, intestinal obstruction which are of deficient cold type may be treated with the variation of this prescription.

(2) The dosage of *Da Huang* should not exceed that of *Fu Zi*.

8.3　Emollient Prescriptions for Causing Laxation

This kind of prescriptions is indicated for constipation due to insufficiency of body fluid or blood deficiency which leads to dry heat in the stomach and intestines.

Ma Zi Ren Wan (Hemp Seed Bolus)

- Source: *Shang Han Lun* (Treatise on Cold-Induced Diseases)

● Ingredients: *Ma Zi Ren* (Fructus Cannabis) 500g.

Shao Yao (Radix Paeoniae Alba) 250g.

Zhi Shi (Fructus Aurantii Immaturus) 250g.

Da Huang (Radix et Rhizoma Rhei) 500g.

Hou Po (Cortex Magnoliae Officinalis) 250g.

Xing Ren (Semen Armeniacae Amarum) 250g.

● Administration: The above drugs are ground into fine powder and then boluses are made out of powdered medicines mixed with honey, just the same size as a parasol seed. Nine grams is taken each time orally with warm boiled water, once or twice a day. These prescriptions may be reduced in proportion to that of the original prescriptions for making decoction.

● Functions: Moisten the intestines to relieve constipation, remove heat and activate *Qi*.

● Indications: Dry heat in the stomach and intestines, marked by constipation, epigastric distention and fullness, abdominal pain, or constipation due to hemorrhoids.

● Explanation:

Ma Zi Ren: the principal drug, sweet in taste, neutral in nature and abundant in lipid, moistening the intestine to relieve constipation.

Xing Ren: bitter in taste and slight warm in nature, moving *Qi* to go downward and moistening the intestines.

Bai Mi (honey) and *Shao Yao*: nourishing *Yin*, moistening dryness and relaxing the intestines.

Da Huang: purging heat and relieving constipation.

Zhi Shi and *Hou Po*: activating *Qi* circulation, breaking the obstruction to removing fullness.

They are assistant and adjuvant drugs.

○ The prescription as a whole plays the effects of moistening intestines, purging heat, circulating *Qi* and relieving constipation.

● Notes:

(1) This is a laxative prescription which is advisable for constipation due to hemorrhoid, anal fissure and habitual constipation belonging to insufficiency of body fluid associated with gastrointestinal dry heat.

(2) It is not advisable for the aged and the weak or pregnant women or those with constipation caused by exhaustion of body fluid and dryness of blood but without heat accumulation.

Zeng Ye Cheng Qi Tang (Purgative Decoction for Increasing Fluid and Sustaining *Qi*)

● Source: *Wen Bing Tiao Bian* (Treatise on Differentiation and Treatment of Epidemic Febrile Diseases)

- Ingredients: *Xuan Shen* (Radix Scrophulariae) 30g.

    Mai Dong (Radix Ophiopogonis) 24g.

    Sheng Di (Radix Rehmanniae) 24g.

    Da Huang (Radix et Rhizoma Rhei) 9g.

    Mang Xiao (Natrii Sulphas) 4.5g.

- Administration: All the drugs should be decocted in water for oral administration. Take the decoction one more time if constipation is not relieved.

- Functions: Nourish *Yin*, produce body fluid, reduce heat and relieve constipation.

- Indications: Retention of dry feces due to insufficiency of *Yin* and accumulation of heat, associated with symptoms of thirst, dry throat, red tongue with yellow and dry coating.

- Explanation:

Xuan Shen, *Mai Dong* and *Sheng Di*: the principal drugs, sweet and salty in taste and cold in nature, nourishing *Yin* and body fluid, clearing away heat, benefiting lung and moistening intestines.

Da Huang and *Mang Xiao*: the assistant and adjuvant drugs, softening hard mass, moistening to relieve dryness, purging heat and relieving constipation.

○ The combination of all the drugs plays the effect of purgation by nourishing *Yin*.

- Notes:

This is a prescription for relieving constipation by producing body fluid with reinforcing and reducing used in combination. Clinically, it is used to treat constipation due to consumption of *Yin* in febrile diseases as well as long-lasting hemorrhoid, or motive intestinal obstruction and acute simple intestinal obstruction belonging to insufficiency of *Yin* due to heat accumulation.

- Appendix:

Xin Jia Huang Long Tang (Newly Added Decoction of Yellow Dragon)

- Source: *Wen Bing Tiao Bian* (Treatise on Differentiation and Treatment of Epidemic Febrile Diseases)

- Ingredients: *Xi Sheng Di* (Radix Rehmanniae) 15g.

    Sheng Gan Xao (Radix Glycyrrhizae) 6g.

    Ren Shen (Radix Ginseng) 4.5g.

    Sheng Da Huang (Radix et Rhizoma Rhei) 9g.

    Mang Xiao (Natrii Sulphas) 3g.

    Xuan Shen (Radix Scrophulariae) 15g.

    Mai Dong (Radix Ophiopogonis) 15g.

    Dang Gui (Radix Angelicae Sinensis) 4.5g.

    Hai Shen (Sea cucumber) 2 pieces.

Jiang Zhi (Juice of Rhizoma Zingiberis) 6 spoonfuls.

● Functions and indications: nourishing *Yin*, benefiting *Qi*, removing accumulation and reducing heat, indicated for interior excess due to heat accumulation and insufficiency of *Qi* and *Yin*, marked by constipation, abdominal distention, fullness and hard mass, lassitude, shortness of breath, dry mouth and throat, parched or chapped lips, dry brown tongue coating or dry black tongue coating with fissures.

8.4 Prescriptions for Eliminating Retained Fluid

This group of prescriptions is indicated for excess syndrome caused by retention of water in the interior.

Shi Zao Tang (Ten Chinese-dates Decoction)

● Source: *Shang Han Lun* (Treatise on Cold-Induced Diseases)
● Ingredients: *Da Zao* (Fructus Ziziphi Jujubae) 10 pcs.

　　　　　　Gan Sui (Radix Euphorbiae Kansui)

　　　　　　Da Ji (Radix Knoxiae)

　　　　　　Yuan Hua (Flos Genkwa)

The above three drugs are in equal dosage.

● Administration: *Gan Sui*, *Da Ji* and *Yuan Hua* are ground into fine powder, and take 0.5-3g of the powder each time, once a day before breakfast, with the decoction of 10 pcs. of *Da Zao*. After the patient got watery diarrhea, a diet of porridge will be recommended to benefit stomach *Qi*.

● Functions: Eliminate retained fluid.

● Indications: *Xuan Yin* (Pleural fluid), marked by water in hypochondriac region, pain in the chest and hypochondrium when coughing or spitting, stuffiness and hardness in the epigastrium, nausea, shortness of breath, headache, dizziness, or difficult respiration due to pain in the thorax and back, wet and slippery coating of the tongue, deep and wiry pulse; as well as the strong patients with edema, distention and big abdomen, difficulty in urination and defecation.

● Explanation:

Gan Sui: draining water-dampness in the meridians.

Da Ji: purging water-dampness in the *Zangfu* organs.

Yuan Hua: removing recurrent water-dampness in the chest and hypochondrium.

These three drugs are drastic drugs and each has its own special effect. The combination of the three drugs can eliminate water and fluid, remove accumulation and reduce edema and abdominal fullness.

Da Zao: reinforcing *Qi*, preventing the injury of the stomach by drastic drugs, and reducing the toxic effect of the other three ingredients.

○ The combination of all the drugs can make drastic purgation without injuring anti-pathogenic *Qi* and play the effect of eliminating water.

● Notes:

(1) It can be used for strong patients with hydrothorax, ascites and general edema caused by hepatic cirrhosis, exudative pleurisy and chronic nephritis.

(2) It is not suitable to use this prescription as decoction. The prescription should be used carefully following the direction. After the adoption of the medicine, if patients have lassitude and poor appetite, the medicine should be stopped even though the water is not thoroughly expelled. Whether another dose is given will be decided after careful consideration of the case.

Summary

5 main purgative prescriptions are selected and they are divided into 4 types according to their functions: purgative prescriptions of cold nature, purgative prescriptions of warm nature, emollient prescriptions for causing laxation and prescriptions for eliminating retained fluid.

(1) Purgative prescriptions of cold nature

Da Cheng Qi Tang is a drastic purgative for removing accumulation of heat and is a main prescription for treating constipation due to gastrointestinal excess heat, indicating for syndromes with distention, fullness, dry feces in the abdomen.

(2) Purgative prescriptions of warm nature

Da Huang Fu Zi Tang can warm meridians, dispel cold, and clear away cold stagnation, used for constipation caused by constitutional *Yang* deficiency and interior accumulation of excess cold.

(3) Emollient prescriptions for causing laxation

Both *Ma Zi Ren Wan* and *Zeng Ye Cheng Qi Tang* can treat constipation due to intestinal dryness. *Ma Zi Ren Wan* moistens intestines to relieve constipation associated with the effect of purging away heat accumulation. It is indicated for constipation caused by gastrointestinal dryness and heat. *Zeng Ye Cheng Qi Tang* nourishes *Yin*, increases fluid, purges away heat and relieving constipation, indicating for constipation due to *Yin* insufficiency and heat accumulation.

(4) Prescriptions for eliminating retained fluid

Shi Zao Tang can eliminate water by purgation, indicating for excess syndrome of edema with abdominal distention as well as "*Xuan Yin*" due to retained water in hypochondrium.

Review Questions

(1) How to classify purgative prescriptions? Please state their representative prescriptions.

(2) What is the compatible significance of *Da Cheng Qi Tang*?

(3) What are the indications and pathology of *Shi Zao Tang*? Why is *Da Zao* used in the prescription?

(4) How to distinguish between the applications of *Ma Zi Ren Wan* and *Zeng Ye Cheng Qi Tang*?

9　Prescriptions for Relieving Both Exterior and Interior Syndromes

This group of prescriptions refers to those which have the effects of treating both exterior and interior syndromes by using drugs for treating exterior syndromes in combination with purgative drugs, heat-clearing drugs or interior-warming drugs.

According to the properties of diseases with both exterior and interior syndromes, prescriptions for relieving both exterior and interior syndromes are divided into three types: the prescriptions for relieving exterior syndrome and making purgation, the prescriptions for relieving exterior syndrome and clearing away interior heat and the prescriptions for relieving exterior syndrome and warming the interior.

When using this group of prescriptions, it is necessary to distinguish cold from heat, deficiency from excess and pay attention to the seriousness of exterior syndrome and interior syndrome in order to balance the proportion of drugs for exterior and drugs for interior.

9.1　Prescriptions for Relieving Exterior Syndrome and Making Purgation

This type of prescriptions is indicated for syndromes with exterior pathogenic factors and interior excess accumulation.

Da Chai Hu Tang (Major Decoction of Bupleurum)

- Source: *Jin Gui Yao Lue* (Synopsis of Prescriptions of the Golden Chamber)
- Ingredients: *Chai Hu* (Radix Bupleuri) 15g.

  Huang Qin (Radix scutellariae) 9g.

  Shao Yao (Radix Paeoniae) 9g.

  Ban Xia (Rhizoma Pinelliae) 9g.

  Zhi Shi (Fructus Aurantii Immaturus Praeparata) 9g.

  Da Huang (Radix et Rhizoma Rhei) 6g.

  Sheng Jiang (Rhizoma Zingiberis Recens) 15g.

  Da Zao (Fructus Ziziphi Jujubae) 5pcs.
- Administration: All the drugs should be decocted in water for oral administration.
- Functions: Treat Shaoyang syndrome by mediation and purge interior heat accumulation.
- Indications: Epigastric distention and fullness with pain when pressing, alternate attacks of chills and fever, depression with slight restlessness, fullness in the chest and hypochondrium, or abdominal fullness, distention and pain, constipation, or fever not reduce with sweat, fullness in gastrium, vomiting and diarrhea, yellow coating of the tongue

and wiry forceful pulse.

● Explanation:

Chai Hu: the principal drug, bitter and pungent in taste and slight cold in nature, dispelling pathogens from *Shaoyang* meridian.

Huang Qin, *Ban Xia* and *Sheng Jiang*: the assistant drugs, helping the principal drug to mediate *Shaoyang*.

Shao Yao, *Da Huang* and *Zhi Shi*: the adjuvant drugs, clearing away heat accumulation from *Shaoyang* meridian.

Da Zao: the guiding drug, calming the middle *Jiao*, and regulating *Ying* and *Wei* in combination with *Sheng Jiang*.

○ The combination of all the drugs plays the effect of mediating *Shaoyang* and purging interior heat accumulation.

● Notes:

(1) The diagnostic points of this prescription are alternate attacks of chills and fever, pain in the chest and abdomen, constipation, yellow tongue coating and wiry pulse. The modified prescription can be used to treat acute simple intestinal obstruction, acute pancreatitis, acute cholecystitis and cholelithes.

(2) Pay attention to the ingredients. There is no *Da Huang* in the original prescription recorded in *Shang Han Lun* (Treatise on Cold-induced Diseases), while there is *Da Huang* in the prescription recorded in *Jin Gui Yao Lue* (Synopsis of Prescriptions of the Golden Chamber).

Fang Feng Tong Sheng San (Miraculous Powder of Ledebouriellae)

● Source: *Xuan Ming Lun Fang* (Precriptions and Expositions of Huangdi's Plain Questions)

● Ingredients: *Fang Feng* (Radix Ledebouriellae) 15g.

　　　　　　　Jing Jie (Herba Schizonepetae) 15g.

　　　　　　　Lian Qiao (Fructus Forsythiae) 15g.

　　　　　　　Ma Huang (Herba Ephedrae) 15g.

　　　　　　　Bo He (Herba Menthae) 15g.

　　　　　　　Dang Gui (Radix Angelicae Sinensis) 15g.

　　　　　　　Chuan Xiong (Rhizoma ligustici Chuanxiong) 15g.

　　　　　　　Chao Bai Shao (Radix Paeoniae Alba Praeparata) 15g.

　　　　　　　Bai Zhu (Rhizoma Atractylodis Macrocephalae) 15g.

　　　　　　　Shan Zhi (Fructus Gardeniae) 15g.

　　　　　　　Da Huang (Radix et Rhizoma Rhei) 15g.

　　　　　　　Mang Xiao (Natrii Salphas) 15g.

　　　　　　　Sheng Shi Gao (Gypsum Fibrosum) 15g.

　　　　　　　Huang Qin (Radix Scutellariae) 30g.

Jie Geng (Radix Platycodi) 30g.

Hua Shi (Talcum) 90g.

Gan Cao (Radix Glycyrrhizae) 60g.

● Administration: Grind the above drugs into powder, and take 6 - 15g each time and add 3 slices of *Sheng Jiang* (Rhizoma Zingiberis) . Decoct them in water for oral use or take 6g each time as pills, twice a day. This prescription may be decocted for internal administration, but the dosage must be reduced in proportion to that of the original prescription.

● Functions: Expel wind, relieve exterior syndrome, reduce heat and promote bowel movement.

● Indications: Excess of pathogenic wind-heat and excess of both exterior and interior, marked by aversion to cold, high fever, headache, vertigo, bitter taste in the mouth, dry and uncomfortable throat, constipation, scanty yellow urine, yellow and greasy coating of the tongue, surging and rapid pulse or wiry and slippery pulse.

● Explanation:

Fang Feng, *Jing Jie*, *Ma Huang* and *Bo He*: expelling wind and relieving exterior syndrome by promoting diaphoresis.

Shi Gao, *Huang Qin*, *Lian Qiao* and *Jie Geng*: clearing away heat from the lung and stomach.

Da Huang and *Mang Xiao*: reducing heat and promoting bowel movement.

Shan Zhi and *Hua Shi*: clearing away heat and removing dampness, relieving internal heat through bowels and urine.

Dang Gui, *Chuan Xiong* and *Bai Shao*: nourishing blood and activating blood.

Bai Zhi: invigorating spleen and drying dampness.

Gan Cao and *Sheng Di*: harmonizing the middle *Jiao*.

○ The prescription as a whole plays the effect of relieving the exterior, dredging the interior, expelling wind and clearing away heat.

● Notes:

(1) The modified prescriptions can treat influenza, acute tonsillitis, furuncles and carbuncles, hematosepsis, cholecystitis, pancreatitis, appendicitis, urticaria and allergic purpura which give rise to the above symptoms. It is also effective to treat difficult headache and migraine of excess type. In addition, it is used for treating obesity and preventing cerebral-vascular accident.

(2) This prescription is the combination of diaphoresis, clearing and purgation methods indicated for syndromes with excess of wind-heat and excess at both exterior and interior.

It is contraindicated for headache of deficient type, deficiency of the spleen and stomach, chills and fever due to internal injury by cold and raw food and drinks.

Appendix:

Shuang Jie San (Powder for Relieving both Exterior and Interior Syndromes)

● Source: *Yang Yi Da Quan* (A Complete Work of External Diseases)

● Ingredients: In *Fang Feng Tong Sheng San*, omit *Ma Huang*, *Mang Xiao*, *Bai Zhu*, *Zhi Zi* and add *Gui Zhi* (Ramulus Cinnamomi).

● Functions and indications: expelling exterior syndrome, clearing away heat and promoting bowel movement, indicating for excessive wind-heat syndrome, marked by the onset of smallpox with unsmooth eruption, constipation, yellow urine, or furuncles due to toxins with both interior and exterior heat.

9.2 Prescriptions for Relieving Exterior Syndrome and Clearing Away Interior Heat

This group of prescriptions is indicated for syndromes with unrelieved exterior syndrome and scorching of interior heat.

Ge Gen Huang Qin Huang Lian Tang (Decoction of Pueraria, Sactellaria and Coptis)

● Source: *Shang Han Lun* (Treatse on Cold-Induced Diseases)
● Ingredients: *Ge Gen* (Radix Puerariae) 15g.
　　　　　　 Zhi Gan Cao (Radix Glycyrrhizae Praeparata) 6g.
　　　　　　 Huang Qin (Radix Scutellariae) 9g.
　　　　　　 Huang Lian (Rhizoma Coptidis) 9g.
● Administration: All the drugs should be decocted in water for oral administration.
● Functions: Relieve exterior syndrome and clear away heat.
● Indications: fever, diarrhea, restlessness, heat sensation in the chest and abdomen, dry mouth, thirst, spontaneous sweating, asthma, red tongue with yellow coating and rapid pulse.
● Explanation:

Ge Gen: the principal drug, sweet and acrid in taste and cold in nature, expelling pathogenic factors from muscles and skin, clearing away heat, helping the clear *Qi* going upward to stop diarrhea.

Huang Qin and *Huang Lian*: the assistang drugs, bitter in taste and cold in nature, clearing away heat, drying dampness and treating diarrhea.

Gan Cao: sweet in taste and mild in nature, harmonizing the middle *Jiao* and regulating the effect of the other drugs.

○ The combination of all the drugs plays the effect of relieving exterior syndrome, clearing away interior heat and stopping diarrhea.

● Notes:

(1) The modified prescription may treat acute enteritis and bacteria dysentery which give rise to the above symptoms.

(2) It is contraindicated for diarrhea of cold-damp type and diarrhea of deficient cold type.

9.3 Prescriptions for Relieving Exterior Syndrome and Warming the Interior

This group of prescriptions is indicated for syndromes with exterior symptoms and interior cold.

Wu Ji San (Powder for Treating Five Kinds of Accumulation)

● Source: Tai Ping Hui Min He Ji Ju Fang (Prescription of Peaceful Benevolent Dispensary)

● Ingredients: Bai Zhi (Radix Angelicae Dahuricae) 90g.

Chuan Xiong (Rhizoma Ligustici Chuanxiong) 90g.

Zhi Gan Cao (Radix Glycyrrhizae Preparata) 90g.

Fu Ling (Poria) 90g.

Dang Gui (Radix Angelicae Sinensis) 90g.

Rou Gui (Cortex Cinnamomi) 90g.

Shao Yao (Radix Paeoniae) 90g.

Ban Xia (Rhizoma Pinelliae) 90g.

Zhi Qiao (Fructus Aurantii) 90g.

Chen Pi (Pericarpium Citri Reticulatae) 180g.

Ma Huang (Herba Ephedrae) 180g.

Cang Zhu (Rhizoma Atractylodis) 720g.

Gan Jiang (Rhizoma Zingiberis) 120g.

Jie Geng (Radix Platycodi) 360g.

Hou Po (Cortex Magnoliae Officinalis) 120g.

● Administration: Grind the drugs into rough powder but Rou Gui and Zhi Qiao should be ground separately. The powder (without Rou Gui and Zhi Qiao) is baked in a frying pan until it changes colour. When the powder is cool, mix it with the powder of Rou Gui and Zhi Qiao. Takes 9g of the mixed powder each time and wrap it in a cloth. Decoct the powder with three slices of Sheng Jiang (Rhizoma Zingberis) in water for oral administration. Or decoct the original drugs for oral dose with the original dosage of the ingredients taken proportionally.

● Functions: Relieve exterior syndrome, dispel cold, regulate Qi, resolve phlegm, activate blood and remove accumulation.

● Indications: exogenous wind-cold with internal injury due to cold, or with five kinds of accumulation as cold, food Qi, blood and phlegm, manifested as fever without sweating, headache and general aching, stiffness and contraction at the nape and back, abdominal fullness, poor appetite, vomiting, abdominal pain, or irregular menstruation of cold type.

● Explanation:

Ma Huang and Bai Zhi: acrid in taste and warm in nature, relieving exterior syndrome by diaphoresis.

Gan Jiang and *Rou Gui*: acrid in taste and hot in nature, warming the interior and dispelling cold.

The above four drugs are principle drugs to remove both interior and exterior cold.

Cang Zhu and *Hou Po*: Drying dampness and invigorating the spleen.

Chen Pi, *Ban Xia* and *Fu Ling*: regulating *Qi* and removing phlegm.

Dang Gui, *Chuan Xiong* and *Bai Shao*: activating and nourishing blood and regulating menstruation to remove blood accumulation.

Zhi Qiao and *Jie Geng*: regulating the ascending and descending of *Qi*, benefiting the chest and the diaphragm to relieve fullness and distention.

The above four groups are assistant and adjuvant drugs.

Zhi Gan Cao: the guiding drug, harmonizing the middle *Jiao*, invigorating the spleen and regulating the effect of other drugs in the prescription.

○ The prescription as a whole plays the effect of relieving exterior syndrome by diaphoresis, warming the interior, expelling cold, treating both *Qi* and blood, and removing both phlegm and food accumulation.

● Notes:

(1) The modified prescription can treat common cold, rheumatic pain of the waist and leg, acute and chronic gastroenteritis, gastric spasm, morbid leukorrhea and menoxenia which give rise to the above symptoms. It is also advisable for cases with cold pain of the waist, leg and lower abdomen, fever without sweeting, slippery wet coating of the tongue and deep slow pulse.

(2) This is a complicated prescription which should be modified according to clinical symptoms. Get rid of drugs for treating exterior syndromes if there is no exterior syndrome. It is contraindicated for cases with yellow coating, thirst, and restlessness and rapid pulse.

Summary

Four main prescriptions for relieving both exterior and interior syndromes are selected. According to the functions, they are divided into three types: the prescriptions for relieving exterior syndrome and making purgation, the prescriptions for relieving exterior syndrome and clearing away interior heat and the prescriptions for relieving exterior syndrome and warming the interior.

(1) The prescriptions for relieving exterior syndrome and making purgation.

Da Chai Hu Tang is a prescription for mediation associated with purgation which treats cases with both *Shaoyang* and *Yangming* syndromes, marked by alternate attacks of chills and fever, epigastric fullness and pain, depression with slight restlessness. *Fang Feng Tong Sheng San* performs the combined effects of three methods: relieving exterior syndrome, clearing away heat and making purgation, and is used for syndromes with excess of wind-heat and excess at both exterior and interior.

(2) The prescriptions for relieving exterior syndrome and clearing away interior heat

Ge Gen Qin Lian Tang has the effects of relieving exterior, clearing away heat and stopping diarrhea, indicating for unrelieved exterior syndrome with diarrhea due to pathogenic heat.

(3) The prescriptions for relieving exterior syndrome and warming the interior

Wu Ji San has the effects of relieving exterior, warming the middle *Jiao* and removing accumulation, which is mainly indicating for syndromes with exogenous wind-cold and internal injury by cold.

Review Questions

(1) How many types can prescriptions for relieving both exterior and interior syndromes be divided into? What are their indications and principles for compatibility?

(2) What are the ingredients, functions and indications of *Ge Gen Huang Qin Huang Lian Tang*?

Why is *Ge Gen* a principle drug in the prescription?

(3) Explain briefly the use of ingredients of *Wu Ji San*?

(4) What are the functions and indications of *Fang Feng Tong Sheng San*?

10　Tonic Prescriptions

Tonic prescriptions are composed of tonifying drugs for treating deficiency syndromes by means of tonfying *Qi*, blood, *Yin* and *Yang* of the human body. Since deficient syndromes have deficiency of *Qi*, deficiency of blood, deficiency of both *Qi* and blood, deficiency of *Yin* and deficiency of *Yang*, tonic prescriptions are divided into five types: prescriptions as *Qi*-tonics, prescriptions as blood-tonics, prescriptions as both *Qi* and blood tonics, prescriptions as *Yin*-tonics and prescriptions as *Yang*-tonics.

Tonic prescriptions are indicated for various kinds of deficient syndromes marked by hypofunction of the body resulting from lingering diseases, insufficiency of *Zang-fu*, *Qi*, blood and body fluid. Pay attention to distinguish the truth or false, the seriousness and the acute or chronic conditions of deficient syndromes in order to apply tonics with mild drugs or tonics with drastic drugs correctly. For cases without deficiency of anti-pathogenic *Qi* but with excess of pathogenic *qi*, tonic prescriptions should not be used in case they may influence the expelling of pathogens.

10.1　Prescriptions as *Qi*-Tonics

This kind of prescriptions is indicated for deficiency of *Qi* of the spleen and lung, marked by lassitude and weak pulse; or prolapse of rectum or prolapse of the uterus due to sinking of the middle *Jiao Qi*.

Si Jun Zi Tang (Decoction of Four Noble Drugs)

● Source: *Tai Ping Hui Min He Ji Ju Fang* (Prescriptions of Peaceful Benevolent Dispensary)

● Ingredients: *Renshen* (Radix Ginseng) 10g.

　　　　　　Bai Zhu (Rhizoma Atractylodis Macrocephalae) 10g.

　　　　　　Fu Ling (Poria) 10g.

　　　　　　Gan Cao (Radix Glycyrrhizae Praeparata) 6g.

● Administration: All the drugs should be decocted in water for oral administration.

● Functons: Benefit *Qi* and invigorate the spleen.

● Indications: *Qi*-deficiency syndrome of the spleen and stomach marked by pale complexion, lassitude, feeble voice, poor appetite, loose stool, pale tongue with thin white coating, forceless and soft pulse.

● Explanation:

Ren Shen: the principal drug, sweet in taste and warm in nature, benefiting *Qi*, tonifying the spleen and nourishing the stomach.

Bai Zhu: the assistant drug, bitter in taste and warm in nature, invigorating the spleen and drying dampness.

Fu Ling: mild sweet in taste, playing the effect of adjuvant drug in combination with *Bai Zhu* to invigorate the spleen and remove dampness.

Zhi Gan Cao: the guiding drug, sweet in taste and warm in nature, benefiting *Qi* and harmonizing the middle *Jiao*.

● The combination of all the drugs plays the effect of benefiting *Qi* and invigorating the spleen.

● Notes:

(1) This is a basic prescription for the treatment of *Qi*-deficiency syndrome of the spleen and stomach. The modified prescription is advisable for *Qi*-deficiency of the spleen and stomach and weakness in transportation and transformation caused by various reasons. In cases of chronic gastroenteritis, dyspepsia, neurasthenia and gastrointestinal dysfunction which have the symptoms of *Qi* deficiency, the modified prescription can be applied.

(2) It is contraindicated for cases with *Yin* deficiency and *Qi* stagnation, and also we should be cautious to treat cases of phlegm-dampness with this prescription.

Shen Ling Bai Zhu San (Powder of Ginseng, Poria and Bighead Atractylodes)

● Source: *Tai Ping Hui Min He Ji Ju Fang* (Prescriptions of Peaceful Benevolent Dispensary)

● Ingredients: *Ren Shen* (Radix Ginseng) 1000g.

Bai Zhu (Rhizoma Atractylodis Macrocephalae) 1000g.

Bai Fu Ling (Poria) 1000g.

Shan Yao (Rhizoma Dioscoreae) 1000g.

Chao Gan Cao (Radix Glycyrrhizae) 1000g.

Bai Bian Dou (Semen Dolichoris Album) 750g.

Lian Zi Rou (Semen Nelumbinis) 500g

Yi Yi Ren (Semen Coicis) 500g.

Sha Ren (Fructus Amomi) 500g.

Jie Geng (Radix Platycodi) 500g.

● Administration: Grind the drugs into fine power. Take 6 grams each time with decoction of Fructus Ziziphi Jujubae. For children, the dosage should be decreased. The drugs can also be prepared as decoction for oral administration but the dosage should be decreased in proportion to the original prescription.

● Functions: Benefit *Qi*, invigorate the spleen, harmonize the stomach, and resolve dampness.

● Indications: Dampness-retention syndrome due to spleen deficiency, marked by weakness of the limbs, lassitude, indigestion, vomiting, or diarrhea, distention and suffocation in the chest and epigastrium, sallow complexion, pale tongue with white greasy coating, forceless and moderate pulse.

● Explanation:

Ren Shen and *Bai Zhu*: the principal drugs, sweet and bitter in taste and warm in nature, tonifying *Qi* and invigorating the spleen.

Shan Yao and *Lian Zi Rou*: sweet in taste and neutral in nature, helping *Ren Shen* to benefit *Qi* and tonify the spleen.

Bai Bian Dou, *Yi Yi Ren* and *Fu Ling*: helping *Bai Zhu* to invigorate the spleen, resolve dampness and stop diarrhea.

The above two groups are assistant drugs.

Sha Ren and *Jie Geng*: the adjuvant drugs, harmonizing the stomach, wakening up the spleen, regulating *Qi* to ease the chest.

Gan Cao: the guiding drug, regulating the effect of other drugs.

● Notes:

(1) The prescription may treat chronic enterogastritis, anemia, chronic nephritis and leukorrhea which belong to retention of dampness due to spleen deficiency. It can also treat chronic cough with profuse sputum caused by weakness of the lung *Qi*. This is "building up the earth to produce metal".

(2) The prescription should be carefully administered to patients with hyperactivity of fire due to *Yin* deficiencys and should be used with discretion for patients associated with deficiency of both *Qi* and *Yin*, or deficiency of *Yin* complicated with deficiency of the spleen.

Bu Zhong Yi Qi Tang (Decoction for Reinforcing Middle-*Jiao* and Replenishing *Qi*)

● Source: *Pi Wei Lun* (Treatise on the Spleen and Stomach)
● Ingredients: *Huang Qi* (Radix Astragali Seu Hedysari) 15g.

    Zhi Gan Cao (Radix Glycyrrhizae praeparata) 5g.

    Ren Shen (Radix Ginseng) 10g.

    Dang Gui (Radix Angelicae Sinensis) 10g.

    Chen Pi (Pericarpium Citri Reticulatae) 6g.

    Sheng Ma (Rhizoma Cimicifugae) 3g.

    Chai Hu (Radix Bupleuri) 3g.

    Bai Zhu (Rhizoma Atractylodis Macrocephalae) 10g.

● Administration: All the ingredients can either be decocted in water for oral administration, or ground into powder for making pills. Take 10 grams of pills each time with warm boiled water, 2-3 times a day.

● Functions: Reinforce the middle *Jiao*, replenish *Qi*, ascend *Yang* and treat *Qi* sinking.

● Indications: Deficiency of the *Qi* of the spleen and stomach, marked by fever, spontaneous sweating, thirst with desire for hot drink, short breath and disinclination to talk, lassitude, weakness of the limbs, pale tongue with thin white coating, forceless and soft pulse, as well as prolapse of anus, hysteroptosis, prolonged diarrhea, prolonged dysentery due to sinking of the middle *Qi*.

● Explanation:

Huang Qi: the principal drug, tonifying the middle *Jiao*, replenishing *Qi*, ascending *Yang* and supporting the exterior.

Ren Shen, *Bai Zhu* and *Zhi Gan Cao*: the assistant drugs, invigorating the spleen and replenishing *Qi*; in combination with the principal drug to tonify the middle *Jiao* and replenish *Qi*.

Chen pi: regulating *Qi* and harmonizing the stomach.

Dang Gui: nourishing blood and tonifying deficiency.

The above five drugs are adjuvant drugs.

Sheng Ma, *Chai Hu*: the guiding drugs, ascending *Yang* to lift sinkness.

○ The combination of all the drugs plays the effect of tonifying the middle *Jiao*, replenishing *qi*, ascending *Yang* and lifting sinkness.

Notes:

(1) The prescription can be modified to treat diseases with *qi*-deficiency of the spleen and stomach seen in such diseases as hypotension, chronic gastroenteritis, myasthenia gravis as well as prolapse of anus, hysteroptosis, gastroptosis, nephroptosis, protracted diarrhea, protracted dysentery and blepharoptosis due to the sinking of spleen *Qi*.

(2) This is a prescription for "removing heat by sweet flavour and warm nature" and also a typical prescription for treating fever due to deficiency of *Qi*. It is prohibited for cases with fever due to *Yin* deficiency and with scorching of internal heat. And it can not be used for those with the impairment of both the body fluid and *Qi* after illness.

(3) *Dang Shen* (Radix Codonopsis Pilosulae) is often used to replace *Ren Shen* in the prescription.

Appendix:

Sheng Xian Tang (Decoction for Treating Sinking of *Qi*)

● Source: *Yi Xue Zhong Zhong Can Xi Lu* (Records of Traditional Chinese and Western Medicine in Combination)

● Ingredients: *Sheng Huang Qi* (Radix Astragali sell Hedysari) 18g.

                Zhi Mu (Rhizoma Anemarrhenae) 10g.

                Chai Hu (Radix Bupleuri) 5g.

                Sheng Ma (Rhizoma Cimicifugae) 3g.

                Jie Geng (Radix Platycodi) 5g.

● Functions and indications: replenishing *Qi* and elevating sinkness, indicating for sinking of *Qi* in the chest, marked by shortness of breath, dyspnea, or even nearly stopping of breath, deep slow and faint pulse or irregular pulse.

Sheng Mai San (Pulse-activating Powder)

- Source: *Nei Wai Shang Bian Huo Lun* (Differentiation on Endogenous and Exogenous Diseases)
- Ingredients: *Ren Shen* (Radix Ginseng) 10g.

  Mai Dong (Radix Ophipogonis) 15g.

  Wu Wei Zi (Fructus Schisandrae) 6g.
- Administration: All the drugs should be decocted in water for oral administration.
- Functions: Replenish *Qi*, produce body fluid, astringe *Yin* and arrest sweat.
- Indications: Impairment of both *Qi* and *Yin*, marked by general lassitude, shortness of breath, disinclination to talk, dryness of the throat, thirst, forceless and weak thready pulse; or deficiency of lung due to chronic cough, dry cough with little sputum, shortness of breath, spontaneous sweating, dryness of the mouth and tongue, forceless and thready pulse.
- Explanation:

Ren Shen: the principal drug, sweet in taste and warm in nature, replenishing *Qi* and tonifying the lung.

Mai Dong: the assistant drug, sweet in taste and cold in nature, nourishing *Yin*, clearing away heat and producing body fluid.

Wu Wei Zi: the adjuvant and guiding drug, sour in taste and warm in nature, controlling sweat, producing body fluid and relieving thirst.

- The combination of all the drugs plays the effect of replenishing *Qi*, producing body fluid, astringing *Yin* and arresting sweat.
- Notes:

(1) The modified prescription can treat heatstroke, chronic bronchitis, lung tuberculosis and heart disease which are caused by deficiency of both *Qi* and *Yin*.

(2) It is neither fit for patients whose exopathogen has not been dispelled, nor for those with excess of summer heat without impairment of *Qi* and body fluid.

10.2 Prescriptions as Blood-Tonics

This kind of prescriptions is indicated for blood deficiency, marked by dizziness, blurred vision, palpitation, pale tongue, and thready and rapid pulse.

Si Wu Tang (Decoction of Four Ingredients)

- Source: *Tai Ping Hui Min He Ji Ju Fang* (Prescription of Peaceful Benevolent Dispensary)
- Ingredienuts: *Shu Di* (Radix Rehmanniae Praeparata) 12g.

  Dang Gui (Radix Angelicae Sinensis) 10g.

  Bai Shao (Radix Paeoniae Alba) 10g.

Chuan Xiong (Rhizoma Ligustici Chuanxiong) 6g.

● Administration: All the drugs should be decocted in water for oral administration.

● Functions: Tonify and regulate blood.

● Indications: Deficiency and stagnation of blood with symptoms as dizziness and vertigo, palpitation, insomnia, lustreless complexion, menstrual disorders, scanty mentruation or amenorrhea, pale tongue, thready wiry or thready choppy pulse; as well as postpartum lochia resulting in a mass or swelling in the abdomen, showing lower abdominal hardness and pain.

● Explanation:

Shou Di: the principal drug, sweet in taste and warm in nature, nourishing *Yin* and tonifying blood.

Dang Gui: the assistant drug, tonifying blood, nourishing the liver, harmonizing blood and regulating menstruation.

Bai Shao: the adjuvant drug, nourishing blood to soften the liver, and harmonizing *Ying* System.

Chuan Xiong: the guiding drug, activating blood, circulating *Qi* and regulating *Qi* and blood.

○ The combination of all the drugs performs the functions of tonifying blood without causing stagnation of blood and circulating blood without harming the blood, and as a result, achieving the result of tonifying and regulating blood.

Notes:

(1) The modified prescriptions are used to treat deficiency and stagnation of blood, seen in diseases as malnutrition, anemia, vegetative nerve functional disturbance, menopausal syndrome, menstrual disorder, prefetal and postpartum diseases.

(2) The prescription is not advisable for patients with spleen and stomach *Yang* deficiency, marked by anorexia and loose stool. It also can not treat fever due to *Yin* deficiency and metrorrhagia with collapse of *Qi*.

Dang Gui Bu Xue Tang (Chinese Angelica Decoction for Replenishing Blood)

● Source: *Nei Wai Shang Bian Huo Lun* (Differentiation on Endogenous and Exogenous Diseases)

● Ingredients: *Huang Qi* (Radix Astragali seu Hedysari) 30g.

　　　　　　Dang Gui (Radix Angelicae Sinensis) 6g.

● Administration: All the drugs should be decocted in water for oral administration.

● Functions: Tonify *Qi* and produce blood.

● Indications: Fever due to blood deficiency, marked by hot sensation of the muscle, redness of the face, severe thirst with desire to drink, surging big pulse which is forceless by heavy pressing. It also treats fever and headache during menstruation or after delivery due to blood deficiency, or treats cases with sores or carbuncles that the diabrotic wound healed very slowly.

● Explanation:

Huang Qi: the principal drug, sweet in taste and warm in nature, tonifying the spleen and lung *Qi* to support the source of the production of *Qi* and blood.

Dang Gui: the assistant drug, sweet and acrid in taste and warm in nature, nourishing blood and regulating *Ying*.

○ The combination of the two drugs signifies that "*Yin* grows while *Yang* is generating" and "vigorous *Qi* will help to produce blood".

● Notes:

(1) The prescription treats various kinds of anemia and allegic purpura due to deficiency of blood and weakness of *Qi*.

(2) It is contraindicated for hectic fever due to *Yin* deficiency.

Gui Pi Tang (Decoction for Invigorating the Spleen and Nourishing the Heart)

● Source: *Ji Sheng Fang* (Prescriptions for Succouring the Sick)
● Ingredients: *Bai Zhu* (Rhizoma Atractylodlis Macrocephalae) 30g.

Fu Shen (Poria cum Ligno Hospite) 30g.

Huang Qi (Radix Astragali seu Hedysari) 30g.

Long Yan Rou (Arillus Longan) 30g.

Suan Zao Ren (Semen Ziziphi Spinosae) (Stir-fried) 30g.

Ren Shen (Radix Ginseng) 15g.

Mu Xiang (Radix Aucklandiae) 15g.

Zhi Gan Cao (Radix Glycyrrhizae Praeparata) 8g.

Dang Gui (Radix Angelicae Sinensis) 3g.

Yuan Zhi (Radix Polygalae) 3g.

● Administration: Grind the drugs into rough powder and take 12 grams each time; or all the drugs, with 5 pcs. of fresh ginger and 3-5 pcs of Chinese dates, are decocted in water for oral administration; or the drugs are made into boluses, 10 grams each, and be taken with warm boiled water.

● Functions: Replenish *Qi* and tonify blood, invigorate the spleen and nourish the heart.

● Indications: Weakness of both the spleen and heart marked by palpitation, amnesia, insomnia, poor appetite, general debility, sallow complexion, pale tongue with thin white coating, thready and moderate pulse, or dysfunction of the spleen in governing the blood, marked by hemafecia, subcutaneous purpura, metrorrhagia and metrostaxis, preceded menstrual period with excessive blood loss in light colour, or continuous dripping of menstruation, pale tongue and thready pulse.

● Explanation:

Ren Shen and *Huang Qi*: the principal drugs, which are sweet in taste and warm in nature, reinforcing *Qi* and invigorating the spleen.

Bai Zhu and *Gan Cao*: reinforcing the spleen and replenishing *Qi* to help the principal drugs to strengthen the source for the production of *Qi* and blood.

Dang Gui: sweet and acrid in taste and warm in nature, nourishing the liver to produce heart blood.

Fu Shen, *Zao Ren* and *Long Yan Rou*: sweet in taste and neutral in nature, nourishing the heart to tranquilize the mind.

The above six drugs are assistant drugs.

Yuan Zhi: the adjuvant drug, relieving mental stress by means of restoring normal coordination between the heart and the kidney.

Mu Xiang: the guiding drug, regulating *Qi* and enlivens the spleen to prevent *Qi*-replenishing drugs and blood tonics from causing stagnation of *Qi*.

○ The prescription as a whole plays the effect of reinforcing both *Qi* and blood and treating both the heart and spleen.

● Notes:

(1) The modified prescription can treat hemorrhage in gastric and duodenal ulceration, disfunctional uterine bleeding, aplastic anemia, thrombocytopenia purpura, neurasthenia and heart diseases which belong to deficiency of the heart and spleen and dysfunciton of the spleen in controlling blood.

(2) It should not be administered to those with pathogenic heat hidden interiorly or those with rapid pulse due to *Yin* deficiency.

Fu Mai Tang (Pulse-Restoring Decoction)

also called *Zhi Gan Cao Tang* (Decoction of Prepared Licorice)
   ● Source: *Shang Han Lun* (Treatise on Cold-Induced Diseases)
   ● Ingredients: *Zhi Gan Cao* (Radix Glycyrrhizae Praeparata) 12g.
      Sheng Jiang (Rhizoma Zingiberis) 10g.
      Gui Zhi (Ramulus Cinnamomi) 10g.
      Ren Shen (Radix Ginseng) 6g.
      Sheng Di (Radix Rehmanniae) 30g.
      E Jiao (Colla Corii Asini) 6g.
      Mai Dong (Radix Ophiopogonis) 10g.
      Ma Ren (Fructus Cannabis) 10g.
      Da Zao (Fructus Ziziphi Jujubae) 10pcs.

   ● Administration: Except for *E Jiao*, all the drugs in the prescription are to be decocted in water and then the liquid part is separated from the residue and mixed with 10ml of rice wine. *E Jiao*, separately melted in boiling water, is divided into two portions and one portion is mixed with half of the decoction for oral administration.

● Functions: Replenish *Qi*, enrich blood, nourish *Yin* and restore pulse.

● Indications: Insufficiency of *Yin* blood and weakness of *Yang Qi*, marked by knotty and intermittent pulse, palpitation, emaciation, shortness of breath, bright and dry tongue with little coating; or consumptive cough, marked by cough with bloody sputum, shortness of breath, insomnia due to vexation, emaciation, spontaneous sweating and night sweating, dryness of the throat and tongue, constipation, and weak and rapid pulse.

● Explanations:

Zhi Gan Cao: the principal drug, sweet in taste and warm in nature, replenishing *Qi*, dredging the meridians and enriching both *Qi* and blood.

Ren Shen and *Da Zao*: replenishing *Qi*, tonifying the spleen and restoring pulse.

Sheng Di, *E Jiao*, *Mai Dong* and *Ma Ren*: nourishing *Yin*, tonifying blood, enriching blood and restoring pulse.

The above six drugs are assistant drugs.

Gui Zhi, *Sheng Jiang* and Rice Wine: the adjuvant drugs, acrid in taste and warm in nature, dispersing with the acrid taste to circulate *Yang Qi* and dredge the meridians.

○ The prescription as a whole plays the effects of nourishing *Yin*, enriching blood, replenishing *Qi* and restoring pulse.

● Notes:

(1) The prescription is suitable for functional arrhythmia, extra systole, coronary heart disease, rheumatic heart disease, viral myocarditis, and hyperthyroidism which pertain to insufficiency of *Yin*-blood and weakness of the heart *Qi*.

(2) It is not applicable for patients with weakness of gastrointestine or with diarrhea.

Appendix:

Jia Jian Fu Mai Tang (Modified Pulse-Restoring Decoction)

● Source: *Wen Bing Tiao Bian* (Treatise on Differentiation and Treatment of Epidemic Febrile Diseaes)

● Ingredients: *Zhi Gan Cao* (Radix Glycyrrhizae Praeparata) 20g.

Gan Di Huang (Radix Rehmanniae) 20g.

Sheng Bai Shao (Radix Paeoniae Alba) 20g.

Mai Dong (Radix Ophiopogonis) 15g.

E Jiao (Colla Corii Asini) 10g.

● Functions and indications: Enriching blood, nourishing *Yin*, producing body fluid and moistening dryness, indicating for deficiency of *Yin*-fluid due to remained pathogenic heat in the later period of febrile diseases, manifested as hot sensation in the palms and soles, dryness of the mouth and tongue, forceless and big pulse.

10.3 Prescriptions as Both *Qi* and Blood-Tonics

This kind of prescriptions is indicated for deficiency of both *Qi* and blood, marked by shortness of breath, lassitude, palpitation, insomnia, pale tongue, and forceless pulse.

Ba Zhen Tang (Eight Precious Ingredients Decoction)

- Source: *Zheng Ti Lei Yao* (Classification and Treatment of Traumatic Diseases)
- Ingredients: *Ren Shen* (Radix Ginseng) 10g.

    Bai Zhu (Rhizoma Atractylodis Macrocephalae) 10g.

    Fu Ling (Poria) 10g.

    Dang Gui (Radix Angelicae Sinensis) 10g.

    Shu Di (Radix Rehmanniae Praeparata) 10g.

    Bai Shao (Radix Paeoniae Alba) 10g.

    Chuan Xiong (Rhizoma Ligustici Chuanxiong) 10g.

    Zhi Gan Cao (Radix Glycyrrhizae Praeparata) 6g.

- Administration: All the drugs, with 3 slices of *Sheng Jiang* (Rhizoma Zingiberis) and 5 pcs. of *Da Zao* (Fructus Ziziphi Jujubae), are to be decocted in water for oral administration.

- Functions: Reinforce both *Qi* and blood.

- Indications: Deficiency of both *Qi* and blood, marked by pale or sallow complexion, dizziness and vertigo, lassitude, shortness of breath, dislike speaking, lassitude, palpitation, poor appetite, thready weak or forceless big pulse.

- Explanation:

Ren Shen and *Shu Di*: the principal drugs, sweet in taste and warm in nature, replenishing *Qi* and nourishing blood.

Bai Zhu and *Fu Ling*: invigorating the spleen, resolving dampness and helping *Ren Shen* to replenish *Qi* and tonify the spleen.

Dang Gui and *Bai Shao*: nourishing blood, harmonizing *Ying* and helping *Shu Di* to reinforce *Yin* blood.

The above four drugs are assistant drugs.

Chuan Xiong: the adjurant drug, activating blood and circulating *Qi*, playing the effect of tonifying without stagnation.

Zhi Gan Cao: the guiding drug, replenishing *Qi*, harmonizing the middle *Jiao* and regulating the effect of all the drugs.

○ The combination of all the drugs plays the effect of reinforcing both *Qi* and blood.

- Notes:

The prescription may treat cases with weakness after illness, anemia, various kinds of chronic diseases, irregular menstruation, uterine bleeding and external diseases such as sores which are difficult to heal, pertaining to deficiency of *Qi* and blood.

- Appendix:

(1) *Shi Quan Da Bu Wan* (Bolus of Ten Powerful Tonics)

- Source: *Tai Ping Hui Min He Ji Ju Fang* (Prescription of Peaceful Benevolent Dispensary)

- Ingredients: *Ba Zhen Tang* plus *Huang Qi* (Radix Astragali seu Hedysari) 10g. and *Rou Gui* (Cortex Cinnamomi) 3g.

- Functions and indications: Warm and tonify *Yi* and blood, indicating for weakness of knees, poor appetite, seminal emission, disunion of sores and carbuncles, and metrorrhagia and metrostaxis.

(2) *Yu Lin Zhu* (Raising Chinese Unicon Pill)

- Source: *Jing Yue Quan Shu* (Complete Works of Zhang Jingyue)
- Ingredients: *Ren Shen* (Radix Ginseng) 60g.

  Chao Bai Zhu (Rhizoma Atractydis Macrocephalae) (Parching) 60g.

  Fu Ling (Poria) 60g.

  Dang Gui (Radix Angelicae Sinensis) 120g.

  Chuan Xiong (Rhizoma Ligustici Chuanxiong) 30g.

  Zhi Gan Cao (Radix Glycyrrhizae Praeparata) 30g.

  Tu Si Zi (Semen Cuscutae) 120g.

  Du Zhong (Cortex Eucommiae) (Parching with wine) 60g.

  Lu Jiao Shuang (Cornu Cervi Degelatinatum) 60g.

  Chuan Jiao (Pericarpium Zanthoxyli) 60g.

- Administration: Grind the above drugs into fine powder, and make the powder into boluses with honey. Take six grams each time with warm boiled water.

- Functions and indications: tonifying *Qi* and blood, nourishing the liver and kidney, strengthening *Chong* and *Ren* meridians, regulating menstruation to help pregnancy, indicated for woman's cases, such as insufficiency of *Qi* and blood, deficiency of both the liver and kidney, irregular menstruation, or delayed menstruation with light color of blood, or scanty menstruation with abdominal pain, or dripping constantly, soreness and weakness in the lumbar region and knees, cold pain in the lower abdoman, hyposexuality and sterility.

10.4 Prescriptions as *Yin*-Tonics

This kind of prescriptions is indicted for *Yin* deficiency, marked by soreness and weakness of waist and knees, hectic fever, night sweating, red tongue with little coating, thready and rapid pulse.

Liu Wei Di Huang Wan (Bolus of Six Drugs Including Rehmannia)

- Source: *Xiao Er Yao Zheng Zhi Jue* (key to Therapeutics of Children's Diseases)
- Ingredients: *Shu Di* (Rhizoma Rehmanniae Praeparata) 24g.

  Shan Yu Rou (Fructus Corni) 12g.

  Shan Yao (Rhizoma Dioscoreae) 12g.

  Ze Xie (Rhizoma Alismatis) 10g.

  Dan pi (Cortex Montan Radicis) 10g.

Fu Ling (Poria) 10g.

● Administration: The above drugs are ground into fine powder and are mixed with honey to make boluses. 15 grams is for one bolus and is taken each time with warm boiled water. 3 times a day. The drugs can also be decocted in water for oral administration.

● Functions: Nourish *Yin* and tonify the kidney.

● Indications: Insufficiency of kidney *Yin* and flaring up of fire, marked by soreness and weakness of waist and knees, dizziness and vertigo, tinnitus, deafness, hectic fever and night sweating, five centers heat, diabetes, seminal emission, dryness of the tongue, sore throat, pain of the heel, loose teeth, dripping urination, red tongue with little coating, and thready and rapid pulse.

● Explanation:

Shu Di: the principal drug, sweet in taste and warm in nature, nourishing *Yin*, tonifying the kidney, supplementing essence.

Shan Yu Rou: warm in nature, tonifying the liver and kidney and astrigenting essence.

Shan Yao: sweet in taste and neutral in nature, tonifying the spleen *Yin* and strengthening essence.

The above two are assistant drugs.

The combination of *Shu Di*, *Shan Yu Rou* and *Shan Yao* is good at tonifying all the three *Yin*, the liver, spleen and kidney, but especially the kidney *Yin*.

Ze Xie: removing turbid dampness and preventing *Shu Di* being too greasy in nature.

Dan Pi: reducing the liver fire and controlling the warm nature of *Shan Yu Rou*.

Fu Ling: resolving dampness from the spleen and helping *Shan Yao* to transport.

The above three drugs are adjuvant and guiding drugs.

○ The combination of all the drugs plays the effects of nourishing *Yin* and tonifying kidney.

● Notes:

(1) The modified prescription can treat cases with syndrome of the liver and kidney *Yin* deficiency, such as chronic nephritis, hypertention, diabetes, lung tuberculosis, renal tuberculosis, hyperthyroidism, central retinitis, climacteric syndrome, amenorrhea, scanty menstruation and infantile dysplasis.

(2) The prescription should be administered carefully to those with weakened function of the spleen in transportation and transformation.

Zuo Gui Wan (Bolus as Kidney-Yin-Tonic)

● Source: *Jing Yue Quan Shu* (Complete Works of *Zhang Jingyue*)
● Ingredients: *Shu Di* (Rhizoma Rehmanniae Praeparata) 24g.
　　　　　　　Shan Yao (Rhizoma Dioscoreae) (parched) 12g.
　　　　　　　Gou Qi (Fructus Lycii) 12g.

Shan Yu Rou (Fructus Corni) 12g.

Niu Xi (Radix Achyranthis Bidentatae et Radix Cyathulae) 12g.

Tu Si Zi (Semen Cuscutae) 12g.

Lu Jiao Jiao (Colla Cornus Cervi) 12g.

Gui Ban Jiao (Colla Plastri Testudinis) 12g.

● Administration: The boluses are made out of the powdered drugs with honey. Each bolus weighs 9g. One bolus is to be taken each time with slightly salty liquid in the early morning and before bedtime on with empty stomach.

● Functions: Nourish *Yin* and tonify kidney.

● Indications: insufficiency of genuine *Yin* (kidney *Yin*), marked by dizziness and vertigo, soreness and weakness of waist and kness, seminal emission or spermatorrhea, spontaneous sweating, night sweating, dryness of the mouth and tongue, red tongue with little coating and thready pulse.

● Explanation:

Shu Di: the principal drug, sweet in taste and warm in nature, nourishing *Yin* and replenishing essence to support genuine *Yin*.

Shan Yao: tonifying the spleen, replenishing *Yin*, nourishing the kidney and strengthening essence.

Gou Qi Zi: tonifying the kidney, replenishing essence, nourishing the liver and brightening eyes.

Shan Yu Rou: nourishing the liver and kidney and controlling essence and perspiration.

Gui Ban Jiao and *Lu Jiao Jiao*: closely related to health, used in combination for replenishing essence and marrow by "seeking *Yin* from *Yang*", with the former tending to nourish *Yin* and the latter tending to tonify *Yang*.

The above five are used as assistant drugs.

Tu Si Zi and *Niu Qi*: tonifying the liver and kidney and strengthening waist and knees, used as adjuvant and guiding drugs.

○ The combination of all the drugs plays the effects of tonifying the kidney and nourishing *Yin*.

● Notes:

(1) The prescription can treat insufficiency of genuine *Yin* occurring in cases of chronic diseases, debilitated constitution due to old age or the recovery stage of febrile diseases.

(2) Prolonged administration of the prescription will easily obstruct the functions of the spleen and stomach. For this reason, it is advisable to add into the prescription *Chen Pi* (Pericarpium Citri Reticulatae), *Sha Ren* (Frutus Amomi) or other drugs so as to regulate *Qi* and enliven the spleen. It should be used carefully for the cases with diarrhea due to deficiency of the spleen.

Yi Guan Jian (Decoction for Nourishing the Liver and kidney)

- Source: *Liu Zhou Yi Hua* (Medical Talks in *Liu Zhou*)
- Ingredients: *Sheng Di* (Radix Rehmanniae) 30g.

    Gou Qi Zi (Fructus Lycii) 12g.

    Sha Shen (Radix Glehniae) 10g.

    Mai Dong (Radix Ophiopogonis) 10g.

    Dang Gui (Radix Angelicae Sinensis) 10g.

    Chuan Lian Zi (Fructus Meliae Toosendan) 5g.

- Administration: All the drugs are decocted in water for oral administration.
- Functions: Nourish *Yin* and regulate the circulation of liver *Qi*.
- Indications: Insufficiency of the liver *Yin* and consumption of gastric fluid with stagnation of *Qi*, marked by thoracic, epigastric and hypochondriac pain, or vomiting bitter fluid, dry throat, red tongue with less fluid on its surface, thready, wiry and forceless pulse.

- Explanation:

Sheng Di: sweet in taste and cold in nature.

Gou Qi Zi: sweet in taste and neutral in nature.

Both are the principal drugs to nourish the liver *Yin*.

Sha Shen, *Mai Dong* and *Dang Gui*: assistant drugs, nourishing blood and softening the liver.

Chuan Lian Zi: the adjuvant and guiding drug, activating the liver *Qi*.

Though bitter in taste and cold in nature, *Chuan Lian Zi* will not consume *Yin* when it is used together with *Yin*-blood-tonifying drugs.

○ The prescription as a whole performs the functions of nourishing *Yin* and soothing the liver.

- Notes:

The modified prescription can treat cases with deficiency of *Yin* and stagnation of *Qi* seen in diseases as primary stage of cirrhosis, chronic hepatitis and chronic gastritis.

10.5　Prescriptions as *Yang*-Tonics

This kind of prescription is indicated for weakness of kidney-*Yang* manifested as soreness and weakness of the waist and knees, dysuria or polyuria, forceless pulse and deep thready in the *Chi* position.

Shen Qi Wan (Bolus for Tonifying Kidney-*Qi*)

- Source: *Jin Gui Yao Lue* (Synopsis of Prescriptions of the Golden Chamber)
- Ingredients: *Gan Di Huang* (Radix Rehmanniae) 24g.

    Shan Yao (Rhizoma Dioscoreae) 12g.

    Shan Zhu Yu (Fructus Corni) 12g.

Ze Xie (Rhizoma Alismatis) 10g.

Fu Ling (Poria) 10g.

Dan Pi (Cortex Moutan Radicis) 10g.

Gui Zhi (Ramulus Cinnamomi) 3g.

Fu Zi (Radix Aconiti Praeparata) 3g.

● Administration: Grind the drugs into very fine powder and then mix them with honey to make boluses. Each bolus weighs 9 grams. The bolus is taken twice a day with warm boiled water. And the drugs can also be decocted in water for oral administration.

● Functions: Warm and tonify the kidney-*Yang*.

● Indications: insufficiency of kidney-*Yang*, marked by soreness and weakness of waist and knees, cold feeling in the lower part of the body, contracture or tension in the lower abdomen, dysuria or polyuria which are severe in the night, impotence and prospermia as well as retention of phlegm fluid, edema, diabetes and beriberi; pale and enlarged tongue, weak pulse with deep thready in the *Chi* position.

● Explanation:

Gan Di Huang: the principal drug, sweet in taste and warm in nature, tonifying the kidney and nourishing *Yin*.

Shan Zhu Yu and *Shan Yao*: tonifying the liver and spleen and nourishing essence and blood.

Fu Zi and *Gui Zhi*: slightly producing the junior fire so as to support kidney *Qi* and warm kidney *Yang*.

The above four are assistant drugs.

Ze Xie, *Dan Pi* and *Fu Ling*: the adjuvant and guiding drugs, removing the turbid substance from the kidney.

○ The prescription in all seeks *Yang* within *Yin* and plays the effects of warming *Yang* and tonifying the kidney.

● Notes:

(1) The modified prescriptions are applied for cases with insufficiency of kidney-*Yang* seen in diseases such as chronic nephritis, diabetes, hypothyroidism, aldosteronism, sexual neurasthenia, hypoadrenalism, chronic bronchial asthma and climacteric syndrome.

(2) It is not advisable for cases with insufficiency of kidnney-*Yin* with flaring-up of deficient fire or consumption of body fluid due to pathogenic dry-heat.

You Gui Wan (The Kidney-*Yang*-Reinforcing Bolus)

● Source: *Jing Yue Quan Shu* (Complete Works of *Zhang Jingyue*)

● Ingredients: *Shu Di* (Rhizoma Rehmanniae Praeparata) 24g.

    Shan Yao (Rhizoma Disocoreae) (Parched) 12g.

    Shan Zhu Yu (Fructus Corni) 9g.

    Gou Qi Zi (Fructus Lycii) 9g.

Tu Si Zi (Semen Cuscutae) 12g.

Lu Jiao Jiao (Colla Cornus Cervi) 12g.

Du Zhong (Cortex Eucommiae) 12g.

Rou Gui (Cortex Cinnamomi) 6g.

Dang Gui (Radix Angelicae Sinensis) 9g.

Zhi Fui Zi (Radix Aconiti Lateralis Praeparata) 6g.

● Administration: Except *Shu Di* which will be well-steamed to make into paste, other drugs are ground into fine powder to be mixed with honey and the paste of *Shu Di* to make bolus. Each bolus weighs 9 grams. One bolus is taken each time with boiled water.

● Functions: Warm and tonify kidney-*Yang* and replenish essence.

● Indications: insufficiency of kidney-*Yang* and decline of life-gate fire, often seen in aged patients or chronic diseases, marked by lassitude, aversion to cold, cold limbs, soreness and weakness of the waist and knees, impotence, seminal emission, or sterility due to deficiency of *Yang*, or poor appetite, or incontinence of urine, pale tongue with white coating, deep and slow pulse.

● Explanation:

Fu Zi and *Rou Gui*: acrid in taste and hot in nature.

Lu Jiao Jiao: sweet in taste and salty in nature, warming and tonifying the primary *Yang* in the kidney and expelling cold.

Shu Di, *Shan Yu Rou*, *Gou Qi Zi* and *Shan Yao*: the assistant drugs, nourishing *Yin*, tonifying the kidney, reinforcing the liver and spleen, and replenishing essence and marrow.

Tu Si Zi and *Du Zhong*: the adjuvant drugs, tonifying the liver and kidney and strengthening waist and kness.

Dang Gui: the guiding drug, nourishing and regulating blood.

○ The prescription as a whole plays the effect of warming *Yang*, tonifying kidney, replenishing essence and nourishing blood so as to reinforce *Yang* within the kidney.

● Notes:

(1) The modified prescriptions are used for cases with insufficiency of kidney *Yang*, seen in diseases such as nephrotic syndrome, senile osteporororosis, sterility due to spermacrasia, anemia and leukopenia, etc.

(2) It is not advisable for cases with deficiency of kidney complicated with turbid-dampness.

Summary

Fourteen tonic prescriptions are selected which are divided into five types according to their functions. They are prescriptions as *Qi*-tonics, prescriptions as blood-tonics, prescriptions as both *Qi* and blood tonics, prescriptions as *Yin*-tonics and prescriptions as *Yang*-tonics.

(1) Prescriptions as *Qi*-tonics

Si Jun Zi Tang, *Shen Ling Bai Zhu San*, *Bu Zhong Yi Qi Tang* and *Sheng Mai San* all have the effect of tonifying *Qi*, indicating for syndromes of *Qi*-deficiency. *Si Jun Zi Tang* is mainly to replenish *Qi* and invigorate the spleen, indicating for deficiency of spleen and stomach *Qi*. It is a basic prescription of tonifying *Qi*. *Shen Ling Bai Zhu San* has the effect of replenishing *Qi* and invigorating the spleen associated with the functions of harmonizing the stomach and removing dampness, indicating for retention of dampness due to deficiency of the spleen. *Bu Zhong Yi Qi Tang* is mainly to replenish *Qi* and raise *Yang*, indicating for impairment of the spleen due to overexertion marked by fever due to *Qi* deficiency and symptoms caused by *Qi* sinking. *Sheng Mai San* mainly replenishes *Qi* and produces body fluid, indicating for consumption of both *Qi* and *Yin* caused by excessive heat which scorches body fluid.

(2) Prescriptions as blood-tonics

Si Wu Tang, *Dang Gui Bu Xue Tang*, *Gui Pi Tang* and *Zhi Gan Cao Tang* all have the effect of tonifying blood. *Si Wu Tang* is mainly to tonify blood and regulate blood, and is a basic prescription for treating blood deficiency. *Dang Gui Bu Xue Tang* is mainly to tonify *Qi* so as to produce blood, indicating for internal injury due to overexertion, failure of *Qi* to produce blood and fever due to blood deficiency. *Gui Pi Tang* mainly replenishes *Qi*, tonifies blood, invigorates spleen and nourishes heart, indicating for deficiency of the heart blood and spleen *Qi*. *Zhi Gan Cao Tang* is mainly to reinforce *Qi*, nourish *Yin* and blood, indicating for insufficiency of *Qi* and blood, marked by knotty and intermittent pulse, palpitation and the consumptive lung disease.

(3) Prescriptions as both *Qi* and blood tonics

Ba Zhen Tang is a typical prescription for tonifying both *Qi* and blood, indicating for great loss of blood or deficiency of both *Qi* and blood.

(4) Prescriptions as *Yin*-tonics

Liu Wei Di Huang Wan, *Zuo Gui Wan*, and *Yi Guan Jian* are all used to nourish *Yin* of the liver and kidney, treating *Yin* deficiency syndromes. *Liu Wei Di Huang Wan* is a representative prescription for tonifying kidney *Yin* and has the function of strengthening the water to control fire, indicating for flaring-up of deficient fire due to insufficiency of kidney-*Yin*. *Zuo Gui Wan* mainly nourishes kidney *Yin* and replenishes essence, treating internal deficiency syndromes such as impairment of genuine *Yin*, essence and marrow. It only has the effect of reinforcing without reducing comparing with *Liu Wei Di Huang Wan*. *Yi Guan Jian* has the function of nourishing *Yin* and activating liver *Qi* and is good at nourishing *Yin* and blood to benefit the liver, indicating for insufficiency of blood of the liver and kidney with unsmooth movement of liver *Qi*.

(5) Prescriptions as *Yang*-tonics

Both *Shen Qi Wan* and *You Gui Wan* have the effect of warming and tonifying kidney *Yang*, indicating for syndrome of insufficiency of kidney *Yang*. *Shen Qi Wan* warms and tonifies kidney *Yang* to produce junior fire. *You Gui Wan* warms and tonifies kidney *Yang* to replenish essence and blood. Comparing the two prescriptions, *You Gui Wan* is a pure tonification recipe which does not have reducing effect, and its effects of reinforcing kidney *Yang* and replenishing essence are stronger than *Shen Qi Wan*.

Review Questions

(1) Please list out the representative prescriptions and their indications according to the classification of tonic prescriptions.

(2) *Gui Pi Tang* can mainly treat severe palpitation and amnesia which belong to the pathology of the upper *Jiao*, but why can it also treat metrorrhagia and metrostaxis which is the problem of the lower *Jiao*?

(3) Why are *Yang*-tonics associated with drugs for nourishing *Yin*? And why are *Yin*-tonics associated with drugs for reinforcing *Yang*? Please give examples.

(4) Why is the dosage of *Huang Qi* five times as much as *Dang Gui* in the prescription *Dang Gui Bu Xue Tang*?

(5) What are the differences in compatibility among *Zuo Gui Wan*, *You Gui Wan*, *Liu Wei Di Huang Wan* and *Shen Qi Wan*? And what are the differences in their functions?

11 Prescriptions for Treating Wind

This type of prescriptions, mainly composed of the wind-dispelling drugs with acrid taste, or wind-calming and convulsion-relieving drugs, having the effect of dispelling exogenous wind or calming endogenous wind, indicating for wind disease, are called prescriptions for treating the wind.

Wind diseases are divided into two categories: exogenous wind and endogenous wind. Dispersing or dispelling method is used for exogenous wind diseases and calming method is used for endogenous wind diseases. Therefore, prescriptions for treating wind are divided into two types: The prescriptions for dispelling exogenous wind and the prescriptions for calming endogenous wind.

11.1 Prescriptions for Dispelling Exogenous Wind

This group of prescriptions is indicated for headache, aversion to wind and numbness of the limbs which are caused by exogenous wind.

Chuan Xiong Cha Tiao San (Chuanxiong Mixture)

● Source: *Tai Ping Hui Min He Ji Ju Fang* (Prescriptions of Peaceful Benevolent Dispensary)

● Ingredients: *Chuan Xiong* (Rhizoma Ligustici Chuanxiong)
　　　　　　　Jing Jie (Herba Schizonepetae)
　　　　　　　Bai Zhi (Radix Angelicae Dahuricae)
　　　　　　　Qiang Huo (Rhizoma seu Radix Notopterygii)
　　　　　　　Zhi Gan Cao (Radix Glycyrrhizae Praeparata)
　　　　　　　　　　　　each of the above 60g.
　　　　　　　Xi Xin (Herba Asari) 30g.
　　　　　　　Fang Feng (Radix Ledebouriellae) 45g.
　　　　　　　Bo He (Herba Menthae) 240g.

● Administration: Grind the drugs into fine powder, take 6 grams each time with tea after meal. It can also be decocted in water for oral administration, but the dosages should be reduced according to the proportion.

● Functions: Dispel wind and relieve pain.

● Indications: Headache due to exogenous wind marked by lateral or vertical headache, aversion to cold, fever, dizziness, stuffy nose, thin white coating of the tongue and floating pulse.

● Explanation:

Chuan Xiong, *Bai Zhi* and *Qiang Huo*: the principal drugs, acrid in taste and warm in nature, dispelling wind and relieving pain.

Among the above drugs, *Chuan Xiong* is effective for *Shaoyang* headache and Jueyin headache (vertical and lateral headache). *Qiang Huo* is for *Taiyang* headache (occipital headache), and *Bai Zhi* is for *Yangming* headache (frontal headache).

Xi Xin: dispelling cold and relieving pain used for *Shaoyin* headache.

Bo He: refreshing the mind, dispelling wind and other pathogens.

Jing Jie and *Fang Feng*: expelling and dispersing wind in the upper part of the body. These three groups are assistant drugs.

Gan Cao: harmonizing the middle *Jiao*, benefiting *Qi* and regulating the effect of other drugs in the prescription.

Taking the medicine with tea is to refresh the mind as well as preventing the excessive warm dryness and the excessive elevating and dispelling actions of the wind-dispelling drugs' which are of acrid taste.

Gan Cao and Tea are used as adjuvant and guiding drugs.

○ The combination of all the drugs plays the effect of dispelling wind and relieving pain.

● Notes:

(1) The modified prescription is advisable for common cold, migraine, nervous headache, headache due to chronic rhinitis, which belong to the attack of exogenous wind.

(2) The prescription is not indicated for headache due to *Qi* deficiency or blood deficiency or hyperactivity of liver- *Yang* or *Yin* deficiency of the liver and kidney or stirring-up of liver-wind.

Qian Zheng San (Powder for Treating Wry-Mouth)

● Source: *Yang Shi Jia Cang Fang* (*Yang*'s Home Collection of Formulas)
● Ingredients: *Bai Fu Zi* (Rhizoma Typhonii)

           Jiang Chan (Bombyx Batryticatus)

           Quan Xie (Scorpio)

These three drugs are in eaqual dosage.

● Administration: Grind the above drugs into fine powder, take 3 grams each time after mixing well with hot wine or warm boiled water. It can also be used as decoction.

● Functions: Dispel wind, remeve phlegm and relieve spasm.

● Indications: Facial paralysis with deviation of the mouth and eyes, caused by wind.

● Explanation:

Bai Fu Zi: the principal drug, acrid and sweet in taste and warm in nature, dispelling wind, removing phlegm, good at treating wind on the head and face.

Jiang Can and *Quan Xie*: the assistant drugs, salty and acrid in taste and neutral in nature, dispelling wind and relieving spasm. *Jiang Can* also removing phlegm and *Quan Xie* dredging the meridians.

Mixed with hot wine, the powdered drugs will have the effect of clearing blood vessels and conducting other drugs to the affected collaterals.

○ The combination of all the drugs plays the effect of dispelling wind, removing phlegm and relieving spasms.

● Notes:

(1) The modified prescription can be used to treat facial paralysis, trigeminal neuralgia and migraine which are caused by obstruction of the meridians by phlegm.

(2) The prescription is not advisable for wry mouth or hemiplegia caused by *Qi* deficiency and blood stasis or stirring-up of the liver-wind.

(3) Dosages as decoction: *Bai Fu* Zi 3-5g. *Quan Xie* 9g. *Jiang Chan* 9g.

Xiao Feng San (Powder for Dispersing Pathogenic Wind)

● Source: *Wai Ke Zheng Zong* (Orthodox Manual of External Diseases)
● Ingredients: *Dang Gui* (Radix Angelicae Sinensis) 6g.

> *Sheng Di* (Radix Rehmanniae) 6g.
> *Fang Feng* (Radix Ledebouriellae) 6g.
> *Chan Tui* (Periostracum Cicadae) 6g.
> *Zhi Mu* (Rhizoma Anemarrhenae) 6g.
> *Ku Shen* (Radix Sophorae Flavescentis) 6g.
> *Hu Ma Ren* (Semen Sesami) 6g.
> *Jing Jie* (Herba Schizonepetae) 6g.
> *Cang Zhu* (Rhizoma Atractylodis) 6g.
> *Niu Bang Zi* (Fructus Arctii) 6g.
> *Shi Gao* (Gypsum Fibrosum) 9g.
> *Mu Tong* (Caulis Akebiae) 4.5g.
> *Gan Cao* (Radix Glycyrrhizae) 4.5g.

● Administration: All the drugs are decocted in water. Take the decoction with empty stomach.

● Functions: Dispel wind, nourish blood, clear away heat and remove dampness.

● Indications: Rubella and eczema, marked by red skin rash or general cloudy spats with pruritus, exudation of fluid after being scratched, white or yellow coating of the tongue, floating rapid pulse.

● Explanation:

Jing Jie and *Fang Feng*: acrid in taste and slight warm in nature.

Niu Bang Zi: acrid and bitter in taste and cold in nature.

Chan Tui: sweet in taste and cold in nature.

The above four drugs are used as principal drugs for expelling wind from the body surface.

Cang Zhu: dispersing wind-dampness.

— 238 —

Ku Shen : clearing away heat and drying dampness.

Mu Tong : removing damp-heat from urine.

Shi Gao and *Zhi Mu* : clearing away heat and reducing fire.

Those five drugs are assistant drugs.

Dang Gui, *Sheng Di* and *Hu Ma Ren* : the adjuvant drugs, nourishing and activating blood, nourishing *Yin* and moistening dryness.

Sheng Gan Cao : the guiding drug, clearing away heat, removing toxins and regulating the effects of other drugs.

○ The prescription as a whole plays the effects of dispelling wind, nourishing blood, clearing away heat and removing dampness.

● Notes:

(1) The modified prescription may treat allergic dermatitis, nervous dermatitis, dermatitis medicamentosa and urticaria which are caused by pathogenic wind-heat.

(2) During the period for taking this medicine, do not take acrid food, fish, strong tea and avoid smoking and drinking in case they will influence the effect of the medicine.

11.2 Prescriptions for Treating Endogenous Wind

The prescriptions for treating endogenous wind are indicated for endogenous wind syndrome. For persistent high fever and convulsions due to internal wind caused by extreme excessive pathogenic heat, or for dizziness, vertigo, pain and hot sensation in the head and even sudden falling down with hemiplegia caused by stirring-up of the liver wind due to hyperactivity of the liver *Yang*, the therapy of calming the liver and stopping the wind will be adopted since they are typical excess syndromes of endogenous wind. Contracture of the muscles and tendons, involuntary movment (shaking) of the four limbs in the later period of febrile disease is internal wind of the deficient type, and the treatment method will be nourishing *Yin* to stop endogenous wind.

Ling Jia Gou Teng Tang (Decoction of Antelope's Horn and Uncaria Stem)

● Source: *Tong Su Shang Han Lun* (Revised Popular Treatise on Cold-induced Diseases)

● Ingredients: *Ling Yang Jiao* (Cornu Saigae Tataricae) 4.5g. (Decocted first)

　　　　　　 Shuang Gou Teng (Ramulus Uncariae Cum Uncis) 9g (Decocted later)

　　　　　　 Sang Ye (Folium Mori) 6g.

　　　　　　 Ju Hua (Flos Chrysanthemi) 9g.

　　　　　　 Xian Sheng Di (Radix Rehmanniae) 15g.

　　　　　　 Bai Shao (Radix Paeoniae Alba) 9g.

　　　　　　 Chuan Bei (Bulbus Fritillariae Cirrhosae) 12g.

　　　　　　 Zhu Ru (Caulis Bambusae in Taenis) (fresh, decocted first with *Ling Yang Jiao* in water) 15g.

Fu Shen Mu (Poria cum Ligno Hospite) 9g.

Sheng Gan Cao (Radix Glycyrrhizae) 3g.

● Administration: All the drugs should be decocted in water for oral administration.

● Functions: Cooling the liver, calming endogenous wind, increasing body fluid and relaxing muscles and tendons.

● Indications: Occurrence of wind due to liver heat, marked by persistent high fever, restlessness, spasm and convulsion of the four limbs, and even coma, dry and deep-red tongue or prickled and parched tongue, wiry and rapid pulse.

● Explanation:

Ling Yang Jiao: salty in taste and cold in nature, cooling the liver and stopping the wind.

Gou Teng: sweet in taste and cold in nature, clearing away heat and relieving convulsions.

They are principal drugs.

Sang Ye and *Ju Hua*: the assistant drugs, acrid in taste and cool in nature, clearing away heat, calming the liver and stopping endogenous wind, used as assistant drugs to strengthen the effect of cooling the liver and calming wind.

Xian Sheng Di, *Bai Shao* and *Sheng Gan Cao*: producing body fluid, nourishing *Yin*, tonifying the liver and relaxing tendons and musles, treating both the root cause and symptoms in combination with *Ling Yang Jiao* and *Gou Teng*.

Bei Mu and *Zhu Ru*: clearing away heat and removing phlegm.

Fu Shen Mu: calming the liver and tranquilizing the mind.

The above 6 ingredients are adjuvant drugs.

Sheng Gan Cao: the guiding drug, regulating the effects of the other drugs.

○ The prescription as a whole performs the functions of cooling the liver, calming endogenous wind, clearing away heat, relieving convulsions, producing body fluid, and relaxing tendons and muscles.

● Notes:

(1) This is a typical prescription for treating wind due to extreme excessive heat. The modified prescription may treat headache, dizziness, vertigo and convulsions seen in diseases such as hypertension, functional disturbance of vegetative nervous system, cerebrovascular accident, hyperthyroidism, epilepsy during pregnancy and epidemic encephalitis B which belong to stirring-up of wind due to live-heat.

(2) It is not advisable for stirring up of wind due to *Yin* deficiency in the later stage of febrile diseases, marked by spasm of the muscles and tendons and involuntary movement of limbs.

(3) *Ling Yang Jiao* now is often used as powder, 0.3-0.6g. each time.

Zhen Gan Xin Feng Tang (Tranquilizing Liver-Wind Decoction)

● Source: *Yi Xue Zhong Zhong Can Xi Lu* (Records of Traditional Chinese and Western Medicine in Combination)

● Ingredients: *Huai Niu Xi* (Radix Achyranthis Bidentatae) 30g.

Sheng Zhe Shi (Ochra Haematitum) (ground into fine powder) 30g.

Sheng Long Gu (Os Draconis Fossilia Ossis Mastodi) (smashed) 15g.

Sheng Gui Ban (Plastrum Testudinis) (Smashed) 15g.

Sheng Hang Shao (Radix Paeoniae Alba) 15g.

Xuan Shen (Radix Scrophulariae) 15g.

Tian Dong (Radix Asparagi) 15g.

Chuan Lian Zi (Fructus Meliae Toosendan) (Smashed) 6g.

Sheng Mai Ya (Fructus Hordei Germinatus) 6g.

Yin Chen (Herba Artemisiae Capillaris) 6g.

Gan Cao (Radix Glycyrrhizae) 4g.

● Administration: All the drugs should be decocted in water for oral adminstration.

● Functions: Suppress liver wind, nourish *Yin* and check adverse-rise of *Yang*.

● Indications: Stirring-up of wind due to *Yang* excess, marked by dizziness, vertigo, distension in the eye, tinnitus, pain and hot sensation in the head, flushed face, restlessness, or frequent belching, or progressive difficulty in moving the limbs, or gradual deviation of the mouth, or dizziness even falling down with loss of consciousness, coming round when moved, but in some cases not as normal as before, wiry and forceful pulse.

● Explanation:

Huai Niu Xi: the principal drug, bitter and sour in taste, conducting blood to descend and tonifying the liver and kidney.

Zhe Shi, *Long Gu* and *Mu Li*: the assistant drugs, discending the upward peversion of *Qi*, suppressing *Yang*, calming the liver and stopping wind.

Gui Ban, *Xuan Shen*, *Tian Dong* and *Bai Shao*: moistening and nourishing *Yin* fluid to check the excess of *Yang*.

Yin Chen, *Chuan Lian Zi* and *Sheng Mai Ya*: promoting and regulating the circulation of liver *Qi*, clearing away heat.

Gan Cao: regulating the effect of the other drugs, combining with *Mai Ya* to harmonize the stomach and regulate the middle *Jiao* to prevent metal and mineral drugs from affecting the functions of the stomach.

They are all adjuvant and guilding drugs.

○ The combination of all the drugs plays the effect of calming the liver, stopping wind, nourishing *Yin* and lowering the ascending of *Yang*.

● Notes:

The modified prescription can treat hypertension, cerebrovascular accident and hypertensive encephalopathy which belong to *Yin* deficiency of the liver and kidney, hyperactivity of the liver *Yang* and disorder of *Qi* and blood.

Tian Ma Gou Teng Yin (Decoctin of Gastrodia and Uncaria)

● Source: *Za Bing Zheng Zhi Xin Yi* (New Standards for Diagnosis and Treatment of Miscellaneous Diseases)

● Ingredients: *Tian Ma* (Rhizoma Gastrodiae) 9g.

      Gou Teng (Ramulus Uncariae Cum Uncis) (decocted later) 12g.

      Shi Jue Ming (Concha Haliotidis) (decocted first) 18g.

      Zhi Zi (Fructus Gardeniae) 9g.

      Huang Qin (Radix Scutellariae) 9g.

      Chuan Niu Qi (Radix Achyranthis Bidentatae) 12g.

      Du Zhong (Cortex Eucommiae) 9g.

      Yi Mu Cao (Herba Leonuri) 9g.

      Sang Ji Sheng (Ramulus Loranthi) 9g.

      Ye Jiao Teng (Caulis Polygoni Multiflori) 9g.

      Fu Shen (Poria cum Ligno Hospite) 9g.

● Administration: All the drugs are to be decocted in water for oral administration.

● Functions: Calm the liver, stop wind, clear away heat, activate blood and tonify liver and kidney.

● Indications: Internal wind caused by hyperactivity of the liver *Yang*, marked by headache, dizziness and vertigo, insomnia, tinnitus, blurred vision, involuntary movement of limbs, or even hemiplegia, red tongue with yellow coating, wiry and rapid pulse.

● Explanation:

Tian Ma: sweet in taste and neutral in nature.

Gou Teng: sweet in taste and cold in nature.

Shi Jue Ming: salty in taste and cold in nature.

The above three are principal drugs which calm the liver and stop wind.

Zhi Zi and *Huang Qin*: the assistant drugs, bitter in taste and cold in nature, clearing away heat from the liver meridian and reducing fire.

Yi Mu Cao: activating blood and inducing diuresis.

Niu Xi: conducting blood to descend.

Du Zhong and *Sang Ji Sheng*: tonifying the liver and kidney.

Ye Jiao Teng and *Fu Shen*: tranquilizing the mind.

The above six ingredients are adjuvant and guiding durgs.

○ The prescription as a whole plays the effect of calming the liver, stopping endogenous wind, clearing away heat, activating blood and tonifying the liver and kidney.

● Notes:

The modified prescription may treat hypertension, cerebrovascular accident, hyperthyroidism, functional disturbance of vegetative nerve, epilepsy, dizziness and vertigo which give rise to wind syndromes caused by hyperactivity of the liver-*yang*.

Da Ding Feng Zhu (Great Pearl for Wind Syndrome)

- Source: *Wen Bing Tiao Bian* (Treatise on Differentiation and Treatment of Epidemic Febrile Diseases)
- Ingredients: *Bai Shao* (Radix Paeoniae Alba) 18g.

    E Jiao (Colla Corii Asini) 9g.

    Gui Ban (Plastrum Testudinis) 12g.

    Sheng Di (Radix Rehmanniae) 18g.

    Ma Ren (Fructus Cannabis) 6g.

    Wu Wei Zi (Fructus Schisandrae) 6g.

    Mu Li (Concha Ostreae) 12g.

    Mai Mei Dong (Radix Opiopogonis) 18g.

    Zhi Gan Cao (Radix Glycyrrhizae Praeparata) 12g.

    Ji Zi Huang (Yolk) (fresh) 2 pcs.

    Bie Jia (Carapax Trionycis) 12g.

- Administration: Decoct all the drugs in water except *E Jiao* which is melted into the decoction after removing the residue. Take it warmly after mixing with yolk.
- Functions: Nourish *Yin* and calm endogenous wind.
- Indications: Endogenous wind in the later stage of febrile diseases, due to *Yin* deficiency, marked by lassitude, twitching of muscles, weak pulse, deep red tongue with little coating, with the tendancy of collapse.
- Explanation:

Ji Zi Huang and *E Jiao*: the principal drugs, sweet in taste and neutral in nature, nourishing *Yin* and body fluid in order to calm endogenous wind.

Bai Shao, *Di Huang* and *Mai Dong*: nourishing *Yin* to soften the liver, strengthening water so as to hold wood.

Gui Ban and *Bie Jia*: nourishing *Yin* and suppressing *Yang*.

These five are the assistant drugs.

Ma Ren: nourishing *Yin* to treat dryness.

Mu Li: calming the liver and suppressing *Yang*.

Wu Wei Zi and *Zhi Gan Cao*: sour and sweet in taste, used to produce *Yin*.

The above 4 ingredients are adjuvant and guiding drugs to strengthen the functions of nourishing *Yin* and calming wind.

○ The prescription as a whole performs the functions of nourishing *Yin* and body fluid, softening the liver and calming the endogenous wind.

- Notes:

(1) The modified prescription may treat palpitation, insomnia, vertigo and involuntary movement of limbs in the later period of epidemic cerebrospinal meningitis and encephalitis B which give rise to wind syndromes due to *Yin* deficiency or failure of blood in nourishing the heart.

(2) The prescription is not advisable for cases with insufficiency of fluid and excess of pathogenic *Qi*.

Di Huang Yin Zi (Rehmannia Decoction)

● Source: *Xuan Ming Lun Fang* (Prescriptions and Expositions of *Huangdi's* Plain Questions)

● Ingredients: *Shu Di* (Radix Rehmanniae Praeparata) 15-30g.

Rou Cong Rong (Herba Cistachis) 10-15g.

Ba Ji Tian (Radix Morindae Officinalis) 10g.

Shan Zhu Yu (Fructus Corni) 10g.

Shi Hu (Herba Dendrobii) 10g.

Mai Dong (Radix Opiopogonis) 10g.

Fu Ling (Poria) 10g.

Pao Fu Zi (Radix Aconiti Lateralis Praeparata) 4.5-6g.

Rou Gui (Cortex Cinnamomi) 3-6g.

Shi Chang Pu (Rhizoma Acori Graminei) 4.5-6g.

Bo He (Herba Menthae) 1.5g.

Sheng Jiang (Rhizoma Zingieris) 3 slic.

Da Zao (Fructus Ziziphi Jujubae) 4 pcs.

● Administration: All the drugs are decocted in water for oral administration in two times.

● Functions: Nourish kidney *Yin*, warm kidney *Yang*, open orifices and remov phlegm.

● Indications: Aphasia in apoplexy due to kidney deficiency, manifested as voiceless, weakness or paralysis of the lower limbs, or impaired movement of the limbs with analgesia, feeble pulse.

● Explanation:

Shu Di: sweet in taste and warm in nature.

Shan Zhu Yu: sour in taste and warm in nature.

They are used to reinforce kidney Yin.

Ba Ji Tian, *Rou Cong Rong*, *Fu Zi* and *Rou Gui*: acrid sweet and salty in taste and warm in nature, warming and reinforcing kidney *Yang*.

All the above ingredients are principal drugs.

Shi Hu, *Mai Dong* and *Wu Wei Zi*: the assistant drugs, nurishing *Yin* and controlling fluid to coordinate *Yin* and *Yang*.

Shi Chang Pu, *Yuan Zhi* and *Fu Ling*: the adjuvant drugs, coordinating the heart and kidney, opening the orifices and removing phlegm.

Sheng Jiang, *Da Zao* and *Bo He*: the guiding drugs, regulating *Ying* and *Wei*.

○ The combination of all the drugs plays the effect of nourishing kidney *Yin*, tonifying kidney *Yang*, opening the orifices and removing phlegm.

● Notes:

(1) The modified prescription may treat aphasia seen in diseases as myelitis, lateral sclerosis, syringomyelia and chronic progressive bulbar paralysis.

(2) The prescription is indicated for cases with voiceless, disabled foot, and paralysis due to serious deficiency. Therefore, it is not advisable for syndromes due to hyperactivity of the liver-*yang*.

(3) In the original prescription, there are equal dosages for every drugs. Grind into powder and take 9g., each time to be decocted in water with 5pc. of *Sheng Jiang*, 1pc. of *Da Zao* and 5-7 leaves of *Bo He*.

Summary

8 main prescriptions for treating wind are selected, which are divided into two types according to their functions: the prescriptions for dispelling exogenous wind and the prescriptions for calming endogenous wind.

(1) Prescriptions for dispelling exogenous wind:

Chuan Xiong Cha Tiao San is good at dispelling wind in the upper part of the body, indicating for migraine and headache caused by attack of pathogenic wind. *Qian Zheng San* is good at eliminating wind and removing phlegm, indicating for deviation of the mouth and eyes due to obstruction of wind phlegm in meridians. *Xiao Feng San* dispels wind, nourishes blood, clears away heat and removes dampness. It is a commonly used prescription for the treatment of urticaria and eczema.

(2) Prescriptions for calming endogenous wind:

Ling Jiao Gou Teng Tang, *Zhen Gan Xi Feng Tang*, and *Tian Ma Gou Teng Yin* can calm the liver and stop endogenous wind. *Ling Jiao Gou Teng Tang* has a strong effect of cooling the liver, clearing away heat and relieving convulsion, indicating for stirring-up of wind due to excessive heat in the liver meridian. *Zhen Gan Xi Feng Tang* has strong effect of suppressing *Yang*, calming the liver and stopping wind, indicating for stirring-up of liver wind caused by hyperactivity of the liver *Yang*. *Tian Ma Gou Teng Yin* is associated with the effect of clearing away heat, activating blood and tranquilizing the mind, indicating for headache, vertigo and insomnia caused by excess of the liver yang and upward disturbance of the liver wind. *Da Ding Feng Zhu* is a prescription for nourishing *Yin* and calming wind, indicating for stirring-up of deficient wind due to damage of true *Yin* by pathogenic heat. *Di Huang Yin Zi* is good at nourishing kidney *Yin*, tonifying kidney *Yang*, opening the orifices and removing phlegm, indicating for aphasia caused by upward peversion of tubid phlegm due to weakness of the kidney.

Review Questions

(1) Please state the significance of ingredients and indications of *Chuan Xiong Cha Tiao Yin* and *Xiao Feng San*.

(2) Both *Ling Jiao Gou Teng Yin* and *Zhen Gan Xi Feng Tang* can calm endogenous wind and treat stirring-up of liver wind. What are the differences of indications and treatment principles between them?

(3) Please state the significance of ingredients and indications of *Tian Ma Gou Teng Yin*.

(4) Please explain the differences and similarities between *Da Ding Feng Zhu* and *Ling Yang Gou Teng Tang* in their ingredients, functions and indications.

(5) Why can *Di Huang Yin Zi* treat aphasia syndrome? What are the features of applying drugs?

12　Prescriptions for Treating Dryness

The prescriptions, consisting of the drugs with acrid and sweet taste and cold nature, having the effect of moistening the dryness by activating lung Qi or by nourishing Yin, being used for dryness syndromes, are called the prescriptions for treating dryness.

According to the etiology of the diseases, dryness syndromes are divided into two types: moistening dryness by activating lung Qi and moistening dryness by nourishing Yin.

The prescriptions for moistening dryness are used for exogenous or endogenous dryness syndromes, and they should not be used for cases with constitutional dampness. For cases with loose stool due to spleen deficiency, Qi stagnation and profuse phlegm, this kind of prescriptions should be used with great care.

12.1　Moistening Dryness by Activating Lung Qi

This type of prescriptions is used to treat exogenous cool-dryness syndrome.

Xing Su San (Powder of Armeniacae Amarum and Perillae)

- Source: *Wen Bing Tiao Bian* (From Detailed Analysis of Seasonal Febrile Diseases)
- Ingredients: *Su Ye* (Folium Perillae) 9g.
  Xing Ren (Semen Armeniacae Amarum) 9g.
  Ban Xia (Rhizoma Pinelliae) 9g.
  Fu Ling (Poria) 9g.
  Qian Hu (Radix Peucedani) 9g.
  Ku Xing Ren (Bitter Radix Platycodi) 6g.
  Ju Pi (Pericarpium Citri Reticulatae) 6g.
  Zhi Qiao (Fructus Aurantii) 6g.
  Gan Cao (Radix Glycyrrhizae) 3g.
  Sheng Jiang (Rhizoma Zingberis Recens) 3 pcs.
  Da Zao (Fructus Ziziphi Jujubae) 3 pcs.
- Administration: The drugs are decocted in water for oral administration.
- Functions: Expel cool-dryness, promote lung Qi to eliminate phlegm.
- Indications: attack of exogenous coolness and dryness, manifested as slight headache, aversion to cold without sweat, cough with thin phlegm, nasal obstruction, dry throat, white tongue coating, and wiry pulse.
- Explanation:

Su Ye: acrid in taste and warm in nature, inducing diaphoresis and promoting lung Qi to eliminate cool-dryness from the body surface.

Xing Ren: bitter in taste and mild warm in nature, promoting lung's function to relieve cough and eliminate phlegm, performing as the principal drug in the prescription.

Qian Hu: expelling wind, desending adverse rising *Qi* and eliminating phlegm.

Jie Geng and *Zhi Qiao*: promoting lung's function in dispersing and descending, used as assistant drugs.

Ban Xia, *Ju Pi* and *Fu Ling*: promoting *Qi* and eliminating phlegm, as the adjuvant drugs.

Sheng Jiang, *Da Zao* and *Gan Cao*: the guiding drugs, regulating *Ying* and *Wei* and coordinating the effects of all the drugs in the prescription.

○ All the above drugs as a whole has the effects of expelling external pathogenic factors, promoting lung function, activating *Qi* to resolve phlegm.

● Notes:

(1) For cases of influenza, bronchitis and pneumonectasis, etc, manifested as cool-dryness syndrome due to invading of exogenous pathogenic factors, this prescription is advisable.

(2) It's not advisable for cases of warm-dryness syndrome.

Sang Xing Tang (Decoction of Mulberry Leaf and Apricot Kernel)

● Source: *Wen Bing Tiao Bian* (Detailed Analysis of Seasonal Febrile Diseases)

● Ingredients: *Sang Ye* (Folium Mori) 6g.

　　　　　　Xing Ren (Semen Armeniacae Amarum) 9g.

　　　　　　Sha Shen (Radix Adenophorae) 12g.

　　　　　　Zhe Bei (Bulbus Fritillariae Thunbergii) 6g.

　　　　　　Dan Dou Chi (Semen Sojae Praeparatum) 6g.

　　　　　　Zhi Zi Pi (Pericarpium Gardeniae) 6g.

　　　　　　Li Pi (Exocarpium Pyrus) 6g.

● Administration: The drugs are decocted in water for oral administration.

● Functions: Expel warm-dryness, moisten the lung to relieve cough.

● Indications: Affection of exogenous warm-dryness, manifested as headache, fever, thirst, dryness of throat and nose, dry cough or with little sticky phlegm, red tongue with thin white and dry coating, and floating and rapid pulse.

● Explanation:

Sang Ye: bitter in taste, cold in nature, expelling dry-heat.

Xing Ren: activating lung *Qi*, moistening dryness to relieve cough.

The above two are used as the principal drugs in the prescription.

Dou Chi: acrid in taste and cool in nature, expelling exogenous pathogenic factors to strengthen the effect of *Sang Ye*.

Bei Mu: clearing heat to resolving phlegm, strengthening the effect of *Xing Ren* to stop cough and eliminating phlegm.

Sha Shen: nourishing the lung, stopping cough and producing fluid.

The above three are used as the assistant drugs.

Zhi Zi Pi: light in nature, entering the upper *Jiao* to clear away lung heat.

Li Pi: clearing away heat and moistening dryness, stopping cough and resolving phlegm.

The above two drugs are used as the adjuvant and guiding drugs.

○ All above drugs as a whole perform the functions of expelling dry-heat, moistening the lung to stop cough.

● Notes:

(1) It's a representative prescription for treating the cases due to external warm-dryness.

The modified prescription is applied for mild cases of exogenous warm-dryness, seen in diseases such as upper respiratory tract infection, acute bronchitis, hemoptysis due to bronchiectasis, whooping cough, etc.

Qing Zao Jiu Fei Tang (Decation for Clearing Away Dryness and Treating Lung Disorders)

● Source: *Yi Men Fa Lu* (Rules for Physicians)

● Ingredients: *Dong Sang Ye* (Folium Mori) 9g.

        Shi Gao (Gypsum Fibrosum) 8g.

        Gan Cao (Radix Glycyrrhizae) 3g.

        Ren Shen (Radix Ginseng) 2g.

        Hu Ma Ren (Semen Sesami, stir-fryed and ground) 3g.

        E Jiao (Colla Corii Asini) 3g.

        Pi Pa Ye (Folium Eriobotryae, baked with honey) 3g.

● Administration: The drugs are decocted in water for oral administration.

● Functions: Clear away dryness and moisten the lung.

● Indications: Damage of the lung by warm-dryness, marked by headache, fever, dry cough, dyspnea, dry throat and nose, thirst, stuffiness in the chest, dry tongue with less coating, forceless, big and rapid pulse.

● Explanation:

Sang Ye: a principal drug, bitter and sweet in taste and cold in nature, clearing away lung dry-heat.

Shi Gao: acrid in taste and cold in nature, clearing away lung heat.

Mai Dong: nourishing *Yin* and moistening lung.

The above three ingredients are the assistant drugs.

Ren Shen and *Gan Cao*: reinforcing *Qi* and regulating middle *Jiao*, building up the "earth" to supplement the "metal".

Ma Ren and *E Jiao*: nourshing *Yin* and moistening the lung.

Xing Ren and *Pi Pa Ye*: the adjuvant drugs, descending the adverse-rising lung *Qi*.

○ All the above drugs as a whole has the functions of clearing away dry-heat, nourishing *Yin* and strengthening *Qi*.

● Notes:

It can be used as a basic prescription to treat the cases of pneumonia, bronchial asthma, acute and chronic bronchitis, pneumonectasis, lung cancer and early stage of pulmonary tuberculosis with cough and less phlegm, which belongs to the type of damage of the lung by warm-dryness and deficiency of both lung *Qi* and *Yin*.

Appendix:

Qiao He Tang (Decoction of Fructus Forsythiae and Folium Nelumbinis)

● Source: *Wen Bing Tiao Bian* (Detailed Analysis of Seasonal Febrile Disease)

● Ingredients: *Bo He* (Herba Menthae) 5g.

Lian Qiao (Fructus Forsythiae) 5g.

Sheng Gan Cao (Radix Glycyrrhizae) (raw) 3g.

Zhi Zi (Fructus Gardeniae) 5g.

Jie Geng (Radix platycodi) 9g.

Lu Dou Pi (Semen Phaseoli Raciatus) (Peel) 6g.

● Functions and indications: slightly dispersing to clear away dry-heat from the upper *Jiao* and the *Qi* system, marked by tinnitus, red eyes, swelling of gum, sore throat, thin yellow and dry coating, and rapid pulse.

12.2　Moistening Dryness by Nourishing *Yin*

The prescriptions of moistening dryness by nourishing *Yin* are advisable to endogenous dryness due to impairment of body fluid.

Yang Yin Qing Fei Tang (Decoction for Nourishing *Yin* and Clearing Away Lung-Heat)

● Source: *Chong Lou Yu Yao* (Jade Key to the Secluded Chamber)

● Ingredients: *Sheng Di* (Radix Rehmanniae) 12g.

Mai Dong (Radix Ophiopogonis) 9g.

Sheng Gan Cao (Radix Glycyrrhizae) 3g.

Xuan Shen (Radix Scrophulariae) 9g.

Bei Mu (Bulbus Fritillariae Thunbergii) (remove the heart) 5g.

Dan Pi (Cartex Moutan Radicis) 5g.

Bo He (Herba Menthae) 3g.

Bai Shao (Radix Paeoniae Alba) 5g.

● Administration: The drugs are decocted in water for oral administration.

● Functions: Nourish *Yin*, clear away lung heat, eliminate toxins, and ease throat.

● Indications: Diphtheria, manifested as white membrane over the pharynx which is difficult to be wiped away, sore throat, dry nose and lips, difficult breathing, rapid forceless or thready rapid pulse.

● Explanation:

Sheng Di: sweet and bitter in taste and cold in nature, nourishing *Yin* and clearing away heat, used as the principal drug in the prescription.

Xuan Shen: bitter, sweet and salty in taste, cold in nature, nourishing *Yin*, promoting the production of the body fluid, reducing fire and removing toxins.

Mai Dong: sweet in taste and cold in nature, nourishing *Yin* and clearing away lung heat.

The above two are as the assistant drugs.

Dan Pi: clearing away heat, cooling the blood and relieving swelling.

Bai Shao: nourishing *Yin* and blood.

Bei Mu: moistening the lung and eliminating phlegm, clearing away heat and dispersing the lumps.

The above three are adjuvant drugs.

Bo He: small dosage for expelling exogenous pathogenic factors and easing throat.

Sheng Gan Cao: reducing fire and removing toxins, coordinating the effects of all the drugs.

These two are used as guiding drugs.

○ All the drugs as a whole plays the functions of nourishing the liver and kidney, relieving swelling, easing the throat, and expelling external pathogenic factors.

● Notes:

It is a basic prescription used to treat *Yin* deficiency with dry-heat seen in cases of acute tonsillitis and pharyngo-laryngitis, nasopharyngeal cancer and chronic bronchitis, etc.

Mai Men Dong Tang (Decoction of Ophiopogonis)

● Source: *Jin Gui Yao Lue* (Synopsis of Prescriptions of the Golden Chamber)
● Ingredients: *Mai Men Dong* (Radix Ophiopogonis) 60g.

        Ban Xia (Phizoma Pinelliae) 9g.

        Ren Shen (Radix Ginseng) 6g.

        Gan Cao (Rdix Glycyrrhizae) 4g.

        Jing Mi (Fructus Oryzae Sativae) 6g.

        Da Zao (Fructus Ziziphi Jujubae) 3pcs.

● Administration: The drugs are decocted in water for oral administration.
● Functions: Nourish the lung and stomach, lower the adverse-rising of *Qi*.
● Indications: "Lung withering syndrome", marked by cough, spitting mucous and saliva, short breath, dry throat, dry and red tongue with less coating, and forceless and rapid pulse.

● Explanation:

Mai Men Dong: sweet in taste and cold in nature, nourishing the *Yin* of the lung and stomach, as the principal drug in the prescription.

Ren Shen, *Gan Cao*, *Jing Mi* and *Da Zao*: sweet in taste and warm in nature, reinforcing *Qi* so as to strengthen the source for the production of body fluid, as the assistant drugs.

Ban Xia: the adjuvant and guiding drug, descending the adverse-rising of *Qi*, with *Mai Men Dong* to prevent the *Qi* of the middle *Jiao* being blocked by *Yin*-tonification drugs.

○ All the above drugs as a whole perform the functions of nourishing *Yin* of the lung and stomach and lowering the rising of *Qi*.

● Notes:

(1) It can be used to treat the cases of chronic bronchitis, bronchiectasis, chronic pharyngitis and laryngitis, silicosis, and pulmonary tuberculosis, etc. belonging to the type of lung *Yin* deficiency and adverse-rise of *Qi* and fire, or the cases of gastroduodenal ulcer, atrophic gastritis with vomiting due to deficiency of stomach *Yin* and adverse-rise of *Qi*.

(2) It is not advisable for cases of "lung withering syndrome" of deficient cold type.

Summary

5 main prescriptions for moistening dryness are chosen and divided into two kinds: moistening dryness by activating the lung and moistening the dryness by nourishing *Yin* according to their effects.

(1) Moistening dryness by activating the lung

Xing Su San, *Sang Xing Tang*, *Qing Zao Jiu Fei Tang* all have the effects of expelling external dryness. *Xing Su San* is a representative prescription for cases attributive to cool-dryness invading the lung. *Sang Xing Tang*, *Qing Zao Jiu Fei Tang* have the effects of expelling warm-dryness for treating the cases due to dry-heat invading the lung. Comparing the two prescriptions, *Sang Xing Tang*'s effect of clearing away heat is not as strong as *Qing Zao Jiu Fei Tang*, therefore, it is advisable for mild cases due to external dry-heat. *Qing Zao Jiu Fei Tang* has a stronger effect of clearing away heat and nourishing *Yin* and is used for serious cases due to external dry-heat.

(2) Moistening dryness by nourishing *Yin*

Yang Yin Qing Fei Tang and *Mai Men Dong Tang* have the effect of nourishing *Ying* to moisten dryness. *Yang Yin Qing Fei Tang* nourishes the lung and kidney as well as disperses exterior pathogens, and is an effective prescription for diphtheria and sore throat due to *Yin* deficiency. *Mai Men Dong Tang* has the effects of nourishing the lung and stomach and descending adverse-rising *Qi*, used for cases of "lung withering syndrome" due to *Yin* deficiency of the lung and stomach, and vomiting due to stomach *Yin* deficiency.

Review Questions

(1) How many types are the prescriptions for treating dryness divided into? What kind of disease are they used for?

(2) What are the differences of the ingredients, functions and indications between *Sang Xing Tang* and *Xing Su San*?

(3) Which book is *Mai Men Dong Tong* from? Write out its ingredients, functions and indications, and explanation of the ingredients.

13 Prescriptions with Sedative Effect

Prescriptions with sedative effect are mainly composed of tranquilizers of heavy nature or drugs for nourishing heart mind. They are indicated for mental disorders due to instability of the mind.

According to the causes, this type of diseases is divided into deficient and excessive syndromes. Therefore, the prescriptions with sedative effect has two kinds: calming the mind with drugs of heavy nature and calming the mind with drugs for nourishing the heart. Usually, instability of the mind is caused by various reasons, deficiency mixed with excess and one causing the other, so heavy sedatives and drugs for nourishing the heart are often used together clinically. Most prescriptions with heavy sedatives are composed of metal and stone drugs which might affect the function of the stomach, so they can't be used for a long time, especially for cases with stomach and spleen deficiency.

13.1 Calming the Mind with Drugs of Heavy Nature

The prescriptions for calming the mind with drugs of heavy nature are advisable for heart *Yang* excess manifested as restlessness, insomnia, palpitation etc.

Zhu Sha An Shen Wan (Pill of Cinnabaris for Tranquilizing the Mind)
　　　　(also named *An Shen Wan*, Pill for Tranqulizing the Mind)

- Source: *Yi Xue Fa Ming* (Inventions of Medicine)
- Ingredients: *Zhu Sha* (Cinnabaris) 15g.
　　　　　　Huang Lian (Rhizoma Coptidis) 18g.
　　　　　　Zhi Gan Cao (Radix Glycyrrhizae Praeparata) 16g.
　　　　　　Sheng Di Huang (Radix Rehmanniae) 8g.
　　　　　　Dang Gui (Radix Angeliae Sinensis) 8g.
- Administration: Make the powder of above drugs into pills. Take 6-9g. each time with water before sleep, or the drugs except *Zhu Sha* are decocted in water, with the dosages reduced in proportion for oral administration. *Zhu Sha* is ground into powder with water and is taken with the decoction.
- Functions: Calm the heart, tranquilize the mind, clear away heat and nourish blood.
- Indications: flaring up of heart fire and damage of *Yin* and blood, manifested as irritability, insomnia, dreaminess, severe palpitation, nausea, chest upset with hot sensation, red tongue, thready and rapid pulse.
- Explanation:

Zhu Sha: slight cold in nature, tranquilizing the mind, calming the heart and reducing heart fire.

Huang Lian: bitter in taste and cold in nature, reducing heart fire, relieving irritability and tranquilizing the mind.

The above two are the principal drugs in the prescription.

Dang Gui, *Sheng Di*: nourishing blood and *Yin*, as the assistant drugs.

Gan Cao: regulating all drugs, as the adjuvant and guiding drug.

○ The prescription as a whole treats both the root cause and symptoms, performing the effects of tranquilizing the mind, reducing the fire and nourishing *Yin*.

● Notes:

(1) It can be used to treat insomnia in neurasthenia, amnesia, palpitation, or trance appearing in depression due to excess of heart fire.

(2) The prescription should not be taken for a long time because *Zhu Sha* (Cinnabaris) is poisonous.

13.2 Calming the Mind with Drugs for Nourishing the Heart

The prescriptions for calming the mind with drugs of nourishing the heart are applicable to the cases with *Yin* deficiency and preponderance of Yang, marked by restlessness, insomnia, palpitation, night sweating, amnesia, nocturnal emission, and red tongue with less coating.

Suan Zao Ren Tang (Decoction of Ziziphi)

● Source: *Jin Gui Yao Lue* (Synopsis of Prescriptions of the Golden Chamber)
● Ingredients: *Suan Zao Ren* (Semen Ziziphi Spinosae) 18g.

        Gan Cao (Radix Glycyrrhizae) 3g.

        Zhi Mu (Rhizoma Anemarrhenae) 10g.

        Fu ling (Roria) 10g.

        Chuan Xiong (Rhizoma Ligustici Chuanxiong) 5g.

● Administration: The drugs are decocted in water for oral administration.

● Functions: Nourish blood to tranquilize the mind, clear away heat to relieve restlessness.

● Indications: Restlessness and insomnia due to deficiency, associated with palpitation, night sweating, vertigo, dry throat and mouth, thready and wiry pulse.

● Explanation:

Suan Zao Ren: the principal drug, sweet in taste and neutral in nature, nourishing the liver-blood, and tranquilizing the mind.

Chuan Xiong: regulating and nourishing the liver-blood.

Fu Ling: calming the heart and tranquilizing the mind.

They are the assistant drugs.

Zhi Mu: clearing away heat due to *Yin* deficiency to relive irritability, as the adjuvant drug.

Can Cao: the guiding drug, clearing away heat and coordinating the effects of all the drugs.

○ All above drugs as a whole perform the effects of nourishing blood, tranquilizing the mind, clearing away heat due to *Yin* deficiency to relieve irritability.

● Notes:

It's applicable to the cases of neurasthenia and climacteric syndrome due to liver blood deficiency or endogenous heat resulting from *Yin* deficiency, manifested as irritability, insomnia, palpitation, night sweating, etc.

Tian Wang Bu Xin Dan (Heavenly King Tonic Pill for Mental Discomfort)

● Source: *She Sheng Mi Pou* (Secret Recipes for Longevity)
● Ingredients: *Sheng Di Huang* (Radix Rehmanniae) 120g.

  Ren Shen (Radix Ginseng) 15g.

  Dan Shen (Radix Salviae Miltiorrhizae) 15g.

  Yuan Shen (Radix Scrophulariae) 10g.

  Fu Ling (Poria) 15g.

  Wu Wei Zi (Fructus Schisandrae) 15g.

  Yuan Zhi (Radix Polygalae) 15g.

  Jie Geng (Radix Platycodi) 15g.

  Dang Gui (Radix Angelicae Sinensis) 60g.

  Tian Men Dong (Radix Asparagi) 60g.

  Mai Men Dong (Radix Ophiopogonis) 60g.

  Bai Zi Ren (Semen Biotae) 60g.

  Suan Zao Ren (Semen Ziziphi Spinosae) 60g.

● Administration: Grind into powder, mixed the powder with honey to produce pills coated with *Zhu Sha* (Cinnabaris) . Take 9g. each time with warm water; or the drugs are decocted in water for oral administration, but the dosages should be reduced proportionally with those in the original prescription.

● Functions: Nourish *Yin* to clear away deficient heat, tonify the heart and tranquilize the mind.

● Indications: Deficiency of *Yin* and blood, manifested as irritability, palpitation, insomnia, amnesia, oral ulcer, constipation, red tongue with less coating, thready and rapid pulse.

● Explanation:

Sheng Di: the principal drug, sweet and bitter in taste and cold in nature, nourishing the kidney water to clear away deficient type heat.

Xuan Shen, *Tian Dong* and *Mai Dong*: sweet and salty in taste and cold in nature, strengthening the functions of the principal drug in nourishing *Yin* and clearing away heat.

Dang Gui and *Dan Shen*: nourishing blood.

The above five drugs are the assistant drugs.

Ren Shen and *Fu Ling*: reinforcing *Qi* and calming the heart.

Suan Zao Ren and *Wu Wei Zi*: controlling the heart *Qi* and tranquilizing the mind.

Bai Zi Ren, *Yuan Zhi* and *Zhu Sha*: tonifying the heart and calming the mind.

The above seven ingredients are the adjuvant drugs.

Jie Geng: the guiding drug, promoting the functions of the lung and heart, conducting the effects of other drugs to ascend.

○ The prescription as a whole treats both the primary cause and symptoms, performing the effects of nourishing *Yin* to clear away deficient heat, tonifying the heart to tranquilize the mind.

● Notes:

It's applicable to the cases of neurasthenia with insomnia and dreaminess or heart disorders due to *Yin* and blood deficiency.

Summary

3 prescriptions are grouped into the following 2 sub-categories: calming the mind with drugs of heavy nature and calming the mind with drugs for nourishing the heart.

(1) Calming the mind with drugs of heavy nature

Zhu Sha An Shen Wan has the effects of calming the heart and tranquilizing the mind, clearing away heat and nourishing blood, applicable to cases with irritability, insomia, palpitation and dreaminess due to excess of heart fire and damage of the *Yin* and blood.

(2) Calming the mind with drugs for nourishing the heart

Suan Zao Ren Tang, *Tian Wang Bu Xin Dan* have the effects of nourishing Yin, blood and the heart to tranquilize the mind. *Suan Zao Ren Tang* is good at nourishing the liver blood, suppressing deficient *Yang* to treat the cases with palpitation, insomnia resulting from deficiency of liver blood and deficiency of *Yin* with hyperactivity of *yang*. While *Tian Wang Bu Xin Dan* stresses on nourishing the *Yin*-blood to enrich the heart and tranquilize the mind, for cases with irritability, insomnia, amnesia resulting from *Yin*-blood deficiency.

Review Questions

(1) Write out the ingredients, functions, indications and explanation of *Zhu Sha An Shen Wan*.

(2) What are the differences between *Suan Zao Ren Tang* and *Tian Wang Bu Xin Dan* in their functions and indications?

14 Prescriptions of Resuscitation

Prescriptions of resuscitation are mainly composed of analeptics with fragrant flavor which have the function of inducing resuscitation and are used in the treatment of the tense syndrome of coma.

Coma is divided into two kinds of syndromes: deficiency and excess. The excess type of coma is called tense syndrome. According to the difference of the syndrome due to heat or cold, the prescriptions of resuscitation are further classified into two kinds: inducing resuscitation with cool drugs and inducing resuscitation with warm drugs.

Prescriptions of resuscitation are only applicable to the tense syndrome of coma, not to the flaccidity syndrome of coma which is characterized by profuse sweating, cold limbs, weak breath, enuresis, opened mouth and closed eyes. For the excess syndrome of *Yang-ming*-fu organs associated with coma and delirium due to disturbance by excessive heat, it is advisable to use prescriptions of cold purgatives but not prescriptions of resuscitation.

Most drugs in the prescriptions of resuscitation are fragrant and can be readily distributed to the whole body. Hence, these prescriptions should be prepared into bolus (or pill) and powder, and take with warm water. Boiling in water for a long time is not advisable. Besides, this type of prescription should be used temporarily and stop using it as soon as the disease is cured.

14.1 Inducing Resuscitation with Cool Drugs

The prescriptions for inducing resuscitation with cool drugs are indicated for the tense syndrome of coma due to seasonal toxic heat invading the pericardium. It also applicable to other type of coma with tense syndrome associated with heat, seen in apoplexy, phlegmatic collapse syndrome, and sudden lose of consciousness attributed to external turbid evil.

An Gong Niu Huang Wan (Bolus of Calculus Bovis for Resuscitation)

● Source: *Wen Bing Tiao Bian* (Treatise on Differentiation and Treatment of Epidemic Febrile Diseases)
● Ingredients: *Niu Huan* (Calculus Bovis) 30g.
　　　　　　　Yu Jin (Radix Curcumae) 30g.
　　　　　　　Xi Jiao (Cornu Rhinocerotis, replaced by Shui Niu Jiao) 30g.
　　　　　　　*Huang Li*an (Rhizoma Coptidis) 30g.
　　　　　　　Huang Qin (Radix Scutellariae) 30g.
　　　　　　　Shan Zhi (Fructus Gardeniae) 30g.
　　　　　　　Zhu Sha (Cinnabaris) 30g.

*Xiong Hu*an (Realgar) 30g.

Bing Pian (Borneolum Syntheticum) 7.5g.

She Xiang (Moschus) 30g.

Zhen Zhu (Margarita) 15g.

Jin Bo Yi (for coating, gold sheet)

● Administration: Grind the drugs into find powder. Make the powder into boluses by mixing it with honey. Each bolus weighs 3g. and be wrapped with thin gold sheet. Take one bolus each time. Reduce the dosage for small child.

● Functions: Clear away heat and toxins, induce resuscitation, and remove phlegm.

● Indications: Seasonal febrile diseases with the pericardium attached by heat, phlegm-heat misting the heart orifices, manifested as high fever, coma, delirum; or apoplexy, or infantile convulsions due to liver heat stagnation.

● Explanation:

Niu Huang, *She Xiang*: bitter, cold and fragrant, clearing away heat and toxins, removing phlegm, inducing resuscitation, as the principal drugs in the prescription.

Shui niu Jiao: salty in taste and cold in nature, clearing the heart, cooling the blood and removing toxins.

Huang Qin, *Huang Lian*, *Shan Zhi*: bitter in taste and cold in nature, clearing away heat, reducing fire and removing toxins.

Bing Pian, *Yu Jin*: fragrant smell, preventing the invasion of turbid evils, and inducing resuscitation and by clearing the orifices.

Above 6 drugs are used as assistant drugs.

Zhu Sha, *Zhen Zhu*: calming the heart and tranquilizing the mind.

Xiong Huang: removing phlegm and toxins.

The above two drugs are the adjuvant drugs.

Honey: the guiding drug, regulating the function of the stomach.

Gold Sheet: tranquilizing the mind with its heavy nature.

○ All drugs as a whole performs the effects of clearing away heat and toxins, removing phlegm and inducing resuscitation.

● Notes:

(1) It is applicable to cases of some acute infectious diseases with high fever and coma, seen in such diseases as encephalitis B, epidemic encephalitis, or coma in cerebral accident, hepatic coma, which belongs to the type of excessive heat.

(2) *Xi Jiao* in the prescription can be replaced by 5-10 times *Shui Niu Jiao* (Cornu Bubali).

Zhi Bao Dan (Bolus of Precious Drugs)

● Source: *Tai Ping Hui Min He Ji Ju Fang* (Prescriptions of Peaceful Benevolent Dispensary)

● Ingredients: *Sheng Wu Xi Xie* (crude, scale, Cornu Rhinocerotis) 30g.

 Sheng Dai Mao Xie (crude, scale, Carapax Eretmochelydis, replaced by Shui Niu Jiao) 30g.

 Hu Bo (Succinum) 30g.

 Zhu Sha (Cinnabaris)(ground, refined with water) 30g.

 Xiong Huang (Realgar)(ground, refined with water) 30g.

 Long Nao (Borneolum Syntheticum) 7.5g.

 She Xiang (Moschus) 7.5g.

 Niu Huang (Calculus Bovis) 15g.

 An Xi Xiang (Benzoinum) 45g.

 Jin Bo (half for coating, half for decoction, gold sheet) 50 pcs.

 Yin Bo (Silver sheet) 50 pcs.

● Administration: Grind the drugs into fine powder, pass the powder through a sieve and make it into boluses with honey, weighing 3g. each. Take one bolus (reduce the dosage for children) daily with water.

● Functions: Resolve turbid substance, induce resuscitation, clear away heat and toxins.

● Indications: Sunstroke, apoplexy and seasonal febrile diseases due to stagnation of phlegmdampness, manifested as coma, delirium, coarse breathing with phlegm, fever, irritability, red tongue with yellowish, greasy and dirty coating, slippery and rapid pulse; also used for infantile convulsion due to stagnation of phlegm-heat.

● Explanation:

She Xiang, *Bing Pian*, *An Xi Xiang*: opening the orifice, eliminating turbid dampness with fragrant flavor.

Shui niu Jiao, *Niu Huang* and *Dai Mao*: clearing away heat and toxins.

Above drugs are the principal drugs in the prescription.

Zhu Sha and *Hu Bo*: calming the heart and tranquilizing the mind.

Xiong Huang: removing phlegm, clearing away toxins.

These three drugs are the assistant drugs.

Jin Bo and *Yin Bo*: together with *Zhu Sha* and *Hu Bo*, strengthening the effect of calming the mind with drugs of heavy nature.

Jin Bo and *Yin Bo* are not used now in the patent medicine.

○ The prescription as a whole performs effects of clearing away heat-toxins, removing phlegm and inducing resuscitation.

● Notes:

(1) It is used to the comatose cases due to heart orifice being attacked by phlegm, seen in diseases such as cerebral accident, hepatic coma, encephalitis B, and epilepsy.

(2) Most drugs in the prescription are acrid, dry and fragrant. It's good for opening the orifice and inducing resuscitation, but it has the disadvantage of damaging *Yin* and body

fluid, therefore it's not advisable to cases of apoplexy due to excess of the liver-*Yang* resulting from *Yin* deficiency.

Zi Xue San (Purple-Snow Powder)

- Source: *Wai Tai Mi Yao* (Clandestine Essentials from the imperial Library)
- Ingredients: *Shi Gao* (Gypsum Fibrosum) 1.5kg.

  Han Shui Shi (Calcitum) 1.5kg.

  Ci Shi (Magnetitum) 1.5kg.

  Hua Shi (Talcum) 1.5kg.

  Xi Jiao Xie (scale, cornu Rhinocerotis, replaced by Shui Niu Jiao) 150g.

  Ling Yang Jiao Xie (scale, Cornu Saigae Tataricae) 150g.

  Qing Mu Xiang (Radix Aristolochiae) 150g.

  Chen Xiang (Lignum Aquilariae Resinatum) 150g.

  Xuan Shen (Radix Scrophulariae) 500g.

  Sheng Ma (Rhizoma Cimicifugae) 500g.

  Gan Cao (Radix Glycyrrhizae) 240g.

  Pu Xiao (Natrii Sulphas) 5kg.

  Xiao Shi (refind, Nitrum) 96g.

  She Xiang (Moschus) 1.5g.

  Zhu Sha (Cinnabaris) 90g.

  Huang Jin (Aurum)(The original prescription is 100 Liang)

  Ding Xiang (Flos Caryophylli) 30g.

- Administration: Prepared into powder for oral administration. Take 1.5-3g. each time, twice a day. Reduce the dosage for children.
- Functions: Clear away heat and toxins, relieve convulsions and induce resuscitation.
- Indications: Febrile diseases that heat entered pericardium, manifested as high fever, irritability, coma, delirium, convulsions, thirst, dry lips, red urine, constipation, infantile convulsion due to heat.
- Explanation:

Shi Gao, *Hua Shi*, *Han Shui Shi*: sweet in taste and cold in nature, clearing away heat.

Shui niu Jiao: clearing the heart and removing toxins.

She Xiang, *Qing Mu Xing* and *Ding Xiang*: activating *Qi* and inducing resuscitation.

Xuan Shen, *Sheng Ma* and *Gan Cao*: clearing away heat and toxins.

Xuan Shen also nourishes *Yin* and promotes production of fluid, and *Gan Cao* regulates the function of the stomach.

Above drugs for clearing heat and reducing resuscitation are the principal drugs in the prescription.

Ling Yang Jiao: salty in taste and cold in nature, clearing the liver heat and relieving convulsions.

Zhu Sha, *Ci Shi* and *Huang Jin*: tranquilizing the mind.

Pu Xiao and *Xiao Shi*: clearing away heat and dissipating masses.

These 6 drugs are the assistant drugs in the prescription.

○ All above drugs as a whole perform the effects of clearing away heat, inducing resuscitation, stopping the wind and relieving convulsions.

● Notes:

(1) It's applicable for cases of epidemic encephalitis, encephalitis B, scarlet fever, and other acute febrile diseases manifested as high fever, coma, convulsions, thirst, dry lips, or infantile convulsions due to stirring of wind resulting from excessive heat.

(2) It is also applicable to the cases of infantile measles due to excess of heat-toxins manifested as deep red papule, retarded appearance of eruptions, high fever, heavy breath, coma, purplish red color of the vein on the radial side of index finger.

(3) Nowdays, *Huang Jin* (gold) is not used any more.

14.2 Inducing Resuscitation with Warm Drugs

The prescriptions for inducing resuscitation with warm drugs are indicated to the cases of windstoke, cold-stroke and phlegm-stroke, which belong to the tense syndrome of coma due to affection of cold, manifested as sudden loss of consciousness, trismus, coma, white coating, slow pulse.

Su He Xian Wan (Bolus of Storax)

● Source: *Tai Ping Hui Min He Ji Ju Fang* (Prescriptions of Peaceful Benevolent Dispensary)

● Ingredients: *Bai Zhu* (Rhizoma Atractylodis Macrocephalae) 60g.

Qing Mu Xiang (Radix Aristolochiae) 60g.

Wu Xi Xie (Scale, Cornu Rhinocerotis, replaced by Shui Niu Jiao) 6g.

Xiang Fu (Rhizoma Cyperi) 60g.

Zhu Sha (Cinnabaris) 60g.

Ke Zi (Fructus Chebulae) 60g.

Bai Tan Xiang (Lignum Santali) 60g.

An Xi Xiang (Benzoinum) 60g.

Cheng Xiang (Lignum Aquilariae Resinatum) 60g.

She Xiang (Moschus) 60g.

Ding Xiang (Flos Caryophylli) 60g.

Bi Bo (Fructus Piperis Longi) 60g.

Long Nao (ground, Borneolum Syntheticum) 30g.

Su He Xiang You (Oleum Storax) 30g.

Ru Xiang (Olibanum) 30g.

● Administration: The drugs are ground into powder and made into bolus with honey (weighing 3g. each bolus) for oral administration. Take one bolus each time, twice a day. Reduce the dosage for children.

● Functions: Induce resuscitation with fragrant drugs, promote *Qi* circulation to stop pain.

● Indications: windstroke, or affection of seasonal pestilential factors, manifested as sudden loss of consciousness, trismus; or obstruction of the *Qi* circulation by cold, manifested as sudden abdominal pain or cardiac pain, even unconsciousness; or coma due to obstruction of Qi by phlegm.

● Explanation:

Su He Xiang, *She Xiang*, *Bing Pian* and *An Xi Xiang*: fragrant in smell, inducing resuscitation, used as the principal drugs in the prescription.

Qing Mu Xiang, *Chen Xiang*, *Ru Xiang*, *Ding Xiang* and *Xiang Fu*: assistant drugs, promoting the circulation of *Qi* and relieving stagnation, expelling cold, eliminating turbidity, removing the obstruction of *Qi* and blood in *Zang-fu* organs.

Bi Bo: together with other fragrant drugs to strengthen the effect of dispersing cold, stopping pain and relieving obstruction.

Shui niu Jiao: clearing away toxins.

Zhu Sha: calming the heart and tranquilizing the mind.

Bai Zhu: strenghtening the spleen and reinforcing the middle *Qi*, drying dampness and removing turbidity.

Ke Zi (baked): warming and astringing *Qi* to prevent the impairment of health *Qi* by the fragrant drugs.

The above five ingredients are used as adjuvant and guiding drugs.

○ The prescription as a whole performs the effects of inducing resuscitation with fragrants, promoting the circulation of *Qi* to relieve pain.

● Notes:

(1) It is applicable for cases of angina pectoris as well as pain in the chest and abdomen due to stagnation of *Qi* and accumulation of cold.

(2) Since the acrid and fragrant drugs may damage the fetus, this prescription should be used cautiously for pregnant women, and they are also not advisable to the flaccidity syndrome of coma.

Summary

The above 4 prescriptions are classified into two types: inducing resuscitation with warm drugs or cold drugs.

(1) Inducing resuscitation with cold drugs

An *Gong Niu Huang Wan*, *Zhi Bao Dan* and *Zi Xue Dan* are the representative prescriptions of inducing resuscitation with cold drugs. They have the effects of clearing away heat and toxins and inducing resuscitation, indicating for the tense syndromes of coma caused by excessive heat. An *Gong Niu Huang Wan* is good at clearing away heat and toxins to treat cases with coma and delirium due to heat attacking the pericardium. *Zhi Bao Dan* is good at eliminating turbidities with fragrant drugs, used to treat coma due to phlegm-heat stagnation. *Zi Xue San* is good at eliminating wind to stop convulsions, especially for coma with convulsions due to heat attacking the pericardium.

(2) Inducing resuscitation with warm drugs

Su He Xiang Wan is a representative prescrition for inducing resuscitation with warm drugs, used in the treatment of tense syndrome of coma caused by cold. It is good at promoting the circulation of *Qi* so as to stop pain, advisable for the cases with pain in chest and abdomen due to stagnation of *Qi* and accumulation of cold.

Review Questions

(1) What are the main points for composing the prescriptions of inducing resuscitation with cold drugs? Explain the differences and similarities of the representative prescriptions in functions and indications.

(2) What are the characteristics of the *Su He Xiang Wan*'s composition? Explain its functions and indications.

15　Prescriptions with Astringent Effect

Prescriptions with astringent effect are mainly composed of astringent drugs. They are indicated for disorders of loss of *Qi*, blood, essence and body fluid.

According to the pathology and the places involved, this kind of prescriptions is divided into five types: strengthening the surface to stop sweating, astringing lung *Qi* to stop cough, astringing the intestines to stop diarrhea, preserving essence and controlling urination and emission, and relieving metrorrhagia and leukorrhagia.

The prescriptions with astringent effect are indicated for cases with health *Qi* deficiency and loss of *Qi*, blood, essence and body fluid. According to the degree of the impairment, relevant tonics will be combined so that to treat the primary and the secondary aspects of the disease at the same time. If external pathogenic factors are still retained in the body, the prescriptions with astringent effect will not be used in case it may "urge the invader to stay by closing the door". This kind of prescription is also not used for cases with profuse sweating in febrile diseases, seminal emission due to disturbance by fire, early stage of dysentery due to heat, diarrhea due to food retention, and uterine bleeding or leukorrhea resulting from excess heat etc.

15.1　Strengthening the Surface to Stop Sweating

The prescriptions for strengthening the surface to stop sweating are indicated for cases of spontaneous sweating and night sweating due to surface weakness.

Yu Ping Feng San (Jade Screen Powder)

- Source: *Dan Xi Xin Fa* (Danxi's Experience on Medicine)
- Ingredients: *Fang Feng* (Radix Ledebouriellae) 30g.

　　　　　　Huang Qi (Radix Astragali seu Hedysari) 30g.

　　　　　　Bai Zhu (Rhizoma Atractylodis Macrocephalae) 60g.
- Administration: Grind the drugs into powder. Take 6-9g. with warm water, twice a day, or prepare the drugs into an oral decoction, with the dosages reduced proportionally.
- Functions: Reinforce *Qi*, strengthen the surface, and stop sweating.
- Indications: surface weakness with failure of the defensive *Qi* in controlling the body fluid, and the body easy to be affected by wind, manifested as spontaneous sweating, profuse sweating, aversion to wind, pale complexion, pale tongue with white coating, and floating and weak pulse.
- Explanation:

Huang Qi: sweet in taste and warm in nature, reinforcing *Qi* and strengthening the surface used as the principal drug in the prescription.

Bai Zhu: the assistant drug, bitter and sweet in taste and warm in nature, reinforcing the spleen *Qi*, strengthening the effects of *Huang Qi*.

The above two drugs together can benefit *Qi* and strengthen the surface to stop sweating and prevent pathogenic factors from invading the body.

Fang Feng: the assistant and guiding drug, expelling wind.

Huang Qi with *Fang Feng* strengthens the surface but not retaining pathogenic factors, and *Fang Feng* with *Huang Qi* eliminates pathogenic factors but not injuring the health *Qi*.

○ The above drugs as a whole perform the effects of reinforcing *Qi*, strengthening the surface to stop sweating.

● Notes:

(1) It is applicable to cases of hidrosis, allergic rhinitis, chronic rhinitis, upper respiratory tract infection due to surface deficiency.

(2) It is not advisable to cases of spontaneous sweating due to external pathogenic factors and night sweating due to *Yin* deficiency.

Mu Li San (Powder of Concha Ostreae)

● Source: *Tai Ping Hui Min He Ji Ju Fang* (Prescriptions of Peaceful Benevolent Dispensary)

● Ingredients: *Huang Qi* (Radix Astragali seu Hedysari) 30g.

              Ma Huang Gen (Radix Ephedrae) 30g.

              Mu Li (Concha Ostreae) 3g.

● Administration: Grind the drugs into granules. Decoct 9g. of the granules with *Fu Xiao Mai* (Fructus Tritici Levis)30g. Take the decoction hot, twice a day, or decocted the original drugs in water for oral administration.

● Functions: reinforce *Qi* and strengthen the surface, astringe *Yin* and stop sweating.

● Indications: Spontaneous sweating, night sweating, palpitation, short breath, restlessness, tiredness, light red tongue, thready and weak pulse.

● Explanation:

Mu Li: the principal drug, salty in taste and cold in nature, astringing *Yin*, suppressing *Yang* and stopping sweating.

Huang Qi: the assistant drug, reinforcing defensive *Qi*, strengthening surface to stop sweating.

Ma Huang Geng: the adjuvant drug, benefiting defensive *Qi* to stop sweating.

Fu Xiao Mai: the guiding drug, reinforcing heart *Qi*, relieving restlessness and stopping sweating.

○ The above drugs together perform the effects of nourishing *Yin*, reinforcing qi, strengthening the suface to stop sweating.

● Notes:

(1) It's applicable to the cases of hyperhidrosis due to dysfunction of autonomic nervous system; spontaneous sweating or night sweating after operation or delivery caused by failure of defensive *Qi* in controlling the surface and fluid take the chance to go away.

(2) It's not advisable to cases of night sweating due to fire resulting from *Yin* deficiency.

(3) In the original prescription, *Mu Li* should be soaked in rice water and cleaned away earth, heat with fire to red.

15.2   Astringing Lung *Qi* to Stop Cough

The prescriptions for astringing lung *Qi* to stop cough are indicated for cases of lung deficiency resulting from chronic cough, and impairment of *Qi* and *Yin*, manifested as cough, asthma, spontaneous sweating, weak and rapid pulse.

Jiu Xian San (Powder Containing Nine Drugs)

- Source: *Yi Xue Zheng Zhuan* (Orthodox Medical Records)
- Ingredients: *Ren Shen* (Radix Ginseng) 10g.

  Kuan Dong Hua (Flos Farfarae) 10g.

  Sang Bai Pi (Cortex Mori Radicis) 10g.

  Jie Geng (Radix Playcodi) 10g.

  Wu Wei Zi (Fructus Schisandrae) 10g.

  Bei Mu (Bulbus Fritillarae Cirrhosae) 5g.

  Ying Shu Qiao (Pericarpium Papaveris) 15g.

- Administration: Grind the drugs into fine powder, and decoct 9g. of the powder with one slice of *Sheng Jiang* (Rhizonma Zingiberis Recens) and one piece of *Da Zao* (Fructus Ziziphi Jujubae). Take the decoction while it is warm.

- Functions: Astringe lung *Qi* to relieve cough, reinforce *Qi* and nourish *Yin*.

- Indications: Deficiency of the lung, manifested as chronic cough, short breath, spontaneous sweating, less and sticky phlegm, weak and rapid pulse.

- Explanation:

Ying Shu Qiao: sour in taste, astringing the lung *Qi* to relieve cough.

Ren Shen: reinforcing the lung *Qi*.

They are as the principal drugs.

E Jiao: nourishing *Yin* and reinforcing the lung.

Wu Wei Zi and *Wu Mei*: astringing lung *Qi* to relieve cough, as the adjuvant drugs.

Kuan Dong Hua and *Sang Bai Pi*: descending *Qi*, eliminating phlegm, relieving cough and asthma.

Bei Mu: relieving cough and eliminating phlegm.

The above three are used as adjuvant drugs.

Jie Geng: activating lung *Qi* and eliminating phlegm, as the guiding drug.

○ All above durgs as a whole performs the effects of astringing lung to relieve cough, reinforcing *Qi* and nourishing *Yin*.

● Notes:

(1) It is applicable to the cases of chronic tracheitis, pneumonectasis with chronic cough due to deficiency of both *Qi* and *Yin* of the lung.

(2) It's not advisable to cases of chronic cough with profuse sputum, or with ex-opathogens at the surface.

(3) The dosage of *Ying Shu Qiao* should be limited and it can't be used for a long time.

15.3　Astringing the Intestines to Stop Diarrhea

The prescriptions for astringing the intestines to stop diarrhea are indicated for cases of persistant diarrhea and dysentery or even incontinence of stool due to deficiency cold of the spleen and kidney, resulting in failure to control defecation.

Zhen Ren Yang Zang Tang (Zhenren Decoction
for Nourishing the Viscera)

● Source: *Tai Ping Hui Min He Ji Ju Fang* (Prescriptions of Peaceful Benevolent Dispensary)

● Ingredients: *Ren Shen* (Radix Ginseng) 6g.

Dang Gui (Radix Angelicae Sinensis) 9g.

Bai Zhu (Rhizoma Atractylodis Macrocephalae) 12g.

Rou Dou Kou (Semen Myristicae) 12g.

Rou Gui (Cortex Cinnamomi) 3g.

Zhi Gan Cao (Radix Glycyrrhizae Preparata) 6g.

Bai Shao (Radix Paeoniae Alba) 15g.

Mu Xiang (Radix Aucklandiae) 9g.

Ke Zi (Fructus Chebulae) 12g.

Ying Shu Qiao (Pericarpium Papaveris) 20g.

● Administration: The drugs are decocted in water for oral administration.

● Functions: Warm and reinforce the spleen and kidney, astringe the intestines to stop diarrhea.

● Indications: Chronic diarrhea and dysentery due to deficient cold of the spleen and kidney, manifested as frequent defecation, or incontinence of stool, or prolapsed of rectum, abdominal pain relieved by warmth and pressure, poor appetite, pale tongue with white coating, deep and slow pulse.

● Explanation:

Ying Shu Qiao: sour in taste, astringing the intestines to stop diarrhea.

Rou Gui: acrid in taste and warm in nature.

They are as the principal drugs in the prescription.

Rou Dou Kou: warming the spleen and the middle *Jiao*, astringing the intestines to stop diarrhea, used as the assistant drug.

Ren Shen and *Bai Zhu*: reinforcing *Qi* and strengthening the spleen.

Dang Gui and *Bai Shao*: nourishing and regulating blood to stop pain.

Mu Xiang: activating qi.

The above three are the adjuvant drugs.

Zhi Gan Cao: regulating all the drugs, as the guiding drug.

○ The drugs as a whole perform the effects of warming and reinforcing the spleen and kidney, astringing the intestines to stop diarrhea.

● Notes:

(1) It is also indicated for cases of chronic enteritis, enterophthisis, chronic dysentery, prolapse of rectum, due to deficiency cold of the spleen and kidney (spleen and kidney *Yang* deficiency).

(2) It is forbidden for cases at early stage of dysentery with stagnation of damp-heat.

Si Shen Wan (Pill of Four Miraculous Drugs)

● Source: *Zheng Zhi Zhun Sheng* (Standards for Diagnosis and Treatment)

● Ingredients: *Rou Dou Kou* (Semen Myristicae) 60g.

        Bu Gu Zhi (Fructus Psoraleae) 120g.

        Wu Wei Zi (Fructus Schisandrae) 60g.

        Wu Zhu Yu (Fructus Euodiae) 30g.

● Administration: Grind the above drugs into fine powder. Take 240g. of *Sheng Jiang* (Rhizoma Zingiberis Recens) and 100 pieces of *Hong Zao* (Fructus Jujubae, stones removed) and boil them in water. Mix the powder with *Hong Zao* to make pills as big as the seed of Chinese parasol. Take 6-9g. of the pill each time before meal; or directly prepare them into an oral decoction, with the dosages reduced proportionally.

● Functions: Warm the kidney and spleen, astringe the intestines to stop diarrhea.

● Indications: Cases due to deficiency cold of the spleen and kidney, manifested as morning diarrhea, poor appetite, indigestion, prolonged diarrhea, abdominal pain, cold limbs, fatigue, pale longue with thin white coating, deep, slow and weak pulse.

● Explanation:

Bu Gu Zhi: acrid and bitter in taste and great warm in nature, strengthening the life-gate fire, warming the kidney *Yang*, used as the principal drug.

Rou Dou Kou: the assistant drug, warming the spleen and stomach, astringing the intestines to stop diarrhea.

Wu Wei Zi: astringing to stop diarrhea.

Wu Zhu Yu: acrid in taste and hot in nature, warming the liver and kidney, dispersing cold, and stopping abdominal pain.

The above two are used as the adjuvant drugs.

Sheng Jiang: warming the stomach to dispel cold.

Da Zao: reinforcing the spleen and nourishing the stomach.

These two are used as guiding drugs.

○ The prescription as a whole performs the effects of warming the kidney and spleen, astringing the intestines to stop diarrhea.

● Notes:

(1) The modified prescriptions are used for cases of prolonged diarrhea seen in diseases as chronic colitis, allergic colitis, chronic dysentery, enterophthisis, which are due to deficient type cold of the spleen and kidney.

(2) It's not advisable to cases of diarrhea due to indigestion or damp-heat stagnation in the intestines and stomach.

Chi Shi Zhi Yu Yu Liang Wan (Pill of Halloysitum Rubrum and Limonitum)

● Source: *Shang Han Lun* (Treaties on Cold-Induced Diseases)
● Ingredients: *Chi Shi Zhi* (Halloysitum Rubrum, broken) 30g.

  Yu Yu Liang (Limonitum, broken) 30g.
● Administration: The drugs are decocted in water for oral administration.
● Functions: Astringe the intestines to stop diarrhea.
● Indications: Prolonged diarrhea, failure in controlling defecation.
● Explanation:

Chi Shi Zhi: sweet and sour in taste, warm and puckery in nature, astringing to stop diarrhea and prolapse, as the principal drug.

Yu Yu Liang: the assistant drug, sweet in taste and puckery in nature, astringing the intestines.

○ The two drugs used together perform the effect of astringing the intestines to stop diarrhea.

● Notes:

It is a prescription for treating the symptoms, indicated for cases of prolonged diarrhea due to failure of *Qi* in controlling defecation, seen in diseases such as chronic colitis and prolapsed of rectum, etc.

15.4 Preserving Essence and Controlling Urination and Emission

The prescriptions for preserving essence and controlling urination and emission are indicated for cases of nocturnal emission or spermatorrhea due to deficiency of the kidney which fails to control the seminal palace, or cases of enuresis or frequent urination due to deficiency of the kidney, which causes the failure of the urinary bladder in controlling the urine.

Sang Piao Xiao San (Powder of Octheca Mantidis)

- Source: *Ben Cao Yan Yi* (Amplified Herbalism)
- Ingredients: *Sang Piao Xiao* (Ootheca Mantidis) 30g.

  Yuan Zhi (Radix Polygalae) 30g.

  Chang Pu (Rhizoma Acori Graminei) 30g.

  Long Gu (Os Draconis) 30g.

  Ren Shen (Radix Ginseng) 30g.

  Fu Shen (Lignum Pini Poriaferum) 30g.

  Dang Gui (Radix Angelicae Sinensis) 30g.

  Gui Jia (Plastrum Testudinis, prepared) 30g.

- Administration: Grind the drugs into powder. Take 6g. of the powder with decoction of *Ren Shen* (Radix Ginseng) before going to bed. The drugs can also be decocted in water for making oral decoction with dosages reduced in proportion.
- Functions: Reinforce the heart and kidney, preserve essence and control involuntary urination.
- Indications: Frequent urination, enuresis or seminal emission due to deficiency of both the heart and kidney, associated with trance, amnesia, dream-disturbed sleep, pale tongue with white coating, thready and weak pulse.
- Explanation:

Sang Piao Xiao: the principal drug, sweat and salty in taste, reinforcing kidney, nourishing essence and controlling involuntary urination.

Long Gu: calming the heart and mind, preserving essence.

Gui Jia: nourishing *Yin* to strengthen the heart and kidney.

They are used as the assistant drugs.

Ren Shen: reinforcing the *Qi* in the middle *Jiao*.

Dang Gui: nourishing the heart blood.

Fu Shen: tranquilizing the mind.

The above three are used as the adjuvant drugs.

Yuan Zhi and *Chang Pu*: the adjuvant and guiding drugs, tranquilizing the mind, resuming the "balance functions" between the heart (fire) and kidney(water).

○ All the drugs as a whole perform the effects of regulating and reinforcing the functions of the heart and kidney, preserving essence and controlling involuntary urination.

- Notes:

(1) It can be used for treating the cases of neurasthenia, diabetes and infantile enuresis due to imbalance between the heart and kidney.

(2) It is not advisable to cases of frequent urination, enuresis and emission due to excess of fire in the lower *Jiao* or disturbance by damp-heat, and frequent and incontinent urination due to *Yang* deficiency of the spleen and kidney.

Suo Quan Wan (Pill for Decreasing Urination)

● Source: *Fu Ren Lian Fang* (The Complete Effective Prescriptions for women)

● Ingredients: *Wu Yao* (Radix Linderae)

                  Yi Zhi Ren (Fructus Alpiniae Oxphyllae)

The above two drugs are in equal dosage.

● Administration: Grind the drugs into powder. Cook the powder of *Shan Yao* (Rhizoma Dioscoreae) with liquor into paste, and mix the powder of the above two drugs with the paste to form boluses which weighs 6-9g. each. Take once or twice a day with warm water. The drugs can also be decocted in water for administration with proper dosage.

● Functions: Warm the kidney to dispel cold, decrease urination to control involuntary urination.

● Indications: Deficient cold due to Lower *Yuan*-primary *Qi* manifested as frequent urination, enuresis, pale tongue, deep and weak pulse.

● Explanation:

Yi Zhi Ren: acrid in taste and warm in nature, warming the spleen and kidney, preserving essence and decreasing urination, used as the principal drug.

Wu Yao: assistant drug, acrid in taste and warm in nature, regulating *Qi* and dispelling cold, eliminating cold in the bladder and kidney, treating frequent urination by preserving essence *Qi*.

Shan Yao: invigorating the spleen and reinforcing kidney, controlling essence *Qi*, used as the assistant and guiding drug.

○ The three drugs as a whole, being warm but not dry, perform the effects of warming the kidney, dispelling cold, decreasing urination to stop enuresis.

● Notes:

The prescription is applied to cases of nervous frequent urination, diabetes insipidus, or excess of nasal discharge due to deficient cold in the spleen and kidney.

Mi Yuan Jian (Decoction for Preserving Yuan Qi)

● Source: *Jing Yue Quan Shu* (Complete Works of *Zhang Jing Yue*)

● Ingredients: *Yuan Zhi* (Radix Polygalae, fried) 2.5g.

              Shan Yao (Rhizoma Dioscoreac, fried) 6g.

              Qian Shi (Semen Euryales) 6g.

              Suan Zao Ren (Semen Ziziphi Spinosae, fried) 6g.

              Jin Ying Zi (Fructus Rosea Laevigatae) 6g.

              Bai Zhu (Rhizoma Atractylodis Macrocephalae, fried) 4.5g.

              Fu Ling (Poria) 4.5g.

              Zhi Gan Cao (Raidx Glycyrrhizae Praeparata) 3g.

              Ren Shen (Radix Ginseng) 3-6g.

Wu Wei Zhi (Fructus Schisandrae) 14 pcs.·

● Administration: The drugs are decocted in water for oral administration.

● Functions: Preserve essence, reinforce the spleen and kidney, regulate the functions of the heart and kidney.

● Indications: Spermatorrhea due to exhaustion of the fire in the lower *Jiao*, marked by prolonged emission, frequent spermatorrhea, soreness and weakness of lower back and knees, deep and thready pulse.

● Explanation:

Yuan Zhi: acrid and bitter in taste, slight warm in nature.

Wu Wei Zi: sour in taste and warm in nature.

Suan Zao Ren: sweet in taste and neutral in nature.

The above drugs, as principal drugs, perform the effects of restraining the mind harmonizing the heart and kidney.

Jin Ying Zi: sour in taste, reinforcing the kidney to preserve essence, relieving spermatorrhea, used as the assistant drug.

Ren Shen, *Bai Zhu*, *Fu Ling* and *Gan Cao*: using *Si Jun Zi Tang* (Decoction of Four Noble Drugs) to invigorate the spleen and reinforce *Qi*.

Shao Yao and *Qian Shi*: with *Si Jun Zi Tang*, preserving the essence *Qi* in the lower *Jiao*, as the adjuvant and guiding drugs.

○ The prescription as a whole plays the effects of preserving essence, strengthening the spleen and kidney, and harmonizing the heart with the kidney.

● Notes:

(1) It is indicated for cases of neurasthenia, orchitis, scrotitis due to disharmony between the heart and kidney.

(2) It is forbidden for cases with damp-heat in the lower *Jiao*, or cases who dislike sour taste.

(3) If there is fire, add *Ku Shen* 3-6g. *Qi* deficiency, add *Huang Qi* 3-9g.

15.5 Relieving Metrorrhagia and Leukorrhagia

The prescriptions for relieving metrorrhagia and leukorrhagia are indicated for cases of metrorrhagia and prolonged leukorrhagia.

Gu Jing Wan (Decoction for Controlling Menstruation)

● Source: *Dan Xi Xin Fa* (*Danxi's* Experiential Therapy)
● Ingredients: *Huang Bai* (Cortex Phellodendri) 6g.

　　　　　　Huang Qin (Radix Scutellariae) 15g.

　　　　　　Chun Gen Pi (Cortex Ailanthi) 12g.

　　　　　　Bai Shao (Radix Paeoniae Alba) 15g.

　　　　　　Gui Ban (Plastrum Testudinis) 15g.

Xiang Fu (Rhizoma Cyperi) 6g.

● Administration: Grind the drugs into powder. Mix the powder with wine to make boluses in size of 9g. each. Take the bolus with warm wine before meal.

● Functions: Nourish *Yin*, clear away heat, and relieve metrorrhagia.

● Indications: Metrorrhagia due to *Yin* deficiency resulting in interior heat, manifested as prolonged menstruation, metrorrhagia, dark blood with clots, discomfort and heat over the chest, abdominal pain, reddish urine, red tongue, wiry and rapid pulse.

● Explanation:

Gui Ban: sweet and salty in taste and cold in nature, reinforcing the kidney, nourishing Yin to reduce fire.

Bai Shao: bitter and sour in taste, slight cold in nature, nourishing *Yin* and blood.

They are as the principal drugs.

Huang Qin: clearing away heat to stop bleeding.

Huang Bai: clearing away heat to preserve *Yin*.

The above two are used as the assistant drugs.

Chun Geng Pi: relieving metrorrhagia.

Xiang Fu: regulating the circulation of *Qi* and blood.

○ The prescription as a whole performs the effects of nourishing *Yin*, clearing away heat, dispersing the stagnated liver *Qi* and relieving metrorrhagia.

● Notes:

The modified prescriptions are used for cases of disfunctional uterine bleeding and chronic adnexitis with metrorrhagia due to blood heat resulting from *Yin* deficiency.

Wan Dai Tang (Decoction for Treating Leukorrhaiga)

● Source: *Fu Qing Zhu Nu Ke* (*Fu Qingzhu's* Obstetrics and Gynecology)

● Ingredients: *Bai Zhu* (Rhizoma Atractylodis Macrocephalae) 30g.

    Shan Yao (Rhizoma Dioscoreae) 30g.

    Ren Shen (Radix Ginseng) 6g.

    Bai Shao (Radix Paeoniae Alba, fried) 15g.

    Che Qian Zi (Semen Plantaginis, fried) 9g.

    Cang Zhu (Rhizoma Atractylodis) 9g.

    Gan Cao (Radix Glycyrrhizae) 3g.

    Chen Pi (Pericarpium Citri Reticulatae) 2g.

    Hei Jie Sui (Herba Schizonepetae) 2g.

    Chai Hu (Radix Bupleuri) 2g.

● Administration: The drugs are decocted in water for oral administration.

● Functions: Strengthen the spleen, promote the circulation of the liver *Qi*, resolve dampness and relieve leukorrhagia.

● Indications: leukorrhagia due to spleen deficiency, manifested as white or light yellow and thin leukorrhea without smell, fatigue, loose stool, pale complexion, pale tongue with white coating, soft and weak pulse.

● Explanation:

Ren Shen, *Bai Zu* and *Shan Yao*: sweet and bitter in taste and warm in nature, reinforcing *Qi* and strengthening the spleen to eliminate dampness, used as the principal drug.

Cang Zhu and *Chen Pi*: drying dampness and regulating the spleen function, activating *Qi* circulation with its fragrant smell to prevent the stagnation of *Qi* by the tonification effect of the principal drugs, and smooth flow of *Qi* helping the removing of dampness.

Che Qian Zi: eliminating dampness from urination.

The above three drugs are the assistant drugs.

Bai Shao: dispersing the stagnation of liver *Qi*.

Chai Hu: ascending *Yang* to prevent dampness from affecting the inner part of the body.

Jie Sui: dispersing wind and eliminating dampness to relieve leukorrhagia.

These three are used as adjuvant drugs.

Gan Cao: regulating effects of all the drugs, as the guiding drug.

○ The prescription as a whole performs the effects of strengthening the spleen, dispersing the stagnation of the liver *Qi*, eliminating dampness and relieving leukorrhagia.

● Notes:

(1) It is indicated for cases of chronic cervicitis, pelvic inflammation with leukorrhagia due to excess of dampness resulting from spleen deficiency.

(2) It is not advisable to cases of leukorrhagia with yellowish or with reddish and whitish discharge due to damp-heat attacting the lower *Jiao*.

Summary

According to the functions, the 8 prescriptions with astringing effect are divided into five types: strengthening the surface to stop sweating, astringing lung *Qi* to stop cough, astringing the intestines to stop diarrhea, preserving essence and controlling urination and emission, and relieving metrorrhagia and leukorrhagia.

(1) Strengthening the surface to stop sweating

Both *Yu Ping Feng San* and *Mu Li San* belong to this type of prescriptions. Compare the two prescriptions, *Yu Ping Feng San* is more effective at reinforcing *Qi* to strengthen the body surface, for cases of spontaneous sweating due to surface deficiency and cases who are often affected by cold; *Mu Li San* is good at astringing sweat, nourishing *Yin* and suppressing *Yang*, advisable to cases of sweating especially during the night resulting from *Yin* deficiency.

(2) Astringing lung *Qi* to relieve cough

Jiu Xian San reinforces *Qi* and benefits the lung, astringes lung *Qi* to stop cough, being applicable to cases of prolonged cough, shortness of breath, spontaneous sweating due to deficiency of the lung *Qi*.

(3) Astringing the intestines to stop diarrhea

Zhen Ren Yang Zang Tang, *Si Shen Wan* all have the effects of warming the kidney *Yang*, astringing the intestines to stop diarrhea. They are applicable to cases of prolonged diarrhea and dysentery due to the deficiency of the spleen and kidney *Yang*. This is to treat the root cause of the disease. *Zhen Ren Yang Zang Tang* is good at strengthening the spleen *Qi* to astringe intestines; *Si Shen Wan* is good at warming the kidney and spleen so as to control the intestines and stop diarrhea. *Chi Shi Zhi Yu Yu Liang Wan*, as a prescription for treating the symptoms (the secondary aspect of the disease), astringes the intestines to stop diarrhea, indicated for cases of prolonged diarrhea and dysentery, or even incontinent defecation.

(4) Preserving essence and controlling urination and emission

Sang Piao Xiao San, *Suo Quan Wan* and *Mi Yuan Jian* all have the functions of preserving essence and coutrolling urination and emission for the cases of seminal emission and enuresis. *Sang Piao Xiao Sang* is good at reinforcing the heart and kidney, preserving essence and controlling involuntary urination, mainly used for cases of frequuency urination, turbid urine, trance, delirium due to deficiency of both the heart and kidney. *Suo Quan Wan* is particularly good at strengthening the kidney and decreasing urination, mainly for enuresis due to kidney deficiency. *Mi Yuan Jian* can preserve essence and reinforce the spleen and kidney. It is a prescription for treating both the root cause and the symptoms of the diseases, indicated for cases of spermatorrhea due to exhaustion of the fire in the lower *Jiao*.

(5) Relieving Metrorrhagia and Leukorrhagia

Gu Jing Wan is particularly good for nourishing *Yin* and clearing away heat, relieving metrorrhagia, maily for cases of metrorrhagia due to heat resulting from *Yin* deficiency. *Wan Dai Tang* reinforces the spleen *Qi* and eliminates dampness to relieve leakorrhagia, applicable to cases of leukorrhagia due to spleen deficiency, liver *Qi* stagnation and dampness.

Review Questions

(1) What are the indications of the prescriptions with astringent effects? Write out the classification and representative prescriptions.

(2) Explain the functions, indications and characteristics of the compatibility of drugs of *Zhen Ren Yang Zang Tang*. What is the function of *Mu Xiang* in this prescription?

(3) What are the indications of *Sang Piao Xiao San*? Explain the compatibility of the prescription.

16 *Qi* **Regulating Prescriptions**

Prescriptions for regulating *Qi* are mainly composed of drugs which have the functions of activating *Qi* or descending adverse rise of *Qi*. They are indicated for diseases due to *Qi* stagnation and adverse flow of *Qi*.

Dysfunction of the *Qi* movement of the *Zang-fu* organs is usually manifested as *Qi* stagnation and adverse rise of *Qi*. The former should be treated by activating *Qi*, and the later by descending adverse rise of *Qi*. With prescriptions for regulating *Qi*, the syndromes of cold or heat, deficiency or excess should be differentiated, the presence or absence of complication should be determined, and the relevant drugs should be added. In addition, most of the drugs for regulating *Qi* are fragrant, acrid and dry, and long-term administration may injure body fluid and consume *Qi*, so overuse should be avoided. It is forbidden for cases with fire of deficient type resulting from *Qi* deficiency or *Yin* deficiency. Particular caution should be taken for the aged, debilitated, pregnant women, and patients with hemorrhage.

16.1 *Qi-*Activating Prescriptions

Prescriptions for activating *Qi* are indicated for cases of abdominal fullness, eructation, acid regurgitation due to spleen and stomach *Qi* stagnation, or fullness and pain in the chest, hernia, irregular menstruation caused by liver *Qi* stagnation.

Chai Hu Shu Gan San (Powder of Bupleuri for Dispersing the Depressed Liver- *Qi*)

- Source: *Jing Yue Quan Shu* (Complete Works of Zhang Jingyue)
- Ingredients: *Chen Pi* (Pericarpium Citri Reticulatae, fried with vinegar) 6g.
  Chai Hu (Radix Bupleuri) 6g.
  Chuan Xiong (Rhizoma Ligustici Chuanxiong) 5g.
  Xian Fu (Rhizoma Cyperi) 5g.
  Zhi Qiao (Fructus Aurantii) 5g.
  Shao Yao (Radix Paeoniae Alba) 5g.
  Zhi Gan Cao (Radix Glycyrrhizae Praeparata) 3g.
- Administration: All the drugs are decocted in water for oral administration.
- Functions: Disperse the stagnated liver *Qi*, activate *Qi* to relieve pain.
- Indications: Stagnation of liver *Qi*, manifested as hypochondriac pain, alternating episodes of chills and fever, eructation, abdominal fullness, wiry pulse.
- Explanation:

Chai Hu: bitter and acrid in taste, light cold in nature, dispersing the stagnated liver

Qi, as the principal drug in the prescription.

Xiang Fu: regulating *Qi* to disperse stagnated liver *Qi*.

Chuan Xiong: activating the flow of *Qi* and blood, dispersing stagnation to relieve pain.

These two are used as the assistant drugs.

Chen Pi: regulating *Qi* to improve appetite.

Zhi Qiao: smoothing the chest to relieve distention.

Shao Yao: nourishing blood to soften the liver.

The above three are as the adjuvant drugs.

Gan Cao: regulating all the drugs as the guide.

○ All above drugs as a whole perform the functions of dispersing the stagnated liver *Qi*, activating the flow of *Qi* to stop pain.

● Notes:

(1) It is applicable to cases of chronic hepatitis, chronic gastritis, intercostal neuralgia due to stagnation of the liver *Qi*.

(2) It is not advisable to cases due to excess of the liver fire or damp-heat in the liver and gallbladder.

Yue Ju Wan (Yue Ju Pill)

● Source: *Dan Xi Xin Fa* (Danxi's Experience on Medicine)
● Ingredients: *Xiang Fu* (Rhizoma Cyperi) 6g.

              Chuan Xiong (Rhizoma Ligustici Chuanxiong) 6g.

              Cang Zhu (Rhizoma Atractylodis) 6g.

              Shen Qu (Massa Fermentata Medicinalis) 6g.

              Zhi Zi (Fructus Gardeniae) 6g.

● Administration: All drugs are ground into fine powder, and prepare the powder into small pills, take 6-9g. each time; or prepare them directly into an oral decoction, with the dosages reduced proportionally.

● Functions: Promote *Qi* circulation and disperse stagnation.

● Indications: Six kinds of stagnation: stagnation of *Qi*, blood, phlegm, fire, dampness and food, manifested as fullness in chest, distension and pain in abdomen, eructation, acid regurgitation, nausea, vomiting, indigestion, white and greasy coating, wiry pulse.

● Explanation:

Xiang Fu: acrid, bitter and sweet in taste, neutral in nature, promoting *Qi* circulation and dispersing stagnation, as the principal drug.

Chuan Xiong: promoting blood circulation to remove blood stasis.

Shan Zhi: clearing away heat and reducing fire.

Cang Zhu: drying dampness and strengthening the spleen, smoothing the chest and eliminating dampness.

Shen Qu : promoting digestive function to relieve stagnation.

They are all as the assistant and adjuvant drugs.

○ The prescription as a whole performs the functions of promoting the flow of *Qi* and relieving all kinds of stagnation.

● Notes:

(1) It is indicated for cases of gastric neurosis, gastroduodenal ulcer, chronic gastritis, cholecystitis, cholelithiasis, hepatitis, intercostal neuralgia, depression, dysmenorrhea, irregular menstruation which have the manifestations of the stagnations.

(2) It is not advisable to deficient type of stagnations.

Gua Lou Xie Bai Bai Jiu Tang (Decoction of Trichosanthis, Allii Macrostemi and Wine)

● Source: *Jin Gui Yao Lue* (Synopsis of Prescriptions of the Golden Chamber)
● Ingredients: *Gua Lou* (Fructus Trichosanthis) 30g.

　　　　　　　Xie Bai (Bulbus Allii Macrostemi) 9g.

　　　　　　　Rice Wine, proper amount.
● Administration: All the above drugs should be decocted in water with wine for oral administration. Take it twice when warm.
● Functions: Activate *Yang* and *Qi*, relieve stagnation and eliminate phlegm.
● Indications: chest *Bi* syndrome, manifested as dull pain in the chest that refers to the back, dyspnea, cough, shortness of breath, white and greasy tongue coating, deep and wiry or tense pulse.
● Explanation:

Gua Lou : sweet in taste and cold in nature, removing phlegm, easing the chest and relieving stagnation, as the prinicipal drug.

Xie Bai : acrid in taste and warm in nature, activating *Yang Qi* to relieve stagnation and stop pain, as the assistant drug.

Bai Jiu : activating *Qi* and promoting blood circulation, strengthening the function of ativating *Yang Qi*, as the adjuvant and guiding drug.

○ All above drugs as a whole performs the functions of activating *Yang Qi* to relieve stagnation and remove phlegm.

● Notes:

(1) It is indicated for cases of heart-stroke, intercostal neuralgia, chronic bronchitis, nonsuppurative inflammation of costal cartilage with the syndrome mentioned above.

(2) Since the prescription is warm in nature, it is not advisable to cases of chest pain due to *Yin* deficiency, or dyspnea, chest pain due to heat and phlegm in the lung. For patients who can't take wine, the wine in the prescription can be reduced or not used.

Appendix:

(1) *Zhi Shi Xie Bai Gui Zhi Tang* (Decoction of Aurantii Immaturus, Allii Macroste-

mi and Cinnamonii)

- Source: *Jin Gui Yao Lue* (Synopsis of Prescriptions of the Golden Chamber)
- Ingredients: *Zhi Shi* (Fructus Aurantii Immaturus) 12g.

  Hou Po (Cortex Magnoliae Officinalis) 12g.

  Xie Bai (Bulbus Allii Macrostemi) 9g.

  Gui Zhi (Ramulus Cinnamomi) 3g.

  Gua Lou (Fructus Trichosanthis) 12g.

- Functions and indications: Activate *Yang*, disperse stagnation, remove phlegm and descend *Qi*, indicated for cases of Chest *Bi* syndrome manifested as fullness and pain in chest, dyspnea, cough, shortness of breath, a sensation of gas flowing from the hypochondrium to the heart, white and greasy tongue coating, deep wiry or tense pulse.

(2) *Gua Lou Xie Bai Ban Xia Tang* (Decoction of Frichosanthis, Allii Macrostemi and Pinelliae)

- Source: *Jin Gui Yao Lue* (Synopsis of Prescriptions of the Golden Chamber)
- Ingredients: *Gua Lou* (Fructus Trichosanthis) 30g.

  Xie Bai (Bulbus Allii Macrostemi) 6g.

  Ban Xia (Rhizoma Pinelliae) 12g.

  Rice Wine (yellow wine) 60ml.

- Functions and indications: The prescription has the functions of activating *Yang*, dispersing stagnation, removing phlegm and easing the chest. It is indicated for cases of chest *Bi* syndrome due to severe phlegm-dampness manifested as fullness and pain in the chest that refers to the back, and inability to lie flat.

16.2 Prescriptions for Descending Adverse-Rising *Qi*

Prescriptions for descending adverse rising *Qi* are indicated for cases of cough, dyspnea, hiccups, vomiting due to adverse rise of the lung and stomach *Qi*.

Su Zi Jiang Qi Tang (Decoction of Perillae for Keeping *Qi* Downwards)

- Source: *Tai Ping Hui Min He Ji Ju Fang* (Prescriptions of Peaceful Benevolent Dispensary)
- Ingredients: *Su Zi* (Fructus Perillae) 9g.

  Ban Xia (Rhizoma Pinelliae) 9g.

  Dang Gui (Radix Angelicae Sinensis) 6g.

  Gan Cao (Radix Glycyrrhizae) 6g.

  Qian Hu (Radix Peucedani) 6g.

  Hou Po (Cortex Magnoliae Officinalis) 6g.

  Rou Gui (Cortex Cinnamomi) 3g.

Sheng Jiang (Rhizoma Zingiberis Recens) 3g.

Su Ye (Folium Perillae) 2g.

Da Zao (Fructus Ziziphi Jujubae) 3pcs.

- Administration: All above drugs are decocted in water for oral administration.

- Functions: Lower adverse rising *Qi*, relieve dyspnea, remove phlegm, and stop cough.

- Indications: For the syndrom of excess in upper apart and deficiency in lower part of the body, manifested as profuse expectoration, dyspnea, cough, short breath, fullness and oppressing in the chest, lower back pain, weak legs, fatigue, white and greasy or smooth tongue coating.

- Explanation:

Su Ye: acrid in taste and warm in nature, descending *Qi*, removing phlegm, relieving cough and dyspnea, as the principal drug.

Ban Xia, *Hou Po* and *Qian Hu*: removing phlegm, descending *Qi*, relieving cough and dyspnea, as the assistant drugs.

Rou Gui: warming the kidney to disperse cold, helping the kidney to receive *Qi* so as to relieve asthma.

Dang Gui: nourishing the liver blood, with *Rou Gui* warming the lower *Jiao* and descending adverse rising *Qi*.

Sheng Jiang and *Su Ye*: activating the lung *Qi* to disperse cold.

The above four drugs are as the adjuvant drugs.

Da Zao and *Gan Cao*: regulating the middle *Jiao* and coordinating the effects of all the drugs, as guiding drugs.

○ The prescription as a whole performs the functions of descending *Qi*, removing phlegm and relieving dyspnea and cough.

- Notes:

(1) This prescription stresses on treating the secondary symptoms in emergency. It can descend adverse rising *Qi* and eliminate phlegm, also warm the kidney *Yang* and help the kidney to receive *Qi*. It is indicated for cases of chronic bronchitis, pneumonectasis, pulmonary heart disease, bronchial asthma with cough, dyspnea which belongs to excess in upper and deficiency in lower part.

(2) It's not advisable to cases of cough, asthma caused by the lung and kidney deficiency, or heat-phlegm in the lung.

Xuan Fu Dai Zhe Tang (Decoction of Inulae and Haematitum)

- Source: *Shang Han Lun* (Treaties on Cold-Induced Diseases)
- Ingredients: *Xuan Fu Hua* (Flos Inulae, wrapped up with cloth) 9g.

    Ren Shen (Radix Ginseng) 6g.

    Sheng Jiang (Rhizoma Zingberis Recens) 10g.

Dai Zhe Shi (Haematitum) 9g.

Zhi Gan Cao (Radix Glycyrrhizae Praeparata) 6g.

Ban Xia (Rhizoma Pinelliae) 9g.

Da Zao (Fructus Ziziphi Jujubae) 4 pcs.

● Administration: All drugs will be decocted in water for oral administration.

● Functions: Descend adverse rising Qi, eliminate phlegm, reinforce Qi and regulate the stomach.

● Indications: Deficiency of the stomach and adverse rise of the stomach Qi, manifested as epigastric fullness, belching, vomiting phlegm fluid with mucous, white and smooth tongue coating, wiry and weak pulse.

● Explanation:

Xuan Fu Hua: bitter, acrid and salty in taste, descending adverse Qi and eliminating phlegm, relieving belching, as the principal drug.

Dai Zhe Shi: descending adverse Qi, eliminating phlegm, relieving vomiting and belching, used as the assistant drug.

Ban Xia: drying dampness and eliminating phlegm, descending adverse-rising of Qi and regulating the stomach.

Sheng Jiang: removing phlegm, dispersing stagnation, descending adverse Qi to stop vomiting.

Above two drugs are used together to strengthen the functions of the principal and assistant drugs.

Ren Shen, Da Zao and Gan Cao: strengthening Qi and reinforcing the middle $Jiao$, preventing the metal and stone drugs from injuring the stomach, used as adjuvant drugs.

Gan Cao: harmonizing the effects of all the other drugs, thus also considered as the guiding drug of the prescription.

○ The prescription as a whole performs the functions of descending adverse Qi, eliminating phlegm, reinforcing Qi, regulating the stomach to stop vomiting.

● Notes:

The modified prescription are applied for cases of gastric neurosis, chronic gastritis, gastroptosis, gastroduodenal ulcer, pyloric uncompleted obsbruction, and nervous hiccups, which has adverserising of Qi due to deficiency of the stomach.

Ding Chuan Tang (Decoction for Relieving Asthma)

● Source: She Sheng Zhong Miao Fang (Wonderful Prescription for Keeping Health)

● Ingredients: Bai guo (Semen Ginkgo) 9g.

Ma Huang (Herba Ephedrae) 9g.

Su Zi (Fructus Perillae) 6g.

Gan Cao (Radix Glycyrrhizae) 3g.

Kuan Dong Hua (Flos Farfarae) 9g.

Xing Ren (Semen Armeniacae Amarum) 9g.

Ban Xia (Rhizoma Pinelliae) 9g.

Sang Bai Pi (Cortex Mori Radicis) 9g.

Huang Qin (Radix Scutellariae) 6g.

- Administration: All drugs will be decocted in water for oral administration.
- Functions: Activate and descend the lung *Qi*, clear away heat and eliminate phlegm.
- Indications: Asthma due to wind-cold attacking superficies and retention of phlegm-heat in the lung, manifested as asthma, cough, profuse and thick yellowish phlegm, shortness of breath, chills and fever, yellowish and greasy tongue coating, smooth and rapid pulse.
- Explanation:

Ma Huang: acrid in taste and warm in nature, activating the lung *Qi*, dispersing pathogenic factor and relieving asthma.

Bai Guo: sweet, bitter, puckery in taste, astringing the lung *Qi*, eliminating phlegm to relieve asthma.

The two drugs act together to enhance the antitussive and antiasthmatic effect and prevent the consumption of the lung *Qi* by *Ma Huang*, used as the principal drugs.

Su Zi, *Xing Ren*, *Ban Xia* and *Kuan Dong Hua*: descending adverse *Qi*, relieving asthma and cough, and eliminating phlegm, as the assistant drugs.

Sang Bai Pi and Huang *Qin*: clearing away lung-heat, relieving cough and asthma, as the adjuvant drugs.

Gan Cao: regulating all the drugs, as the guiding drug.

○ All above drugs as a whole perform the functions of activating lung's dispersing and descending function, eliminating phlegm and relieving asthma.

- Notes:

(1) It is indicated for cases of chronic bronchitis, bronchial asthma due to retention of phlegm-heat in the lung.

(2) It's forbidden to cases attacked by wind-cold without interior phlegm-heat characterized by anhidrosis and asthma, or prolonged asthma with *Qi* deficiency marked by weak pulse.

Si Mo Yin (Decoction of Four Powdered Drugs)

- Source: *Cheng Fang Bian Du* (Handy Prescriptions)
- Ingredients: *Ren Shen* (Radix Ginseng) 3g.

  Bin Lang (Semen Arecae) 9g.

  Chen Xiang (Lignum Aquilariae Resinatum) 3g.

  Wu Yao (Tiantai Radix Linderae) 9g.
- Administration: All drugs will be decocted in water for oral administration.
- Functions: Activate *Qi*, descend adverse *Qi*, ease the chest and disperse stagnation.

● Indications: *Qi* stagnation and adverse-rising of *Qi*, characterized by fullness and restlessness in the chest, shortness of breath, epigastric fullness, and poor appetite.

● Explanation:

Wu Yao: acrid in taste and warm in nature, activating and relieving the liver *Qi* stagnation. *Chen Xiang*: acrid and bitter in taste and warm in nature, regulating *Qi* and descending adverse-rising of *Qi* to relieve asthma.

Bin Lang: activating *Qi* to relieve stagnation and fullness sensation.

Ren Shen: reinforcing *Qi* and building up body resistance, preventing the damage of health *Qi* by other drugs.

○ The four drugs together, descending and ascending, reducing and reinforcing, perform the functions of dispersing stagnate liver *Qi* and regulating the stomach and lung.

● Notes:

(1) It is indicated for cases of bronchial asthma, pneumonectasis with the syndrome of adverserising of *Qi*.

(2) *Ren Shen* can be replaced by 6g. of *Dang Shen*.

Shen Zhe Zhen Qi Tang (Decoction of Radix Ginseng and Haematitum)

● Source: *Yi Xue Zhong Zhong Can Xi Lu* (Recordds of Traditional Chinese and Western Medicine in Combination)

● Ingredients: *Ye Tai Shen* (Radix Ginseng) 12g.

　　　　　　　Sheng Zhe Shi (Raw, Haematitum, powder) 12g.

　　　　　　　Sheng Qian Shi (Raw, Semen Euryales) 15g.

　　　　　　　Shan Yao (Rhizoma Dioscoreae) 15g.

　　　　　　　Yu Rou (Fructus Corni) 18g.

　　　　　　　Sheng Long Gu (Raw, Os Draconis) 18g.

　　　　　　　Sheng Mu Li (Raw, Concha Ostreae) 18g.

　　　　　　　Hang Shao (Radix Paeoniae Alba) 12g.

　　　　　　　Su Zi (Fructus Perillae) 6g.

● Administration: The above drugs will be decocted in water for oral administration.

● Functions: Reinforce and astringe *Qi*, suppress adverse ascendant *Qi* to relieve asthma.

● Indications: Deficiency of both *Yang* and *Yin*, adverse arise of the lung and stomach *Qi*, marked by asthma, shortness of breath, or kidney losing the control with upward running of the *Chong* meridian *Qi*, fullness sensation due to adverse rise of the stomach *Qi*, floating and rapid and weak pulse.

● Explanation:

Tai Shen: sweet and warm, reinforcing the *Qi* in the middle *Jiao*.

Zhe Shi: with heavy nature, suppressing adversely ascendant *Qi* to relieve asthma.

They are as the principal drugs.

Shao Yao, *Shan Yu Rou*, *Bai Shao* and *Qian Shi*: nourishing the liver and kidney to astringe the kidney *Qi*.

Long Gu and *Mu Li*: descending floating Yang caused by Yin deficiency, restoring collapse, as the assistant drugs.

Su Zi: eliminating phlegm and descending adverse *Qi* to relieve asthma, as the adjuvant drug.

○ All drugs as a whole perform the functions of reinforcing and astringing *Qi*, suppressing adversely ascendant *Qi* to relieve asthma.

● Notes:

It is indicated for cases of chronic bronchitis, pulmonary dilatation, gastroduodenal ulcer which has the symptoms mentioned above.

Summary

These 8 main *Qi* regulating prescriptions being selected are divided into the following two kinds:

(1) Prescriptions for activating *Qi*

This kind of prescriptions has the effect of activating *Qi* and be used for the *Qi* stagnation syndrome. *Chai Hu Shu Gan San* is particularly for dispersing the stagnation of the liver *Qi* and indicated for cases with pain and fullness sensation caused by stagnation of the liver *Qi*. *Yue Ju Wan* is for activating *Qi* to relieve stagnation, indicated for the stagnation syndromes, especially for *Qi* stagnation syndrome. *Gua Lou Xie Bai Bai Jiu Tang* has the effects of activating *Qi* to relieve pain, promoting *Yang* and eliminating phlegm accumulation. It's applicable to chest *Bi* syndrome due to deficiency of *Yang* in the chest with stagnation of the phlegm and dampness.

(2) Prescriptions for descending *Qi*

They are all having the effects of suppressing adverse-rising *Qi*, and indicated for the syndrome of adverse flow of *Qi*. *Su Zi Jiang Qi Tang*, *Ding Chuan Tang* are particularly helping the lung *Qi* to descend so as to relieve asthma. *Su Zi Jiang Qi Tang* also has the effect of warming to eliminate cold phlegm and treat cases of asthma due to cold dampness and phlegm in the upper (excess) and deficiency in the lower part of the body. *Ding Chuan Tang* is used to promoting the functions of the lung in dispersing and descending and resolving phlegm, treating case of asthma due to invasion of wind-cold and stagnation of phlegm-heat. *Si Mo Yin* can descend and activate *Qi* to treat cases due to adverse rise and stagnation of *Qi*. *Xuan Fu Dai Zhe Tang*, descending adverse rising of *Qi*, eliminating phlegm and reinforcing *Qi*, for cases of vomiting, hiccups due to deficiency of the stomach *Qi* and stagnation of phlegm. *Shen Zhe Zhen Qi Tang* has the effects of reinforcing *Qi* and stopping the rising of *Qi*, applicable to cases of adverse-rising of Qi of the lung and stomach due to deficiency of both *Yin* and *Yang*.

Review Questions

(1) Which one is the principal drug of *Yue Ju Wan*? Why?

(2) Both *Su Zi Jian Qi Tang* and *Ding Chuan Tang* can descend *Qi* and relieve asthma, what are the differences between them?

(3) Try to explain the composition and functions of *Xuan Fu Dai Zhe Tang*?

17 Prescriptions for Regulating Blood

This kind of prescriptions is composed of drugs for regulating blood and has the functions of activating blood and removing stasis or stopping bleeding to treat syndromes of blood stasis or haemorrhage.

Blood diseases can be classified into cold or heat and deficiency or excess syndromes, thus, there are extensive therapeutic methods for blood syndromes. In this part, the prescriptions are divided into two types: activating blood and removing stasis method for syndromes of blood stagnation and stopping bleeding method for syndromes of bleeding.

Blood syndromes are complicated. When prescriptions for regulating blood are applied, it is important to seek for the reasons of the disease and distinguish whether it is root cause or symptoms, acute or chronic case in order to treat the root cause of the disease when it is acute and treat the symptoms when it is chronic, or treat both root cause and symptoms by using reinforcement and elimination in combination. Pay attention that strong elimination of stasis may damage blood, while long-term administration of stasis-eliminating drugs tends to damage health *Qi*. In these cases, *Qi*-tonification drugs and blood-nourishing drugs should be added so as to prevent the damage of health *Qi* while eliminating stasis. Stopping bleeding too early may cause retention of blood stasis, so a small dosage of drugs for activating blood and removing stasis may be added in bleeding-stopping prescriptions or selecting hemostatic drugs which are associated with the effects of activating blood and removing stasis. In addition, prescriptions for activating blood and removing stasis belong to elimination method which can be used only for a short time as soon as the disease is cured. Besides, these prescriptions are drastic in property and easily to stir up bleeding and cause abortion, therefore, they should be cautiously used for patients with menorrhagia and pregnant women.

17.1 Activating Blood and Removing Stasis

This group of prescriptions is indicated for syndrome of blood retention and syndrome of blood stasis.

Shi Xiao San (Wonderful Powder for Relieving Blood Stagnation)

- Source: *Tai Ping Hui Min He Ji Ju Fang* (Prescription of Peaceful Benevolent Dispensary)
- Ingredients: *Wu Ling Zhi* (Faeces Trogopterorum)

    Pu Huang (Pollen Typhae)

These two drugs are of the same dosage.

- Administration: Grind the two drugs into powder and mix two *Qian* (about 6g.) of the powder with vinegar and boil it until it become paste. Add a cup of water and decoct it until about 7/10 of the water remains. Take the decoction warmly before meals.

Modern administration: Grind the drugs into fine powder and mix them with yellow wine or vinegar. Six grams is taken each time. Or take 6-12 grams of the powder each day (wrapped with a piece of cloth) and decoct in water for oral administration.

● Functions: Activate blood, remove stasis, dispel masses and relieve pain.

● Indications: Retention of stagnant blood marked by severe pain in the abdomen, or postpartum retention of lochia, or irregular menstruation with acute pain in the lower abdomen.

● Explanation:

Wu Ling Zhi: the principal drug, bitter and sweet in taste and warm in nature, activating blood, removing stasis and relieving pain.

Pu Huang: the assistant drug, sweet in taste and neutral in nature, circulating blood, removing stasis and relieving pain.

Vinegar or Yellow Wine: activating blood circulation, removing stagnant blood and strengthening the effects of drugs in activating blood and stopping pain.

○ The prescription as a whole plays the effects of activating blood, removing stasis and relieving pain.

● Notes:

(1) This is a common prescription for treating pain caused by blood stasis. The cases with retention of stagnant blood seen in such diseases as coronary heart disease, angina pectoris, ectopic pregnancy can be treatd with the prescription by adding other drugs.

(2) Since *Wu Ling Zhi* has fishy and foul smell which may damage the stomach, it should be cautiously used for patients with weakness of stomach *Qi* and is contraindicated for pregnant women.

Appendix:

Shou Nian San (Powder Picking up with Hand)

● Source: *Qi Xian Liag Fang* (Prescriptions of Magic Effects)

● Ingredients: *Yan Hu Suo* (Rhizoma Corydalis)

                Wu Ling Zhi (Faeces Trogopterorum)

                Cao Guo (Fructus Tsaoko)

                Mo Yao (Myrrha)

● Administration: They are in equal dosage and grounded into powder. Six grams is taken each time with warm boiled water.

● Functions and indications: It has the effects of activating blood, removing stasis, circulating *Qi* and relieving pain, indicating for epigastric and abdominal pain caused by stagnation of *Qi* and blood.

Xue Fu Zhu Yu Tang (Decoction for Removing Blood Stasis in the Chest)

● Source: *Yi Lin Gai Cuo* (Corrections on the Errors of Medical Works)

- Ingredients: *Tao Ren* (Semen Persicae) 12g.

  Hong Hua (Flos Carthami) 9g.

  Dang Gui (Radix Angelicae Sinensis) 9g.

  Sheng Di Huang (Radix Rehmanniae) 9g.

  Chuan Xiong (Rhizoma Ligustici Chuanxiong) 5g.

  Chi Shao (Radix Paeoniae Rubra) 6g.

  Niu Xi (Radix Achyranthis Bidentatae) 9g.

  Jie Geng (Radix Platycodi) 5g.

  Chai Hu (Radix Bupleuri) 3g.

  Zhi Qiao (Fructus Aurantii) 6g.

  Gan Cao (Radix Glycyrrhizae) 3g.

- Administration: All the drugs should be decocted in water for oral administration.
- Functions: Activate blood, remove stasis, circulate *Qi* and relieve pain.
- Indications: Blood stasis in the chest, marked by headache and long-lasting sharp pain in the chest with fixed location, or hiccup and nausea, or irrascibility, or dream-disturbed sleep and insomnia, or palpitation, or fever in the night, dark-red tongue with ecchymoses or purple spots, and choppy pulse.
- Explaination:

Tao Hong Si Wu Tang (Decoction of Four Ingredients Adding Peach Kernel and Safflower): activating blood, removing stasis and nourishing blood.

Si Ni San (Powder for Treating Cold Limbs): circulating *Qi*, harmonizing blood and promoting the circulation of the liver *Qi*.

Jie Geng: promoting lung's function in dispersing and descending and carrying the drugs to go upward.

Jie Geng with *Zhi Qiao* are used together to regulate the ascending and descending of *Qi* in the upper *Jiao* so as to ease the chest.

Niu Xi: clearing the vessels, promoting the circulation of blood, and conducting the blood to descend.

○ The prescription as a whole plays the effect of activating blood, circulating *Qi*, removing stasis and relieving pain.

- Notes:

(1) Coronary heart disease, angina pectoris, rheumatic heart disease, chest pain due to thoracic contusion or costal chondritis, as well as headache and dizziness in sequela of concussion of brain and emotional depression pertained to blood stasis can be treated by the modified prescription.

(2) The prescription is mostly composed of drugs of activating blood and removing stasis, it is not advisable for cases without blood stagnation and is contraindicated for pregnant women.

Appendix:

(1) *Tong Qiao Huo Xue Tang* (Decoction for Clearing the Orifices and Activating Blood Circulation)

- Source: *Yi Lin Gai Cuo* (Corrections on the Errors of Medical Works)
- Ingredients: *Chi Shao* (Radix Paeoniae Rubra) 3g.

  Chuan Xiong (Rhizoma Ligustici Chuanxiong) 3g.

  Tao Ren (Semen Persicae) 9g.

  Hong Hua (Flos Carthami) 9g.

  Lao Cong (Bulbus Allii Fistulosi) 3g.

  Hong Zao (Fructus Ziziphi Jujubae) 5g.

  She Xiang (Moschus) 1.5g.

  Huang Jiu (Yellow Wine) 250g.

- Functions and indications: The prescription has the functions of activating blood and dredging orifices, indicating for headache, dizziness due to blood stasis in the head, or prolonged deafness or loss of hair, green-purplish complexion, or rosacea, or vertigo as well as emaciation due to blood disorders and infantile malnutrition marked by emaciation, big abdomen with veins appearing and hectic fever.

(2) *Ge Xia Zhu Yu Tang* (Decoction for Dissipating Blood Stasis under Diaphram)

- Source: *Yi Lin Gai Cuo* (Corrections on the Errors of Medical Works)
- Ingredients: *Wu Ling Zhi* (Faeces Trogopterorum) 9g.

  Dang Gui (Radix Angelicae Sinensis) 9g.

  Chuan Xiong (Rhizoma Ligustici Chuanxiong) 6g.

  Tao Ren (Semen Persicae) 9g.

  Dan Pi (Cortex Moutan Radicis) 6g.

  Chi Shao (Radix Paeoniae Rubra) 6g.

  Wu Yao (Radix Linderae) 6g.

  Yan Hu Suo (Rhizoma Corydalis) 3g.

  Gan Cao (Radix Glycyrrhizae) 9g.

  Xiang Fu (Rhizoma Cyperi) 3g.

  Hong Hua (Flos Carthami) 9g.

  Zhi Qiao (Fructus Aurantii) 5g.

- Functions and indications: The prescription has functions of activating blood, removing stasis, circulating *Qi* and relieving pain, indicating for masses under diaphragm due to blood stasis, or infantile mass, or abdominal pain with a fixed location, or a feeling of abdominal falling as if there were something heavy in it when lying on bed.

(3) *Shao Fu Zhu Yu Tang* (Decoction for Removing Blood Stagnation in the Lower Abdomen)

- Source: *Yi Lin Gai Cuo* (Corrections on Errors of Medical Works)
- Ingredients: *Xiao Hui Xiang* (Fructus Foenicuii) 1.5g.

  Gan Jiang (Rhizoma Zingiberis) 3g.

Yan Hu Cuo (Rhizoma Corydalis) 3g.

Dang Gui (Radix Angelicae Sinensis) 9g.

Chuan Xiong (Rhizoma Ligustici Chuanxiong) 3g.

Guan Gui (Cortes Cinnamomi) 3g.

Chi Shao (Radix Paeoniae Rubra) 6g.

Pu Huang (Pollen Typhae) 9g.

Wu Ling Zhi (Faeces Trogopterorum) 6g.

● Functions and indications: The prescription has the functions of activating blood, removing stasis, warming meridians and relieving pain, indicating for masses with pain or no pain due to blood stasis in the lower abdomen, or only pain without mass, or distention and fullness in the lower abdomen, or lumbar soreness and abdominal distention during menstruation, or 3 to 5 times occurrence of menstruation in a month with constant bleeding, purplish or dark color of blood, or with clots, or metrorrhagia and metrostaxis with pain in the lower abdomen.

Bu Yang Huan Wu Tang (Decoction of Invigorating *Yang* for Recuperation)

● Source: *Yi Lin Gai Cuo* (Corrections on Errors of Medical Works)
● Ingredients: *Huang Qi* (Radix Astragali Seu Hedysari) 120g.

Dang Gui (Radix Angelicae Sinensis) 6g.

Chi Shao (Radix Paeoniae Rubra) 6g.

Di Long (Lumbricus) 3g.

Chuan Xiong (Rhizoma Ligustici Chuanxiong) 3g.

Hong Hua (Flos Carthami) 3g.

Tao Ren (Semen Persicae) 3g.

● Administraton: All the drugs should be decocted in water for oral administration.
● Functions: tonify *Qi*, activate blood and dredge collaterals.
● Indications: Sequelae of appoplexy, marked by hemiplegia, deviation of the mouth and eye, intricate and obscure speech, involuntary salivation from the mouth, flaccidity of lower limbs, frequent urination or enuresis, white tongue coating and slow pulse.
● Explanation:

Sheng Huang Qi: the principal drug, sweet in taste and warm in nature, tonifying the primary *Qi* to assist the movement of blood.

Dang Gui: the assistant drug, activating blood in order to remove stasis without damage of blood.

Chi Shao, *Chuan Xiong*, *Tao Ren* and *Hong Hua*: helping *Dang Gui* to activate blood and harmonize *Ying*.

Di Long: dredging the meridians and smoothing the circulation in collaterals.

○ The prescription as a whole plays the effects of tonifying the primary *Qi*, activating blood and dredging collaterals.

● Notes:

(1) The prescription is mainly used to treat hemiplegia after apoplexy with pale tongue, white coating, slow and forceless pulse as its diagnostic points. The modified recipe can treat paralysis of *Qi* deficiency and blood stasis seen in the sequelae stage of cerebrovascular accident or poliomyelitis.

(2) The dosage for *Huang Qi* is 120g. in the original prescription. It should be reduced in clinical use. Usually the dosage is from 30-60g.

Sheng Hua Tang (Decoction for Postpartum Troubles)

● Source: *Fu Qing Zhu Nu Ke* (Fu Qing Zhu's Obstetrics and Gynecology)
● Ingredients: *Quan Dang Gui* (Radix Angelicae Sinensis) 25g.

  Chuan Xiong (Rhizoma Ligustici Chuanxiong) 9g.

  Tao Ren (Semen Persicae) 6g.

  Gan Jiang (Rhizoma Zingiberis) 2g.

  Gan Cao (Radix Glycyrrhizae Praeparata) 2g.

● Administration: All the drugs should be decocted with equal dosage of yellow rice wine and infantile urine.

Modern administration: all the drugs are to be decocted in water or together with proper amount of yellow rice wine for oral administration.

● Functions: Activate blood, remove stasis, warm meridians and relieve pain.

● Indications: Attack of cold after childbirth due to blood deficiency, marked by retention of locia and cold pain in the lower abdomen.

● Explanation:

Dang Gui: the principal drug, sweet and acrid in taste and warm in nature, tonifying and activating blood, removing stasis and producing fresh.

Chuan Xiong: acrid in taste and warm in nature, activating blood and circulating *Qi*.

Tao Ren: bitter in taste and neutral in nature, activating blood and removing stasis.

The above two drugs are assistant drugs.

Pao Jiang: dispelling cold from the blood, warming the meridians and relieving pain.

Yellow Rice Wine: warming and dredging blood vessels to strengthen the effect of the drugs.

Infantile Urine: replenishing *Yang*, resolving stasis and conducting putrid blood to go downward.

They are adjuvant drugs.

Zhi Gan Cao: coordinating the effects of other drugs.

● Notes:

It is a commonly-used prescription for women after childbirth. With warm property, it is fit for cases with congealing of cold and stasis of blood after childbirth. The modified recipe can treat abdominal pain due to retention of placenta and postpartum uterine attraction. It is not advisable for cases with blood stagnation associated with heat.

Tao He Cheng Qi Tang (Decoction of Peach Kernel for Activating *Qi*)

- Source: *Shang Han Lun* (Treatise on Cold-Induced Diseases)
- Ingredients: *Tao Ren* (Semen Persicae) 12g.

  Da Huang (Radix et Rhizoma Rhei) 12g.

  Gui Zhi (Ramulus Cinnamomi) 6g.

  Gan Cao (Radix Glycyrrhizae) 6g.

  Mang Xiao (Natrii Sulphas) 6g.
- Administration: Decoct the drugs with water and remove the remainer. Take the decoction warmly after *Mang Xiao* is mixed inside.
- Functions: Eliminate blood stasis.
- Indications: Retention of blood in the lower *Jiao*, manifestd as distention and fullness in the lower abdomen with pain refused to be pressed, normal urination, delirium, severe thirst, fever during night, maniacal behavor, deep and forceful pulse.
- Explanation:

Tao Ren: bitter in taste and neutral in nature, eliminating blood stasis.

Da Huang: bitter in taste and cold in nature, removing stasis and reducing heat.

The combination of the two drugs reduces both stasis and heat and is used as principal drugs.

Gui Zhi: dredging blood vessels and helping *Tao Ren* to eliminate blood stasis.

Mang Xiao: clearing away heat, softening masses and helping *Da Huang* to remove stasis and reducing heat.

They are the assistant drugs.

Zhi Gan Cao: replenishing *Qi*, harmonizing the middle *Jiao* and relieving drastic properties of the other drugs, used as adjuvant and guiding drug.

- Notes:

(1) The modified prescription may treat cases with traumatic injury, retention of stagnant blood, failure to turn the body due to pain, difficult urination and bowel movement and constipation, or pain and distention of head, redness of eyes and toothache caused by vigorousness of fire which depresses blood in the upper part of the body, or epistaxis and hematemesis in purplish dark color caused by quick movement of blood due to pathogenic heat, or postpartum retention of lochia, hard mass and pain in the lower abdomen, asthma and distention which nearly cause to death, etc.

(2) If the case is with unrelieved exterior syndrome, reliving the exterior syndrome first and then eliminating stasis.

(3) It is contraindicated for pregnant women because of its drastic effect in eliminating blood stasis.

Wen Jing Tang (Decoction for Warming Meridians)

● Source: *Jin Gui Yao Lue* (Synopsis of Prescriptions of the Golden Chamber)

● Ingredients: *Wu Zhu Yu* (Fructus Evodiae) 9g.

     Dang Gui (Radix Angelicae Sinensis) 9g.

     Shao Yao (Radix Paeoniae) 6g.

     Chuan Xiong (Rhizoma Ligustici Chuanxiong) 6g.

     Ren Shen (Radix Ginseng) 6g.

     Gui Zhi (Ramulus Cinnamomi) 6g.

     E Jiao (Colla Corii Asini) 9g.

     Mu Dan Pi (Cortex Moutan Radicis) 6g.

     Sheng Jiang (Rhizoma Zingiberis Recens) 6g.

     Gan Cao (Radix Glycyrrhizae) 6g.

     Ban Xia (Rhizoma Pinelliae) 6g.

     Mai Dong (Radix Ophiopogonis) 9g.

● Administration: All the drugs should be decocted in water for oral administration.

● Functions: Warm meridians, dispel cold, remove stasis and nourish blood.

● Indications: Deficiency-cold in the *Chong* and *Ren* meridians with obstruction of stagnant blood, marked by persistent metrostaxis, irregular menstruation, preceded or delayed occurrence of menstruation, twice a month or no occurence in a month, associated with nightfall fever, feverish sensation in the palms, dryness of the lips and mouth, lower abdominal spasm and fullness, as well as failure to conceive for a long time.

 ● Explanation:

Wu Zhu Yu: acrid and bitter in taste and hot in nature.

Gui Zhi: acrid and sweet in taste and warm in nature.

Both are principal drugs to warm meridians, disperse cold and dredge blood vessels.

Dang Gui, *Chuan Xiong*, *Shao Yao* and *E Jiao*: the assistant drugs, nourishing blood, regulating menstruation, removing stasis and producing the fresh.

Dan Pi: helping *Gui Zhi*, *Dang Gui* and *Chuan Xiong* to activate blood circulation, remove stasis and to clear away heat from the Blood system.

Ren Shen, *Gan Cao* and *Mai Dong*: replenishing stomach *Qi*, nourishing stomach *Yin* to make abundant of middle *Qi* in order to produce blood.

Ban Xia: stopping the rising of stomach *Qi*.

Sheng Jiang: warming the liver and calming the stomach, as well as relieving the toxicity of Ban Xia.

Those are the adjuvant drugs.

Gan Cao: coordinating the effect of all the drugs, used as the guiding drug.

 ○ The prescription as a whole plays the effects of warming the meridians, dredging vessels, nourishing blood and removing stasis.

● Notes:

The prescription can treat dysfunctional uterine bleeding and chronic inflammation of pelvis pertaining to deficiency cold in the *Chong* and *Ren* meridians with obstruction of stagnant blood.

17.2 Stopping Bleeding

Hemostatic prescriptions are indicated for various kinds of heorrhagic syndromes caused by quick mevement of blood out of vessels such as hematemesis, epistasis, haemoptysis, bloody stool and metrorrhagia and metrostaxis.

Xiao Ji Yin Zi (Small Thistle Decoction)

● Source: *Ji Sheng Fang* (Prescriptions for Succouring the Sick)
● Ingredients: *Sheng Di Huang* (Radix Rehmanniae) 30g.

Xiao Ji (Herba Cephalanoploris) 15g.

Hua Shi (Talcum Pulveratum) 15g.

Mu Tong (Caulis Akebiae) 9g.

Pu Huang (Pollen Typhae) 9g.

Ou Jie (Nodus Nelumbinis Rhizomatis) 9g.

Dan Zhu Ye (Herba Lophatheri) 9g.

Dang Gui (Radix Angelicae Sinensis) 6g.

Shan Zhi Zi (Fructus Gardeniae) 9g.

Zhi Gan Cao (Radix Glycyrrhizae Praeparata) 6g.

● Administration: All the drugs should be decocted in water for oral administration.
● Functions: Cool the blood, stop bleeding, induce diuresis and treat stranguria.
● Indications: Stagnant heat in the lower Jiao, markd by stranguria with hematuria, frequent urination, painful and dribbling urination or haematuria, red tongue and rapid pulse.
● Explanation:

Xiao Ji: sweet in taste and cool in nature, cooling the blood, stopping bleeding, removing stasis and producing the fresh.

Sheng Di: sweet and bitter in taste and cold in nature, clearing away heat, cooling the blood, stopping bleeding and removing stasis.

They are the principal drugs.

Pu Huang and *Ou Jie*: sweet and astringent in taste and neutral in nature, stopping bleeding by astringency, circulating blood and removing stasis, used as assistant drugs.

Hua Shi, *Mu Tong* and *Dan Zhu Ye*: clearing away heat, inducing diuresis and treating stranguria.

Zhi Zi: clearing away accumulated heat in the lower *Jiao* from the urine.

Dang Gui: removing stasis and producing the fresh, clearing away heat and inducing diuresis without damaging blood.

Those are the adjuvant drugs.

Zhi Gan Cao: relieving spasm to stop pain, coordinating the effects of all the drugs, used as the guiding drug.

○ The prescription as a whole plays the effects of cooling the blood, stopping bleeding, inducing diuresis and treating stranguria.

● Notes:

(1) The modified prescription can treat acute urinary system infection and stone disease in the urinary system.

(2) The drugs in this prescription are cold or cool diuretics, they are only suitable for excess syndromes and heat syndromes. For patients suffering from stranguria with hematuria for a long time and with weakness of anti-pathogenic *Qi*, the original prescription should not be used.

Jiao Ai Tang (Ass-Hide Glue and Argyi Leat Decoction)

● Source: *Jin Gui Yao Lue* (Synopsis of Prescriptions of the Golden Chamber)
● Ingredients: *Chuan Xiong* (Rhizoma Ligustici chuanxiong) 6g.

     E Jiao (Colla Corii Asini) 9g.

     Ai Ye (Folium Artemisae) 9g.

     Gan Cao (Radix Glycyrrhizae) 6g.

     Dang Gui (Radix Angelicae Sinensis) 9g.

     Shao Yao (Radix Paeoniae) 12g.

     Gan Di Huang (Radix Rehmanniae) 18g.

● Administration: Decoct the drugs in 2/3 water and 1/3 yellow rice wine. Remove the residue and get the decoction, then melt *E Jiao* with the decoction and take it warm.

● Functions: Nourish blood, regulate menstruation, prevent abortion and stop metrostaxis.

● Indications: Deficiency and injury of the *Chong* and *Ren* meridians of women, marked by metrorrhagia and metrostaxis, menorrhagia without stopping or ceaseless bleeding due to miscarriage, or vaginal bleeding occurring during pregnancy with abdominal pain.

● Explanation:

E Jiao: sweet in taste and neutral in nature, tonifying blood and stopping bleeding.

Ai Ye: bitter and sweet in taste and warm in nature, warming the meridians and stop bleeding.

Both are the principal drugs.

Shu Di, *Dang Gui*, *Bai Shao* and *Chuan Xiong*: the assistant and adjuvant drugs, tonifying blood, activating blood circulation and regulating menstruation.

Gan Cao: coordinating the effects of all the drugs.

Yellow rice wine: strengthening the effects of other drugs.

They are the guiding drugs.

○ The prescription as a whole plays the effects of nourishing blood, regulating menstruation, preventing abortion and stopping metrostasis.

● Notes:

(1) Patients of persistent haemorrhage seen in dysfunctional uterine bleeding, threatened abortion, and habitual abortion due to deficiency and injury of the *Chong* and *Ren* meridians and blood deficiency associated with cold can be treated by this prescription.

(2) It is not advisable for cases with menorrhagia and metrostaxis or vaginal bleeding during pregnancy caused by heat in Blood system.

Ke Xue Fang (Decoction for Treating Hemoptysis)

● Source: *Dan Xi Xin Fa* (Danxi's Experiential Therapy)
● Ingredients: *Qing Dai* (Indigo Naturalis) 6g.

Hai Shi (Os Costaziae) 9g.

Shan Zhi Zi (Fructus Gardeniae) 9g.

Ke Zi (Fructus Chebulae) 6g.

● Administration: All the drugs should be decocted in water for oral administration.

● Functions: Clear away fire, remove phlegm, astringe lung *Qi* and relieve cough.

● Indications: Invasion to lung by liver fire, marked by cough with sticky and bloody sputum which is difficult to spit out, or irrascibility, sharp pain in the chest and hypochondriac region, red cheeks, constipation, red tongue with yellow coating, wiry and rapid pulse.

● Explanation:

Qing Dai and *Zhi Zi*: the principal drugs, bitter and salty in taste and cold in nature, clearing away liver fire and cooling blood.

Gua Lou Ren and *Hai Shi*: the assistant drugs, clearing away heat, reducing the fire, moistening dryness and resolving phlegm.

Ke Zi: the adjuvant and guiding drug, clearing away heat, astringing lung *Qi*, and lowering the rising of lung *Qi* to stop cough and resolve phlegm.

○ The prescription as a whole plays the effects of clearing away liver fire and astringing lung *Qi*.

● Notes:

(1) The modified prescription can treat cases with the above symptoms such as haemoptysis caused by bronchiectasis and lung tuberculosis, etc.

(2) For cases with haemoptysis caused by liver fire attacking the lung, drugs for clearing the lung and nourishing *Yin* should be added for preventing the injury of Yin.

Huai Hua San (Sophora Powder)

● Source: *Ben Shi Fang* (Effective Prescriptions for Universal Relief)

- Ingredients: *Huai Hua* (Flos Sophorae, baked) 12g.

  Bai Ye (Cacumen Biotae, baked) 12g.

  Jing Jie Sui (Spica Schizonepetae, baked) 6g.

  Zhi Qiao (Fructus Aurantikii, baked) 6g.

- Administration: Grind the above ingredients into fine powder. Take 6 grams each time with boiled water or rice soup. The drugs can also be decocted in water for oral administration with the dosages reducd in proportion to those of the original prescription.

- Functions: Clear the intestines, stop bleeding, expel wind and circulate *Qi*.

- Indications: Hemotochezia caused by wind and toxic heat in the large intestine, marked by bleeding before or after passing stools, or fresh blood in the stools as well as hemorrhoidal bleeding in fresh red color or dark color.

- Explanation:

Huai Hua: the principal drug, bitter in taste and slight cold in nature, clearing damp-heat from the large intestine, cooling blood and stop bleeding.

Ce Bai Ye: helping Huai Hua to cool blood and stop bleeding.

Jing Jie: being parched, expelling wind, entering the Blood system to stop bleeding.

The above two drugs are the assistant drugs.

Zhi Qiao: the adjuvant and guiding drug, descending *Qi* and clearing the large intestine.

○ The prescription as a whole plays the effects of cooling blood, stopping bleeding, clearing the intestines and expelling wind.

- Notes:

(1) This is a commonly-used prescription for treating hemotochezia due to wind and toxic heat in the large intestine as well as hemorrhoidal bleeding.

(2) Drugs in the prescription with cold and cool nature can not be taken for a long time. It is not advisable for patients with bloody stools for a long time associated with *Qi* deficiency or *Yin* deficiency.

Summary

Ten main prescriptions for regulating blood are selected and divided into two types according to their functions: prescriptions for activating blood and removing stasis and prescriptions for stopping bleeding.

(1) Prescriptions for activating blood and removing stasis

This kind of prescriptons all has the functions of activating blood and removing stasis, indicating for syndrome of unsmooth circulation of blood or internal accumulation of stagnant blood. Among them, *Xue Fu Zhu Yu Tang* can activate blood, remove stasis, circulate *Qi* and relieve pain, indicating for various pain syndorme caused by stagnant blood in the chest. *Tao He Cheng Qi Tang* can eliminate blood stasis, remove stagnant heat, indicating for syndrome of retention of blood in the lower *Jiao* due to accumulation of blood heat. *Bu Yang*

Huan Wu Tang is good at tonifying *Qi*, activating blood, removing stasis and dredging the collaterals, indicating for syndrome of hemiplegia caused by obstructron of meridians due to *Qi* deficiency and blood stasis. *Shi Xiao San*, *Wen Jing Tang* and *Sheng Hua Tang* are all commonly used prescriptions for gynaecological diseases. *Shi Xiao San* mainly activates blood, removes stasis and relieves pain, indicating for irregular menstruation, or acute pain in the lower abdomen due to postpartum retention of lochia. *Wen Jing Tang* is good at warming meridians, expelling cold, nourishing blood and removing stasis and is a commonly used prescripton for treating irregular menstruation or sterility caused by deficiency cold in the *Chong* and *Ren* meridians and internal obstruction of stagnant blood. *Sheng Hua Tang* has the functions of activating blood, removing stasis, warming meridians and relieving pain, indicating for postpartum retention of lochia and pain in the lower abdomen due to cold.

(2) Prescriptions for stopping bleeding

This group of prescriptions has the functions of stopping bleeding, indicating for hemorrhagia syndrome. *Xiao Ji Yin Zi*, *Ke Xue Fang* and *Huai Hua San* are prescriptions for cooling blood and stopping bleeding, indicating for haemorrhage syndrome due to quick circulation of blood resulting from heat. *Xiao Ji Yin Zi* is associated with the effects of inducing diuresis and treating stranguria, indicating for stranguria with hematuria. *Ke Xue Fang* is associated with the functions of clearing away fire and resolving phlegm, indicating for haemoptysis due to invasion to lung by liver fire. *Huai Hua San* is good at clearing intestines and expelling wind, indicating for hematocheia due to wind in large intestine. *Jiao Ai Tang* is a prescription for warming and tonifying blood and stopping bleeding as well as regulating menstruation and preventing abortion, indicating for metrorrhagia, metrostaxis and vaginal bleeding during pregnancy due to deficiency and injury of the *Chong* and *Ren* meridians.

Review Questions

(1) Why are prescriptions for activating blood and removing stasis often associated with *Qi*-circulating drugs or *Qi*-tonics? And why are hemostatics often associated with stasis-removing drugs?

(2) Please state the ingredients, significance of compatibility and indications of *Xue Fu Zhu Yu Tang*.

(3) What are the compatibility characteristics of *Bu Yang Huan Wu Tang*? And say its functions and indications.

(4) Both *Wen Jing Tang* and *Sheng Hua Tang* are common prescriptions for treating gynaecological diseases. What are the differences between them?

(5) Which kind of haemoptysis does *Ke Xue Fang* treat? And why is bleeding stopped without using hemostatics?

18 Prescriptions for Resolving and Removing Accumulation

The prescriptions for resolving and removing accumulation are chiefly made up of digestive and resolvents with the effects of promoting digestion, resolving stagnation, removing accumulation and eliminating masses, used to treat stagnation of food and masses in the abdomen.

Most of the prescriptions of this kind have mild resolving and dispersing effects and are indicated for retention of food in the epigastrium and gradual formation of masses. They are grouped into two kinds: the prescriptions for promoting digestion and resolving stagnation and the prescriptions for eliminating masses and removing accumulation.

This kind of prescriptions is used to attack the pathogenic evils, and they should not be used for syndromes of pure deficiency without accumulation. For those with constitutional weakness of the spleen and stomach, or prolonged accumulation and stagnation which consume the anti-pathogenic Qi, drugs for supporting anti-pathogenic Qi and invigorating the spleen should be properly added to play the effect of both removing and tonifying so as not to damage anti-pathogenic Qi when removing accumulation, and at the same time while supporting the anti-pathogenic Qi the pathogenic factors will be removed. Furthermore, attention should be paid to the proper dosage of the drugs in the prescription, and stop using the drugs as soon as the disease is cured.

In addition, internal accumulation and stagnation may impair the movement of Qi, therefore, drugs for regulating Qi are often used in the prescriptions to remove the accumulation by activating the circulation of Qi.

18.1 Prescriptions for Promoting Digestion and Resolving Stagnation

This group of prescriptions is indicated for diseases with accumulation of food.

Bao He Wan (Pill for Promoting Digestion)

- Source: *Dan Xi Xin Fa* (Danxi's Experiential Therapy)
- Ingredients: *Shan Zha* (Fructus Cratae qi) 180g.

  Shen Qu (Massa Fermentata Medicinalis) 60g.

  Ban Xia (Rhizoma Pinelliae) 90g.

  Fu Ling (Poria) 90g.

  Chen Pi (Pericarpium Citri Reticulatae) 30g.

  Lian Qiao (Fructus Forsythiae) 30g.

  Luo Bo Zi (Semen Raphani) 30g.

● Administration: Grind all the above drugs into very fine powder first and then mix the powder with water to make it into pills. Take 6-9g. each time with warm boiled water or *Chao Mai Ya Tang* (Decoction of Parched Fructus Hordei Germinatus). The drugs can also be decocted in water for oral administration with the dosage reduced in proportion with the original prescription.

● Functions: Promote digestion and harmonize the stomach.

● Indications: Retention of food, marked by fullness, distention and pain in the epigastrium and abdomen, eructation, acid regurgitation, poor appetite, nausea, or diarrhea, thick and greasy coating of the tongue and slippery pulse.

● Explanation:

Shan Zha: the principal drug, sour and sweet in taste and slightly warm in nature, removing accumulation of greasy food.

Shen Qu: sweet and acrid in taste and warm in nature, promoting digestion, harmonizing the stomach and removing accumulated food due to over-drinking.

Luo Bo Zi: acrid and sweet in taste, making the *Qi* to go downward, removing accumulated grain food, easing the chest and diaphragm and relieving fullness.

The above two are assistant drugs.

Ban Xia: acrid in taste and warm in nature, drying dampness, removing phlegm, making the *Qi* going downward to help the dispersing of stagnancy.

Chen Pi: acrid and bitter in taste and warm in nature, drying dampness, removing phlegm, regulating *Qi* and harmonizing the middle *Jiao*.

Fu Ling: sweet in taste and neutral in nature, invigorating the spleen, harmonizing the middle *Jiao*, removing phlegm and resolving dampness.

Lian Qiao: bitter in taste, cold in nature and fragrant in smell, dispersing the stagnation and clearing away heat.

○ The combination of all the drugs plays the effects of promoting digestion and harmonizing the stomach.

● Notes:

This is a prescription for promoting digestion and removing accumulation, indicating for retention of food in the epigastrium without deficiency of anti-pathogenic *Qi*. The prescription can treat cases with retention of accumulated food such as acute gastroenteritis and infantile indigestion.

Zhi Zhu Wan (Pill of Immature Bitter Orange and Bighead Atractylodes)

● Source: *Pi Wei Lun* (Treatise on the Spleen and Stomach), Zhang Yuansu's prescription

● Ingredients: *Zhi Shi* (Fructus Aurantii Immaturus) 30g.

　　　　　　 Ba Zhu (Rhizoma Atractylodis Macrocephalae) 60g.

● Administration: The pills are made out of the above ingredients. 6-9 grams is taken each time with decoction of *He Ye* (Folium Nelumbinis) or warm boiled water. The drugs together with *He Ye* can also be decocted in water for oral administration. The dosage is reduced in proportion to the original prescription.

● Functions: Invigorate the spleen and stomach and relieve fullness.

● Indications: Retention of food due to deficiency of the spleen and stagnation of *Qi*, marked by fullness in the chest and epigastrium, poor appetite, loose stool or difficult defecation.

● Explanation:

Bai Zhu: the principal drug, bitter and sweet in taste and warm in nature, invigorating spleen's transporting function and removing dampness.

Zhi Shi: the assistant drug, bitter and acrid in taste and slightly cold in nature, making *Qi* to descend, resolving stagnation and removing distention and fullness.

He Ye: the adjuvant and guiding drug, tonifying the spleen and stomach in order to help the ascending of the clear part of food.

○ The combination of all the drugs plays the effects of ascending the clear, descending the turbid, regulating *Qi*, harmonizing the stomach, invigorating the spleen, eliminating accumulation and relieving fullness.

● Notes:

The prescription may treat cases with deficiency of the spleen and stagnation of *Qi*, seen in such diseases as gastroptosis, gastromyasthenia, gastroneurosis and chronic gastritis, etc.

Jian Pi Wan (Pill for Invigorating the Spleen)

● Source: *Zheng Zhi Zhun Sheng* (Standards of Diagnosis and Treatment)
● Ingredients: *Bai Zhu* (Rhizoma Atractylodis Macrocephalae) 75g.

　　　　　Mu Xiang (Radix Aucklandiae) 22g.

　　　　　Huang Lian (Rhizoma Coptidis) 22g.

　　　　　Gan Cao (Radix Glycyrrhizae) 22g.

　　　　　Bai Fu Ling (Poria) 60g.

　　　　　Ren Shen (Radix Ginseng) 45g.

　　　　　Shen Qu (Massa Fermetata Medicinalis) 30g.

　　　　　Chen Pi (Pericarpium Citri Reticulatae) 30g.

　　　　　Sha Ya (Fructus Amoni) 30g.

　　　　　Mai Ya (Fructus Hordei Germinatus) 30g.

　　　　　Shan Zha (Fructus Crataegi) 30g.

　　　　　Shan Yao (Rhizoma Dioscoreae) 30g.

　　　　　Rou Dou Kou (Semen Myristicae) 30g.

● Administration: Make pills with starch paste or water out of powdered drugs. Take 6-9 g. each time with warm boiled water twice a day. The drugs can also be decocted in water for oral administration.

● Functions: Invigorate the spleen, harmonize the stomach, promote digestion and relieve diarrhea.

● Indications: Retention of food due to weakness of the spleen and stomach, marked by poor appetite, indigestion, distention and fullness in the epigastrium and abdomen, loose stool, greasy coating of the tongue with light yellow color, and forceless or weak pulse.

● Explanation:

Si Jun Zi Tang (Decoction of Four Noble Drugs): They are principal drugs to tonify *Qi*, invigorate the spleen, resolve dampness and relieve diarrhea.

Shan Yao and *Rou Dou Kou*: helping the principal drugs to invigorate the spleen and relieve diarrhea.

Shan Zha, *Shen Qu* and *Mai Ya*: promoting digestion and removing stagnation.

The above five drugs are assistant drugs.

Mu Xiang, *Sha Ren* and *Chen Pi*: regulating *Qi* and harmonizing stomach.

Huang Lian: clearing away heat and drying dampness.

These four are adjuvant and guiding drugs.

○ The combination of all the drugs plays the effect of invigorating the spleen, removing accumulation and relieving diarrhea.

● Notes:

This is a prescription with reinforcement and elimination in combination. It is used to treat chronic gastritis, functional indigestion and chronic heptitis which pertain to retention of food due to weakness of the spleen and stomach, marked by fullness in the epigastrium and abdomen and diarrhea.

18.2 Prescriptions for Eliminating Masses and Removing Accumulation

This group of prescriptions is indicated for syndromes with masses.

Zhi Shi Xiao Pi Wan (Pill with Immature Bitter Orange for Disintegrating Masses and Relieving Stuffiness)

● Source: *Lun Shi Mi Cang* (Secret Record of the Chamber of Orchids)
● Ingredients: *Gan Sheng Jiang* (Rhizoma Zingiberis) 3g.

    Zhi Gan Cao (Radix Glycyrrhizae Praeparata) 6g.

    Mai Ya Qu (Fructus Hordei Germinatus) 6g.

    Bai Fu Ling (Poria) 6g.

    Bai Zhu (Rhizoma Atractylodis Macrocephalae) 6g.

    Ban Xia Qu (Rhizoma Pinelliae) 9g.

    Ren Shen (Radix Ginseng) 9g.

    Hou Po (Cortes Magnoliae Oflcinalis) 12g.

Zhi Shi (Fructus Aurantii Immaturus) 15g.

Huang Lian (Rhizoma Coptidis) 15g.

● Administration: Make pills with water or starchy paste out of the powdered drugs. The pills are to be taken 6-9 grams each time with boiled water, twice a day. Alternatively, the drugs may be decocted in water for oral administration.

● Functions: Eliminate masses, remove fullness, invigorate the spleen and harmonize the stomach.

● Indications: Deficency of the spleen with stagnation of *Qi*, mixture of cold with heat, marked by epigastric masses and fullness, poor appetite, lassitude, tiredness, and irregular bowel movement.

● Expanation:

Zhi Shi: the principal drug, bitter and acrid in taste and cold in nature, activating *Qi* and eliminating masses.

Hou Po: the assistant drug, bitter and acrid in taste and warm in nature, activating *Qi* and relieving fullness.

Huang Lian: clearing away heat, drying dampness and removing masses.

Ban Xia Qu: acrid in taste and warm in nature, dispelling accumulation and harmonizing the stomach.

Gan Jiang: warming the middle Jiao and expelling cold.

The combination of the above three drugs plays the effect of dispersion with acrid property and purgation with bitter property to help the principal and assistant drugs to activate the circulation of *Qi* and remove masses.

Ren Shen, *Bai Zhu*, *Fu Ling* and *Zhi Gan Cao*: tonifying *Qi* and invigorating the spleen.

Mai Ya: promoting digestion and harmonizing the stomach.

The above eight drugs are used as adjuvant and guiding drugs.

○ The prescription as a whole plays the effects of eliminating masses and removing accumulation, by using drugs with effects of both reinforcing and reducing and drugs with nature of both cold and hot.

● Notes:

(1) The modified prescription may treat chronic heptitis, early cirrhosis of liver and chronic gastritis which give rise to the above symptoms.

(2) It is not advisable for cases with accumulated food of excess type or of deficient cold type.

Summary

Four prescriptions for resolving and removing accumulation are selected and divided into two types according to their functions: the prescriptions for promoting digestion and resolving stagnation and the prescriptions for eliminating masses and removing accumulation.

(1) Prescriptions for promoting digestion and resolving stagnation

Bao He Wan promotes digestion and harmonizes the stomach and is a general prescription for promoting digestion and removing accumulation, indicating for all kinds of accumulation of food. Both *Zhi Zhu Wan* and *Jian Pi Wan* are the prescriptions with reinforcement and elimination in combination. *Zhi Zhu Wan* invigorates spleen and promotes the circulation of *Qi*, indicating for retention of food caused by deficiency of spleen and stagnation of *Qi*, While *Jian Pi Wan* invigorates spleen and promotes digestion, indicating for stagnation of food syndrome due to spleen deficiency.

(2) Prescriptions for eliminating masses and removing accumulation

Zhi Shi Xiao Pi Wan promotes the circulation of *Qi*, eliminates masses, invigorates the spleen and harmonizes the stomach, playing reinforcing effect within elimination, indicating for syndromes with masses and fullness due to stagnation of *Qi* and accumulation of dampness, manifested as association of deficiency with excess and mixture of cold with heat.

Review Questions

(1) Why is *Lian Qiao* used in *Bao He Wan* which is a prescription for promoting digestion and harmonizing the stomach?

(2) Why is *Zhi Zhu Wan* considered a prescription having reinforcing effect rather than elimination?

(3) What are the ingredients and indications of *Jian Pi Wan*?

(4) What are the functions and indications of *Zhi Shi Xiao Pi Wan*?

19 Prescriptions for Expelling Parasites

Prescriptions for expelling parasites are composed of anthelmintics to treat parasites in the human body.

The prescriptions often consist of *Wu Mei* (Fructus Mume), *Chuan Jiao* (Pericarpium Zanthoxyli), *Lei Wan* (Onphalia), *Shi Jun Zi* (Fructus Quisqualis), *Ku Lian Pi* (Cortex Meliae) and other drugs. Since syndromes caused by parasites have differences in cold, heat, deficiency and excess, different drugs should be associated with according to the syndrome.

Stool examination should be done in advance to find ova and then give medicine according to the differentiation. During the treatment, greasy food should be avoided and it is necessary to administer the drug with an empty stomach.

Wu Mei Wan (Black Plum Pill)

- Source: *Shang Han Lun* (Treatise on Cold-Induced Diseases)
- Ingredients: *Wu Mei* (Fructus Mume) 480g.

  Xi Xin (Herba Asari) 180g.

  Gan Jiang (Rhizoma Zingiberis) 300g.

  Huang Lian (Rhizoma Coptidis) 480g.

  Dang Gui (Radix Angelicae) 120g.

  Fu Zi (Radix Aconiti Lateralis Praeparata) 150g.

  Shu Jiao (Pericarpium Zanthoxyli) 120g.

  Gui Zhi (Ramulus Cinnamomi) 180g.

  Ren Shen (Radix Ginseng) 180g.

  Huang Bai (Radix Phellodendri) 180g.
- Administration: Soak *Wu Mei* into 50% vinegar for a night and break it into pieces after getting rid of the pit. Mix it with other drugs which will be dried up and ground into powder. Mix the powder with honey for making pills. 9 grams is taken each time. One to tree doses a day on an empty abdomen with warm boiled water. The drugs can also be decocted in water for oral administration with the dosages reduced in proportion to those of the original prescription.
- Functions: Warm *Zang* organs and relieve colic caused by ascaris.
- Indications: Syndrome of colic caused by ascaris, marked by restlessness and vomiting which come and go at times, vomiting ascaris after taking food, cold limbs, abdominal pain, as well as chronic dysentery and chronic diarrhea.
- Explanation:

Wu Mei: sour in taste, controlling ascaris.

Huang Lian: bitter in taste, eliminating ascaris.

Chuan Jiao: acrid in taste, killing parasites and expelling ascaris.

The three drugs are principal drugs.

Xi Xin, *Gui Zhi*, *Gan Jiang* and *Fu Zi*: warming *Zang* organs and expelling cold.

Huang Bai: helping *Huang Lian* to clear away heat and dry dampness.

Ren Shen and *Dang Gui*: tonifying *Qi* and blood, supporting anti-pathogenic *Qi*.

○ The prescription as a whole, combining both cold and heat drugs and taking care of both root cause and symptoms, plays the effects of warming *Zang* organs and relieving colic caused by ascaris.

● Notes:

It is a representative prescription for treating biliary ascariasis and intestinal ascariasis. It can teat chronic colitis and chronic dysentery due to weakness of the intestines and stomach and mixture of cold and heat.

Hua Chong Wan (Anthelmintic Pill)

● Source: *Tai Ping Hui Min He Ji Ju Fang* (Prescription of Peaceful Benevolent Dispensary)

● Ingredients: *Hu Fen* (or Qian Fen) (Basic Lead Carboniate) 1500g.

              He Shi (Fructus Carpesii) 1500g.

              Bin Lang (Semen Arecae) 1500g.

              Ku Lian Gen Pi (Cortex Meliae) 1500g.

              Bai Fan (Alumen) 370g.

● Administration: The above drugs are ground into fine powder and to be sifted, and then made into pills with water, the size of which is as big as hemp seed. Five pills are given to one-year-old child on an empty abdomen with rice soup.

● Functions: Expel and kill all kinds of parasites in the intestines.

● Indications: Intestinal ascaris and other kinds of parastites, marked by abdominal pain with alternate up-and-down attacks, and even pain with vomiting of clear water, or vomiting of ascaris.

● Explanation:

He Shi: bitter and acrid in taste and neutral in nature, slight poisonous, expelling and killing ascaris.

Ku Lian Gen Pi: bitter in taste and cold in nature, poisonous, killing parasites and relieving abdominal pain.

Bin Lang: expelling parasites.

Bai Fan: detoxicating and controlling parasites.

Qian Fen: poisonous, removing turbidness and expelling parasites.

○ The prescription as a whole plays the strong effect of expelling and killing all kinds of parasites.

● Notes:

(1) The prescription can expel and kill ascaris, oxyurid, trichomonas, bladder warm and fasciolopsis, etc.

(2) The drugs are poisonous and stop taking the drugs as soon as the disease is cured. After expelling parasites, some drugs for regulating and reinforcing the spleen and stomach should be given to recover the anti-pathogenic *Qi*. When the prescription is used as decoction, omit *Qian Fen*.

Summary

Two prescriptions for expelling parasites are selected. *Wu Mei Wan* has the functions of warming the *Zang* organs, tonifying deficiency, clearing away heat and relieving colic caused by ascaris, indicating for syndrome of colic caused by cascaras due to mixture of upper heat and lower cold. *Hua Chong Wan* has stronger effects in expelling and killing parasites and is a general prescription for treating various kinds of intestinal parasites.

Review Question

Please state the ingredients, functions, indications and explanation of *Wu Mei Wan*.

20 Prescriptions for Treating Carbuncles

These prescriptions refer to those that mainly consist of the drugs having the effects of clearing away heat and toxins, promoting pus discharge, or warming *Yang* and dissolving masses, with the functions of removing toxic substances and subducing inflammation, they are applied to the treatment of large carbunle, cellulitis, nail-like boil and furuncle.

Carbuncle has a wide range, but is generalized as two kinds, internal and external. Therefore, the prescriptions are subdivided into the prescriptions for treating external carbuncles and the prescriptions for treating internal carbuncles.

20.1 Prescriptions for Treating External Carbuncles

Prescriptions for treating external carbuncles are applied for carbuncles appearing at the body surface.

Xian Fang Huo Ming Yin (Fairy Decoction for Treating Cutaneous Infections)

● Source: *Jiao Zhu Fu Ren Liang Fang* (The Revised Complete Effective Prescriptions for Diseases of Women)

● Ingredients: *Bai Zhi* (Radix Angelicae Dahuricae) 3g.

Bei Mu (Bulbus Fritillariae) 3g.

Fang Feng (Radix Ledebouriellae) 3g.

Chi Shao Yao (Radix Paeoniae Rubra) 3g.

Dang Gui Wei (Radix Angelicae Sinensis) 3g.

Gan Cao Jie (Radix Glycyrrhizae) 3g.

Zao Jiao Ci (Spina Gleditsiae) 3g.

Chuan Shan Jia (Squama Manitis Praeparata) 3g.

Tian Hua Fen (Radix Trichosanthis) 3g.

Ru Xiang (Resina Olibani) 3g.

Mo Yao (Myrrha) 3g.

Jin Yin Hua (Flos Lonicerae) 3g.

Chen Pi (Pericarpium Citri Reticulatae) 9g.

● Administration: All the drugs are to be decocted in water or in half water and half wine for oral administration.

● Functions: Clear away heat and toxin, subduce swelling and resolve masses, activate blood and relieve pain.

● Indications: Primary pyogenic infections of skin and subcutaneous tissues, caused by excessive toxic heat and stagnation of *Qi* and blood, marked by swelling and pain in the affected part, or fever with aversion to cold, thin white or yellow coating of the tongue, rapid and forceful pulse.

● Explanation:

Jin Yin Hua: the principal drug, sweet in taste and cool in nature, clearing away heat and having detoxication effect, used to subbduce and dispel carbuncles.

Fang Feng and *Bai Zhi*: expelling wind, promoting evacuation of pus and subducing swelling.

Gui Wei and *Chi Shao*: activating blood and dredging the meridians.

Ru Xiang and *Mo Yao*: dispelling stasis and relieving pain.

Chen Pi: regulating *Qi* and removing stagnation.

The above drugs are assistant drugs.

Bei Mu and *Hua Fen*: clearing away heat, dispelling accumalation and subducing swelling.

Gan Cao: reducing fire and having detoxication effect.

They are used as adjuvant drugs.

Chuan Shan Jia and *Zao Jiao Ci*: subducing swelling and dissolving masses.

Wine: activating blood circulation and dredging the meridians to help the forces of other drugs.

Those are the guiding drugs.

○ The prescription as a whole plays the effects of clearing away heat and toxic substances, subducing swelling, dissolving masses, activating blood and relieving pain.

● Notes:

(1) This is a commonly-used prescription for treating inflammations and swellings of *Yang* syndrome. Phlegmon, mastitis and various suppurative inflammations without diabrosis can be treated by the prescription.

(2) It is not advisable for cases with diabrotic carbuncles and is avoided by carbuncles of *Yin* type. For patients with congenital deficiency of the spleen and stomach and insufficiency of *Qi* and blood, the prescription should be cautiously used.

Si Miao Yong An Tang (Decoction of Four Wonderful Drugs for Quick Restoration of Health)

● Source: *Yan Fang Xin Bian* (New Compilation of Proved Recipes)
● Ingredients: *Jing Yin Hua* (Flos Lonicerae) 90g.
　　　　　　　Xuan Shen (Radix Scrophulariae) 90g.
　　　　　　　Dang Gui (Radix Angelicae Sinensis) 30g.
　　　　　　　Gan Cao (Radix Glycyrrhizae) 15g.
● Administration: All the drugs are to be decocted in water for oral administration and ten continous doses(without changing the ingredients)will be necessary for achieving the effect.
● Functions: Clear away heat and toxins, activate blood and relieve pain.

● Indications: Gangrene of the extremities due to excessive toxic heat, marked by dark redness, slight swelling with burning sensation at the affected extremities, ulceration with foul smell, severe pain, or accompanied by fever, thirst, red tongue with rapid pulse.

● Explanation:

Jin Yin Hua: the principal drug, sweat in taste and cool in nature, clearing away heat and toxins.

Xuan Shen: reducing fire and removing toxins.

Dang Gui: activating blood, removing stasis.

Gan Cao: associated with *Jin Yin Hua* to strength the functions of clearing away heat and toxins.

Those are used as assistant and adjuvant drugs.

○ The prescription as a whole plays the effects of clearing away heat, removing toxins, activating blood and dredging meridians.

● Notes:

(1) Thromboangitis obliterans of *Yang* syndrome marked by scorching of toxic heat and fire as well as other diseases due to vascular occlusion can be treated with the prescription.

(2) It is not advisable for patients with vascular oculsion of *Yin*-cold or of deficient *Qi* and blood.

Tou Nong San (Powder for Promoting Pus Discharge)

● Source: *Wai Ke Zheng Zong* (Orthodox Manual of External Diseases)
● Ingredients: *Sheng Huang Qi* (Radix Astragali seu Hedysari) 12g.
　　　　　　 Dang Gui (Radix Angelicae Sinesis) 6g.
　　　　　　 Chuan Shan Jia (Squama Manitis) 3g.
　　　　　　 Zao Jiao Ci (Spina Gleditsiae) 5g.
　　　　　　 Chuan Xiong (Rhizoma Ligustici Chuanxiong) 9g.

● Administration: All the drugs are to be decocted in water for oral administration. One cup of wine may be added while taking the decoction.

● Functions: Clear the toxin and remove pus.

● Indications: Carbuncles, swelling and pain due to deficiency of antipathogenic *Qi* which fails to remove toxins, manifested by formation of pus inside which is hardly to ulcer outside, with endless swelling, or with soreness, distention, hot and pain sensation.

● Explanation:

Sheng Huang Qi: the principal drug, sweat in taste and warm in nature, replenishing *Qi* and removing toxins.

Dang Gui and *Chuan Xiong*: nourishing blood and activating blood.

Chuan Shan Jia and *Zao Jiao Ci*: subducing, dispelling and penetrating, used to soften masses and promote pus discharge.

Those are the assistant drugs.

With little Wine: strengthening the functions of circulating and activating blood, used as the adjuvant and guiding drug.

○ The prescription as a whole plays the effects of removing toxins and promoting pus discharge.

● Notes:

The prescription is indicated for cases with unrelieved carbuncle or swelling with difficulty forming pus and incision is also not suitable.

Yang He Tang (Decoction of Warming Yang)

● Source: *Wai Ke Quan Sheng Ji* (Complete Cure for Surgical Diseases)
● Ingredients: *Shou Di* (Radix Rehmaniae Praeparatae) 30g.
  Rou Qui (Cortx Cinnamomi) 3g.
  Ma Huang (Herba Ephedrae) 2g.
  Lu Jiao Jiao (Colla Cornus Cervi) 9g.
  Bai Jie Zi (Semen Sinapis Albae) 6g.
  Pao Jiang (Baked Ginger) 2g.
  Sheng Gan Cao (Radix Glycyrrhizae) 3g.
● Administration: All the drugs will be decocted with water for oral adminstration.
● Functions: Warm *Yang*, nourish blood, disperse cold and remove stagnation.
● Indications: *Yin* type carbuncle, bone carbuncle, multiple abscesses, subcutaneous nodule, arthroncus of knee joint, attributive to deficiency of *Yang* and stagnation of cold, manifested as local and not well-demarcated swelling, mild aching, no change of colour and temperature, no thirst, pale tongue with white coating, deep and thready pulse.

● Explanation:

Shou Di: sweat in taste and warm in nature, warming and nourishing the *Ying*-blood, as the principal drug.

Lu Jiao Jiao: sweet and salty in taste and warm in nature, reinforcing essence and marrow, strengthening the tendon and bone, helping *Shou Di* to nourish blood.

Pao Jiang, *Rou Gui*: warming *Yang*, dispersing cold and clearing the meridians. They are as the assistant drugs.

Ma Huang, *Bai Jie Zi*: dispersing cold, relieving blood stasis, as the adjuvant drugs.

Sheng Gan Cao: clearing toxin and regulating all the drugs in the prescription, as the guiding durg.

○ All above drugs as a whole perform the functions of warming and tonifying blood, dispersing cold and removing blood stasis.

● Notes:

It is indicated for chronic deficient *Yin* type carbuncle, such as bone tuberculosis, tuberculosis of peritoneum, thromboangiitis obliterans, and chronic abscess in deep part due to deficient cold.

Xiao Jin Dan (Xiao Jin Pellet)

- Source: *Wai Ke Quan Sheng Ji* (Complete Cure for Surgical Diseases)
- Ingredients: *Bai Jiao Xiang* (Resina Liquikdmbaris) 150g.

  Cao Wu (Radix Aconiti Kusnezoffii) 150g.

  Wu Ling Zhi (Faeces Trgropterori) 150g.

  Di Long (Lum Bricus) 150g.

  Mu Bie (Semen Momordicae) 150g.

  Ru Xiang (Olibanum) 75g.

  Mo Yao (Myrrha) 75g.

  Gui Shen (Radix Angelicae Sinensis) 75g.

  She Xiang (Moschus) 30g.

  Mo Tan (Carbonized Chinese Ink) 12g.

- Administration: The above drugs will be made into find powder except *She Xiang*. *She Xiang* will be ground separately into find powder and mixed with the drug powder. Sieve the powder and mix with starch (100g of drug powder with 25g of starch). Using the thin paste which is made with another 5g of starch to make the drug powder into pills. Dry them without sunlight or dry them with a machine of lower temperature. Take 2-5 pills each time, twice a day, reduce the dosage for children.

- Functions: Eliminate phlegm and dampness, remove blood stasis to smooth the meridian.

- Indications: Muliple abscess, subcutaneous nodule, scrofula, carcinoma of breast, supprative ostemylitis due to stagnation of cold phlegm-dampness, manifested as swelling and pain without color change at the local part in early stage.

- Explanation:

Cao Wu: acrid and bitter in taste, warm in nature, taking away wind dampness, warming the meridians to disperse cold, used as the principal drug.

Wu Ling Zhi, *Ru Xiang* and *Mo Yao*: promoting blood circulation to remove the stasis, reducing swelling and pain, as the assistant drugs.

Dang Gui: regulating blood circulation.

Di Long: clearing the collaterals.

Bai Jiao Xiang: regulating *Qi* and blood, eliminating carbuncle and deep-rooted carbuncle.

Mu Bie: eliminating phlegm and toxins, relieving swelling.

Mo Tan: eliminating swelling and phlegm.

She Xiang: going to the collaterals to disperse stagnation.

They are as the adjuvant and guiding drugs.

○ All the above drugs as a whole perform the functions of dispersing cold, clearing the collaterals, eliminating dampness and phlegm, removing blood stasis to relieve pain.

● Notes:

(1) Bone tuberculosis, tuberculous mesenteric lymphadenitis, cold type abscess can also be treated with the prescription.

(2) It is forbidden to pregnant women, and cautiously used for weak patients.

Xi Huang Wan (Bolus of Calculus Bovis)

● Source: *Wai Ke Quan Sheng Ji* (Complete Cure for Surgical Diseases)

● Ingredients: *Xi Huang* (good class of Calculus Bovis) 15g.

She Xiang (Moschus) 75g.

Ru Xiang (Olibanum) 500g.

Mo Yao (Myrrha) 500g.

Huang Mi Fan (Cooked Millet) 350g.

● Administration: Grind all the drugs into fine powder, pound it with *Huang Mi Fan* into paste. Make the paste into pills and take with yellow wine 9g each time.

● Functions: Clear toxins and relieve carbancls, eliminate phlegm and disperse stagnation, promote blood circulation to remove blood stasis.

● Indications: Carcinoma of breast, scrofula, subcutaneous nodule, multiple abscesses, lung abscess, pyogenic infection of small intestine.

● Explanation:

Xi Huang: Bitter in taste and cool in nature, clearing heat and toxins, eliminating phlegm and dispersing stagnation, used as the principal drug.

She Xiang: acrid and warm, dredging the meridians and relieving stagnation, as the assistant drug.

Ru Xiang, *Mo Yao*: Activating blood circulation and removing blood stasis, relieving swelling and pain, as the adjuvant drugs.

Huang Mi Fan: regulating the stomach *Qi*.

Take the pills with yellow wine can promote blood circulation and make the drugs to perform the functions fast, as the guiding drug.

○ All drugs in the prescription play the functions of clearing heat and toxin, promoting blood circulation, removing blood stasis and phlegm, and dispersing stagnation.

● Notes:

(1) It is applicable to cases of lymphadenitis, mastitis, carcinoma of breast, multiple abscess, also for esophageal cancer, cardiac cancer.

(2) It's forbidden for patients who suffer from patency abscess, and cases due to deficiency of *Qi* and blood, or *Yin* deficiency leading to hyperactivity of fire.

20.2 Prescriptions for Treating Deep-sited Abscess

Prescriptions for treating deep-sited abscess are indicated for abscess happened in the internal *Zang Fu* organs.

Wei Jing Tang (Decoction of Phagmitis)

- Source: *Bei Ji Qian Ji Yao Fang* (Valuable Prescriptions for Emergency)
- Ingredients: *Wei Jing* (Rhizoma Phragmitis) 30g.

  Yi Yi Ren (Semen Coicis) 30g.

  Dong Gua Zi (Semen Beninasae) 24g.

  Tao Ren (Semen Periscae) 9g.
- Administration: All the drug will be decocted in water for oral administration.
- Functions: Clear away lung heat, eliminate phlegm, remove blood stasis and pus.
- Indications: Pulmonary abscess with cough, lower fever, expectoration of foul, purulent and bloody sputum, slight pain in the chest, squamous and dry skin, red tongue with yellow, greasy coating, slippery and rapid pulse.
- Explanation:

Wei Jing: sweet and cold, clearing lung heat, as the principal drug.

Yi Yi Ren: sweet and slight cold, clearing heat, eliminating dampness and phlegm, excreting pus.

Dong Gua Zi: sweet and cold, clearing heat, removing phlegm and excreting pus.

They are as the assistant drugs.

Tao Ren: moistening the lung to relieve cough, removing blood stasis and dispersing stagnation, as the adjuvant and guiding drug.

○ All of them together play the functions of clearing heat, eliminating phlegm, removing blood stasis and excreting pus.

- Notes:

It is a common prescription for treating pulmonary abscess in all stage. It is also used for bronchitis, pulmonitis, whooping cough due to phlegm heat.

Da Huang Mu Dan Pi Tang (Decoction of Rhei and Moutan Radicis)

- Source: *Jin Gui Yao Lue* (Synopsis of the Prescriptions of the Golden Chambar)
- Ingredients: *Da Huang* (Radix et Rhizoma Rhei) 12g.

  Mu Dan Pi (Cortex Moutan Radicis) 9g.

  Tao Ren (Semen Persicae) 12g.

  Dong Gua Zi (Semen Benincasae) 30g.

  Mang Xiao (Natrii Sulfas) 9g.
- Administration: All the drugs will be decocted in water for oral administration.
- Functions: Clear away heat, remove blood stasis, disperse stagnation and relieve swelling.

● Indications: Early stage of appendicitis, manifested as pain and tenderness over the right lower abdomen, fever, spontaneous sweating, chills, limited extensis of the right leg, thin, greasy and yellow tongue coating, slow and tense pulse.

● Explanation:

Da Huang: bitter in taste and cold in nature, clearing away toxins caused by stagnation of damp-heat and blood stasis in the intestines.

Mu Dan Pi: bitter and acrid in taste, slight cold in nature, clearing heat, cooling the blood and removing blood stasis.

They are as the principal drugs.

Mang Xiao: salty and cold, clearing away heat and removing the obstruction, softening the hardness and dissipating mass, helping Da Huang to relieve intestinal obstruction.

Tao Ren: good at activating blood circulation to remove blood stasis, strengthening *Mu Dan Pi's* function of activating blood circulation and removing stasis, also for promoting bowel movement to relieve constipation.

These two drugs are used as the assistant drugs.

Dong Gua Zi: excreting pus and dispersing stagnation, as the adjuvant drug.

○ All drugs in the prescription perform the functions of clearing heat-toxin, loosing bowel and removing stasis, dispersing stagnation and relieving swelling.

● Notes:

(1) It's indicated for cases of acute appendicitis, acute pelvic inflammation or adnexa inflammation due to stagnation of heat-dampness.

(2) It's not advisable to cases of chronic recurrent appendicitis, acute pyogenic pyodema appendicitis, as well as the aged, pregnant women, weak cases.

Yi Yi Fu Zi Bai Jiang San (Powder of Coix Seed, Aconite Root and Patrinia)

● Source: *Jin Gui Yao Lue* (Synopsis of Prescriptions of the Golden Chamber)

● Ingredients: *Yi Yi Ren* (Semen Coicis) 30g.

               Fu Zi (Radix Aconiti Preaparata) 6g.

               Bai Jian Cao (Herba Patriniae) 15g.

● Administration: All the drugs will be decocted in water for oral administration.

● Functions: Excrete pus and relieve swelling.

● Indications: Appendicitis with pus, non-fever, squannous and dry skin, soft and distend abdomen, rapid pulse.

● Explanation:

Yin Yi Ren: sweet, mild and slight cold, eliminating dampness and relieving swelling, as the principal drug.

Bai Jiang Cao: acrid, bitter and slight cold, discharging pus and promoting blood circulation, used as the assistant drug.

Fu Zi: acrid in taste and heat in nature, dispersing stagnation, activating *Yang Qi*.

○ All drugs in the prescription as a whole perform the functions of excreting pus and relieving swelling.

● Notes:

The prescription is also used for case of chronic appendicitis with pus.

Summary

The 8 prescriptions, being selected for treating pyogenic infection and ulceration of skin, are divided into two categories:

(1) Prescriptions for treating pyogenic infections appearing on body surface

Xian Fang Huo Ming Yin and *Si Miao Yong An Tang* can all be used to clear away heat and toxins. The first one is good to expel external evils, indicating for early stage of pyogenic infection and ulceration of the skin, which belongs to the dispelling therapy. *Si Miao Yong An Tang* is specially used for reducing fire and dispelling stagnation, indicating for cases of gangrene of toe due to excess of heat-toxins. *Xi Huang Wang* has the functions of clearing away toxins and eliminating phlegm, dispersing stagnation and relieving swelling, mainly for treating carbuncle and deep-rooted carbuncle, scrofula, multiple abscess. *Tou Nong San*, promoting pus drainage and strengthening the health *Qi*, for cases of carbuncle, pyogenic infection and ulceration with pus inside. Both *Yang He Tang* and *Xiao Jin Dan* are for treating *Yin*-type abscess: *Yang He Tong*, for warming *Yang* and nourishing blood, expelling cold and dispersing stagnation, while *Xiao Jin Dan*, warming to eliminate cold-dampness, removing phlegm and dredging the meridians.

(2) Prescriptions for treating deep-sited abscess

Wei Jing Tang has the functions of clearing lung heat, eliminating phlegm and excreting pus, for treating lung abscess. Both *Da Huang Mu Dan Pi Tang* and *Yi Yi Fu Zi Bai Jiang San* are used for treating appendicitis. The former is particularly for clearing away heat and removing blood stasis, indicating for cases of appendicitis with pus formed inside, and the later is used to get out pus and stop swelling.

Review Questions

(1) In the prescriptions for treating pyogenic infection and ulceration of skin, which are the representative prescriptions belonging to the promoting pus drainage therapy and dispelling therapy? Explain the ingredients, functions and indications of them?

(2) Explain the ingredients and indications of *Wei Jing Tang* and *Da Huang Mu Dan Tang*.

(3) What are the characteristics of *Si Miao Yong An Tang* in dosage and administration?

(4) What are the differences between *Yang He Tang* and *Xian Fang Huo Ming Yin* in clinical application?

Index (According to Chinese Phonetics)